Pathogen Genomics

Infectious Disease

SERIES EDITOR: *Vassil St. Georgiev*
National Institute of Allergy and Infectious Diseases
National Institutes of Health

Innate Immunity, edited by *R. Alan B. Ezekowitz,* MBChB
  and Jules A. Hoffman, PhD, 2003
Pathogen Genomics: *Impact on Human Health,* edited by *Karen Joy Shaw,* PhD, 2002
Immunotherapy for Infectious Diseases, edited by *Jeffrey M. Jacobson,* MD, 2002
Retroviral Immunology: *Immune Response and Restoration,* edited by *Giuseppe
  Pantaleo,* MD and *Bruce D. Walker,* MD, 2001
Antimalarial Chemotherapy: *Mechanisms of Action, Resistance, and New
  Directions in Drug Discovery,* edited by *Philip J. Rosenthal,* MD, 2001
Drug Interactions in Infectious Diseases, edited by
  Stephen C. Piscitelli, PharmD and *Keith A. Rodvold,* PharmD, 2001
Management of Antimicrobials in Infectious Diseases: *Impact of Antibiotic
  Resistance,* edited by *Arch G. Mainous III,* PhD and *Claire Pomeroy,* MD, 2001
Infectious Disease in the Aging: *A Clinical Handbook,* edited by
  Thomas T. Yoshikawa, MD and *Dean C. Norman,* MD, 2001
Infectious Causes of Cancer: *Targets for Intervention,* edited by
  James J. Goedert, MD, 2000

Pathogen Genomics

Impact on Human Health

Edited by

Karen Joy Shaw, PhD

Johnson and Johnson Pharmaceutical Research and Development, L. L. C.
San Diego, CA

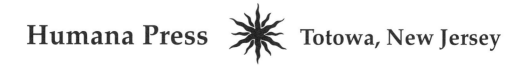

Humana Press Totowa, New Jersey

© 2002 Humana Press Inc.
999 Riverview Drive, Suite 208
Totowa, New Jersey 07512

www.humanapress.com

This publication is printed on acid-free paper. ∞

ANSI Z39.48-1984 (American National Standards Institute) Permanence of Paper for Printed Library Materials.

Cover design by Patricia F. Cleary.

Production Editor: Adrienne Howell

For additional copies, pricing for bulk purchases, and/or information about other Humana titles, contact Humana at the above address or at any of the following numbers: Tel: 973-256-1699; Fax: 973-256-8341; E-mail: humana@humanapr.com or visit our website at http://humanapress.com

Printed in the United States of America.   10 9 8 7 6 5 4 3 2 1

Library of Congress Cataloging-in-Publication Data

Pathogen Genomics: impact on human health / edited by Karen Joy Shaw
          p. ; cm. -- (Infectious disease)
     Includes bibliographical references and index.
     ISBN 1-58829-026-3 (alk. paper)
     1. Microbial genetics. 2. Gene expression. 3. Fungal gene expression. 4. DNA microarrays. 5. Pathogenic microorganisms. I. Shaw, Karen Joy. II. Infectious disease
     (Totowa, N.J.)
     [DNLM: 1. Microbiologic Phenomena--genetics. 2. Genomics QH 307.2 P297 2002]
QH434 .P384 2002
579'.165--dc21   2002017200

Dedication

To the memories of Claire M. Berg and Marion Himes—who set my feet upon this path, gave wise counsel, and always believed in my journey.

Preface

Since the advent of microbial genome sequencing and the development of algorithms to compare and annotate genomes, an enormous wealth of information has become available to the scientific community. This information is further extended by technologies such as DNA microarrays that use sequence information to analyze genomic expression patterns, proteomics to analyze the translation of these patterns into protein products, and a variety of methods of functional analysis to determine the ultimate phenotypic manifestation of the genes themselves. The analysis of this treasure trove is far from complete, but initial findings have already revolutionized the field of microbiology. Microbiologists have made strong inroads into utilizing this information for drug discovery, vaccine development, and diagnostics. This information continues to be an integral part of the study of the fundamentals of pathogenesis, how organisms interact with each other and with their host environment, and will undoubtedly point to places where intervention will have a significant positive impact on human health. *Pathogen Genomics: Impact on Human Health* is intended to review recent developments in this unfolding story.

The utility of genomics extends from the smallest viral genomes to larger more complex organisms, including humans. Although significant progress has been made studying diverse collections of microorganisms, including plant pathogens, thermophilic Archaebacteria, and other organisms thriving in extreme environments, the scope of this book has been limited to pathogenic organisms that interact with a human host. Clearly, the genomics of all sequenced human pathogens could not be addressed in a single volume, but rather organisms were chosen to give a balanced presentation of viruses, bacteria, fungi, and protozoa. The goal is to bridge these disciplines and to explore the impact genomics has had on the discovery and choice of drug targets, selection of antigenic determinants for vaccine development, diagnostics, and our understanding of pathogenesis. Common sets of tools, such as genomic comparisons and microarray analysis, are used to explore many of these organisms. The findings from these analyses offer unique insights into the fundamental nature of each pathogen, as well as common strategies adopted by diverse pathogens to be successful in the human host.

Genomic comparisons and computational data mining have been used to identify the metabolic capabilities of specific pathogens and have revealed how they have adapted to unusual host environments. They have pointed to pathways that are unique to an organism, and have identified pathways that are shared among all prokaryotes, are particular to fungi or protozoa, or are common to all life. The analysis of these data has had a significant impact on the identification and selection of targets for antibacterial, antifungal, and antiparasitic drug discovery, as well as providing candidates for the development of diagnostic tools and vaccines. Some of these findings are reviewed in Chapters 5, 7, 11–14, and 17. Chapter 9 explores the changing nature of epidemiological analysis, from plasmid fingerprinting through sequence-based typing, where advancements in genomic analysis have driven the technological development of new investigative tools for identifying the nature of nosocomial outbreaks.

In silico comparisons of strain-to-strain variations can be used to generate historical genealogies of infectious diseases. In Chapter 6, Behr and Gordon discuss comparisons of genomes of attenuated and virulent strains of organisms such as *Mycobacterium tuberculosis*. These types of analyses are critical to our understanding of the genetic basis of the evolution of virulence, and provide candidate genes whose inactivation may lead to the development of improved live attenuated vaccine strains or may serve as components of subunit vaccines. The use of genomic comparisons for the identification of fungal virulence determinants and vaccine candidates is reviewed in Chapters 15 and 16. Similarly, the identification of proteins involved in the pathogenicity of *Entamoeba histolytica* and *Borrelia burgdorferi*, or with possible utility as vaccine candidates, is explored in Chapters 10 and 18.

Genome analysis using microbial DNA microarrays began with the first eukaryotic genome sequenced, *Saccharomyces cerevisiae (1)*. The yeast arrays have been used extensively for exploring changes in expression profiles resulting from changes in growth conditions, in addition to other microarray applications such as mapping gene cross-over events *(2)*. Microarrays have aided our fundamental understanding of metabolic pathways that are important for antifungal drug discovery, as well as antifungal drug resistance. Chapter 12 reviews microarray analyses of yeast, with particular emphasis on the studies of the effect of inhibitors on ergosterol synthesis in both *Saccharomyces cerevisiae* and *Candida albicans*.

More recently, bacterial arrays have become readily available in the form of hybridization filters (Sigma-Genosys, The Woodlands, TX) for organisms such as *Escherichia coli*, *Helicobacter pylori*, and *Bacillus subtilis*. DNA microarrays containing open reading frames derived by PCR, or oligonucleotides representing these ORFs, continue to be developed and are especially useful in studying pathogenic organisms. One important application of this technology is the examination of the response to a variety of treatments, including antimicrobial drug addition. Chapter 8 reviews the development and utility of bacterial microarray technologies.

Viral microarray technology has taken a two-pronged approach: examination of viral-encoded genes on DNA chips and examination of the host cell response to viral infection. The goal of both approaches is to determine the full complement of genes that are critical to viral propagation, virulence, or control of latency. Chapters 1, 2, and 3 focus on Herpesviruses, Human Papilloma Virus, and Human Immunodeficiency Virus, exploring the utility of microarrays for the identification of novel antiviral drug targets and analysis of viral/host interactions. An additional chapter in the viral section covers the rational design of gene therapeutics for HIV/AIDS, based upon the sequence of HIV-1 subtypes and identification of useful RNA sites that can be targeted by ribozymes (Chapter 4).

Analysis of microbial genomes has revealed that a significant portion of each genome is of unknown function. Entire operons can be identified that are common to bacterial pathogens, yet the functions of these genes have yet to be elucidated. Through genomics one can identify them and using deletion analysis one can show that they are essential to bacterial survival. Functional genomics can begin to provide clues as to what their role is, thus providing information on how to set up high throughput screens to identify novel classes of inhibitors. Several technologies can be utilized to explore the function of unknown proteins, including the use of protein comparisons to define motifs and domains similar to known proteins and threading algorithms for finding similarities in the 3D structure. Other methods, such as the yeast two-hybrid system, seek to find binding partners that may provide a clue to function. High throughput phenotypic microarrays have also been used to simultaneously test a large number of cellular phenotypes and allow novel functions to be assigned to genes *(3)*. Although it is often important to ascribe a function to a target prior to high throughput screening, several methods have been developed to find ligands that bind to proteins, with the idea that amongst the molecules that bind will be inhibitors of function. These types of screens provide the raw materials for further drug development. Many of these technologies are discussed in Chapters 5, 7, 8, 11, 12, 13, 14, 15, and 16.

As a result of the explosion of pathogen and host genomic information, a new era is at hand. The fundamental nature of target evaluation and drug discovery has been radically changed. The wealth of information available will add significant insights to our knowledge of protein function and pathogen physiology, and the exploitation of these findings for the discovery of novel agents to combat pathogenic organisms will continue in the exciting years ahead.

Karen Joy Shaw, PhD

1. Lashkari DA, DeRisi JL, McCusker JH, et. al. Yeast microarrays for genome wide parallel genetic and gene expression analysis. Proc Natl Acad Sci USA 1997; 94:13057–13062.
2. Winzeler EA, Richards DR, Conway AR, et. al. Direct allelic variation scanning of the yeast genome. Science 1998; 281:1194–1197.
3. Bochner, BR, Gadzinski, P, Panomitros, E. Phenotypic microarrays for high-throughput phenotypic testing and assay of gene function. Gen Res 2001; 11:1246–1255.

Contents

Preface .... *vii*

Contributors .... *xiii*

PART I VIRUSES

1 Antiviral Drug Target Discovery with DNA Microarrays
   Klaus Früh and Peter Ghazal *1*

2 Chipping Away at HIV Pathogenesis
   *Steffney Elise Rought, Roman Sasik, Davey Mitchell Smith,
   and Jacques Corbeil* *13*

3 Microarray Analysis of Human Papillomavirus Pathogenesis
   Yijan Elaine Chang and Laimonis A. Laimins *25*

4 Ribozymes as Gene Therapeutic Agents for HIV/AIDS:
   A Potential Paradigm Shift
   Gregory C. Fanning, Janet L. Macpherson, and Geoff Symonds *39*

PART II BACTERIA

5 Genomics and New Technologies Applied to Antibacterial
   Drug Discovery
   Donald T. Moir *53*

6 Genomics of the *Mycobacterium tuberculosis* Complex
   and BCG Vaccines
   Marcel A. Behr and Stephen V. Gordon *69*

7 Bacterial "Genes-to-Screens" in the Post-Genomic Era
   Michael J. Pucci, John F. Barrett, and Thomas J. Dougherty *83*

8 DNA Microarray Expression Analysis in Antibacterial
   Drug Discovery
   Brian J. Morrow and Karen Joy Shaw *97*

9 The Influence of Genomics on the Molecular Epidemiology
   of Nosocomial Pathogens
   Richard V. Goering *113*

10 *Borrelia* Genomics as a Tool for Studying
     Pathogenesis and Vaccine Development
     Alireza Shamaei-Tousi and Sven Bergström *133*

PART III FUNGI

11 Antifungal Target Discovery and Evaluation: *Lessons from*
     Saccharomyces cerevisiae
     Beth DiDomenico and Scott S. Walker *155*

12 Antifungal Drug Discovery: *Old Drugs, New Tools*
     Marianne D. De Backer, Walter H. M. L. Luyten,
        and Hugo F. Vanden Bossche *167*

13 *Cryptococcus neoformans: A Molecular Model for the Study*
        of Fungal Pathogenesis and Drug Discovery in the Genomic Era
     Jennifer K. Lodge and John R. Perfect *197*

14 Antifungal Target Selection in *Aspergillus nidulans*:
        Using Bioinformatics to Make the Difference
     Rosanna Pena-Muralla, Patricia Ayoubi, Marcia Graminha,
        Nilce M. Martinez-Rossi, Antonio Rossi, and Rolf A. Prade *215*

15 Functional Genomics of *Histoplasma capsulatum*:
        Dimorphism and Virulence
     Glenmore Shearer, Jr. *231*

16 Gene Finding in *Coccidioides immitis*:
        Searching for Immunogenic Proteins
     Theo N. Kirkland and Garry T. Cole *247*

PART IV PROTOZOA

17 *Toxoplasma gondii: A Model for Evolutionary Genomics*
        and Chemotherapy
     Jessica C. Kissinger, Michael J. Crawford, David S. Roos,
        and James W. Ajioka *255*

18 The Molecular Biology and Pathogenicity of *Entamoeba histolytica*
     Barbara J. Mann and Brendan J. Loftus *281*

     Index *303*

Contributors

JAMES W. AJIOKA, PhD • *Department of Pathology, University of Cambridge, Cambridge, UK*

PATRICIA AYOUBI, PhD • *Department of Biochemistry and Molecular Biology, Oklahoma State University, Stillwater, OK*

JOHN F. BARRETT, PhD • *Merck Research Laboratories, Merck and Company, Rahway, NJ*

MARCEL A. BEHR, PhD • *Division of Infectious Diseases and Medical Microbiology, McGill University Health Centre, Montreal, Quebec, Canada*

SVEN BERGSTRÖM, MD • *Department of Molecular Biology, Umeå University, Umeå, Sweden*

YIJAN ELAINE CHANG, PhD • *Department of Microbiology-Immunology, Northwestern University Medical School, Chicago, IL*

GARRY T. COLE, PhD • *Department of Microbiology and Immunology, Medical College of Ohio, Toledo, OH*

JACQUES CORBEIL, PhD • *Department of Pathology and Medicine, University of California San Diego; Veterans Medical Research Foundation, San Diego, CA*

MICHAEL J. CRAWFORD, PhD • *Department of Biology, University of Pennsylvania, Philadelphia, PA*

MARIANNE D. DE BACKER, PhD • *Department of Gastrointestinal Emerging Diseases, Johnson and Johnson Pharmaceutical Research and Development, L. L. C., Beerse, Belgium*

BETH DIDOMENICO, PhD • *Schering-Plough Research Institute, Kenilworth, NJ*

THOMAS J. DOUGHERTY, PhD • *Pfizer Global Research and Development, Groton, CT*

GREGORY C. FANNING, DPhil • *Johnson and Johnson Research Pty Limited, Sydney, Australia*

KLAUS FRÜH, PhD • *Vaccine and Gene Therapy Institute, Oregon Health Sciences University, Beaverton, OR*

PETER GHAZAL, PhD • *University of Edinburgh, Summerhall, Edinburgh, UK*

RICHARD V. GOERING, PhD • *Department of Medical Microbiology and Immunology, Creighton University School of Medicine, Omaha, NE*

STEPHEN V. GORDON, PhD • *Veterinary Laboratories Agency, Surrey, UK*

MARCIA GRAMINHA, MS • *Department of Genetics, Faculty of Medicine of Ribeirão Preto, University of São Paulo, Ribeirão Preto, Brazil*

THEO N. KIRKLAND, MD • *Department of Pathology and Medicine, University of California San Diego; Department of Veterans Affairs Medical Center, San Diego, CA*

JESSICA C. KISSINGER, PhD • *Department of Biology, University of Pennsylvania, Philadelphia, PA*

LAIMONIS A. LAIMINS, PhD • *Department of Microbiology-Immunology, Northwestern University Medical School, Chicago, IL*

JENNIFER K. LODGE, PhD • *Edward A. Doisy Department of Biochemistry and Molecular Biology, Saint Louis University School of Medicine, St. Louis, MO*

BRENDAN J. LOFTUS, PhD • *The Institute of Genomic Research, Rockville, MD*

WALTER H.M.L. LUYTEN, MD, PhD • *Janssen Research Foundation, Beerse, Belgium*

JANET L. MACPHERSON, PhD • *Johnson and Johnson Research Pty Limited, Sydney, Australia*

BARBARA J. MANN, PhD • *Departments of Internal Medicine and Microbiology, University of Virginia, Charlottesville, VA*

NILCE M. MARTINEZ-ROSSI, PhD • *Department of Genetics, Faculty of Medicine of Ribeirão Preto, University of São Paulo, Ribeirão Preto, Brazil*

DONALD T. MOIR, PhD • *Genome Therapeutics Corporation, Waltham, MA*

BRIAN J. MORROW, PhD • *Department of Infectious Diseases, Johnson and Johnson Pharmaceutical Research and Development, L. L. C., San Diego, CA*

ROSANNA PENA-MURALLA, PhD • *Department of Microbiology and Molecular Genetics, Oklahoma State University, Stillwater, OK*

JOHN R. PERFECT, MD • *Division of Infectious Disease, Duke University Medical Center, Durham, NC*

ROLF A. PRADE, PhD • *Department of Microbiology and Molecular Genetics, Oklahoma State University, Stillwater, OK*

MICHAEL J. PUCCI, PhD • *Achillion Pharmaceuticals, Inc., New Haven, CT*

DAVID S. ROOS, PhD • *Department of Biology, University of Pennsylvania, Philadelphia, PA*

ANTONIO ROSSI, PhD • *Department of Biochemistry and Immunology, Faculty of Medicine of Ribeirão Preto, University of São Paulo, Ribeirão Preto, Brazil*

STEFFNEY ELISE ROUGHT, PhD • *Department of Pathology and Medicine, University of California San Diego; Veterans Medical Research Foundation, San Diego, CA*

ROMAN SASIK, PhD • *Department of Pathology and Medicine, University of California San Diego, CA*

ALIREZA SHAMAEI-TOUSI, PhD • *Department of Molecular Biology, Umeå University, Umeå, Sweden*

KAREN JOY SHAW, PhD • *Department of Infectious Diseases, Johnson and Johnson Pharmaceutical Research and Development, L. L. C., San Diego, CA*

GLENMORE SHEARER, JR., PhD • *Center for Molecular and Cellular Biosciences, Department of Biological Sciences, Center for Molecular and Cellular Biosciences, University of Southern Mississippi, Hattiesburg, MS*

DAVEY MITCHELL SMITH, MD • *Departments of Pathology and Medicine, University of San Diego, San Diego, CA*

GEOFF SYMONDS, PhD • *Johnson and Johnson Research Pty Limited, Sydney, Australia*

HUGO F. VANDEN BOSSCHE • *Former (Retired) Senior Director of Anti-Infectives Research, Janssen Pharmaceutica, Beerse, Belgium*

SCOTT S. WALKER, PhD • *Schering-Plough Research Institute, Kenilworth, NJ*

I VIRUSES

1

Antiviral Drug Target Discovery with DNA Microarrays

Klaus Früh and Peter Ghazal

SUMMARY

Global expression analysis with DNA microarrays is exquisitely suited to monitor changes in mRNA levels arising from disturbances of the cellular environment. Viral infections are among the most dramatic perturbations a cell can undergo. Therefore, this functional genomics tool promises new insights into the interaction between the virus and host cell. The interface of virus and host can be targeted for drug discovery, as shown by several recent studies demonstrating that inhibiting host-cell proteins can prevent viral infection. Although these results were obtained by hypothesis-driven research, many laboratories have embarked on data-driven approaches based on the systematic analysis of virus-induced changes in the gene-expression profile of the host cell. Based on these results, it is now possible to determine the relevance of cellular genes that change upon viral infection. Cellular gene products that are essential for viral replication represent novel molecular targets for drug discovery, thus expanding target discovery in virology—an area thus far limited to genes encoded by viral genomes.

INTRODUCTION

All possible drug targets for the treatment of human diseases are encoded in the human genome sequence (1,2), except for the infectious diseases attributable to pathogens, which contain their own genomes. Thus, the entire universe of possible targets for the treatment of infectious diseases is represented by the genomes of both the pathogen and the host. A systematic, functional genomic approach to antiviral drug discovery should therefore attempt to reveal the changes that take place in the transcriptomes and proteomes of both the pathogen and host genomes. Proteomics has already been applied to study bacterial and fungal organisms (3). However, this tool is still in development for the much more complex proteome expressed by higher eukaryotic cells, including virally infected cells. By contrast, DNA microarrays are sufficiently advanced to study changes in the transcriptome of both the virus and the host cell. High-density DNA arrays are generated by spotting DNA fragments, usu-

From: *Pathogen Genomics: Impact on Human Health*
Edited by: K. J. Shaw © Humana Press Inc., Totowa, NJ

ally derived by polymerase chain reaction (PCR), or synthetic oligonucleotides onto solid surfaces such as glass slides or filter membranes *(4)*. Alternatively, oligonucleotide probes are directly synthesized on glass wafers, using photolithography *(5)*. The deposition of thousands of probes on solid support surfaces allows the simultaneous monitoring of expression levels of the corresponding messenger RNAs isolated from various sources. This technology is particularly useful for the analysis of host-pathogen interactions *(6)*, since well-controlled experiments are made possible through comparison of the mRNA populations of infected cells to noninfected cells. Also, the genetic manipulation of infectious organisms allows the comparison of profiles obtained from wild-type or mutant forms. Moreover, changes in cellular gene-expression levels in response to pathogen insult can be assessed in infectious disease models by specifically inhibiting host gene products to determine their significance in the virus life cycle.

This chapter reviews some of this work, with particular emphasis on herpesviruses. Herpesviruses are large DNA viruses that encode from 80 to 220 genes. The expression of virus genes upon infection is temporally regulated. The first genes to be expressed (immediate-early, IE), are independent of viral *de novo* protein synthesis, and encode either regulatory trans-acting factors or immune inhibitory proteins. The next set of genes expressed (early, E) requires the presence of viral regulatory proteins and contributes an essential source of factors, including viral DNA replication, repair enzymes, and other nonstructural proteins, such as those that serve in signal transduction and immune evasion. Late (L) genes are essentially expressed after the onset of DNA replication, and contribute primarily to assembly, morphogenesis, and egress of virions. Thus, the time of viral gene expression during infection provides an important clue to its functional role. Given the complexity of the herpesviral genomes, DNA microarrays that display all viral open reading frames (ORFs) are now applied to the study of the viral transcriptome, as discussed in the following section.

Herpesviruses have co-evolved with, and are highly adapted to, their host species. Infections with herpesviruses are usually asymptomatic, yet cause disease in immunosuppressed individuals. In the normal host, the virus is controlled so that life-long infections are established, one of the hallmarks of this virus family. As a result of such latent asymptomatic infections, herpesviruses often reach remarkably high prevalence rates in the human population. The highly successful adaptation of these viruses to their host implies that they are masters in manipulating the host-cell environment to their advantage. Although this intricate interplay between the products of the viral genome and gene products of the host genome has been an area of intense investigation for many years, most interactions are still unknown. Functional genomics tools allow a fresh look at these virus-induced changes, and these studies reveal novel and unexpected connections. Some of these changes are the result of a host response designed to eliminate or thwart the viral attacker. Other changes are bystander effects, which are neutral with respect to fostering or inhibiting viral replication. Notably, some of the virus-induced changes in the host-cell program are essential for viral replication. The task ahead is therefore to first catalog the viral and host-cell gene-expression program, and then to validate the importance of these genes for the success of viral infection.

VIRUS DNA ARRAYS

Microarray Analysis of a Virus Transcription-Replication Cycle

The genomes of herpesviruses are among the most complex viral genomes, with 80–220 ORFs in the case of herpes simplex virus (HSV) and human cytomegalovirus (HCMV), respectively. DNA arrays are therefore useful to simultaneously monitor the global transcriptional pattern of herpesviruses. The first generation of a viral DNA chip for genome-wide expression measurements was reported for the HCMV genome, the largest member of the herpesvirus family *(7)*. In this study, an HCMV DNA chip was used to catalog the temporal class of viral gene expression and characterize the profile of virus transcription upon drug inhibition. Prior to this study, less than 30% of the genome had been transcriptionally mapped. A strong correlation between temporal expression class and assigned function was observed. Subsequently, the viral DNA microarray approach was successfully applied to the functional analysis of the well-established HSV, *(8),* and the newly discovered Kaposi's sarcoma-associated herpesvirus (KSHV; human herpesvirus 8) *(9)*. In the case of KSHV, only a few genes have been previously characterized, and the correlation between gene expression and function has provided key clues for the role of many KSHV genes yet to be characterized. The genome-wide mapping of temporal gene expression also provides important information to help understand and dissect the regulatory pathways of particular virulent genes. For instance, with HCMV, sequence compositional analysis of the 5′ non-coding DNA sequences of the temporal classes—using algorithms that automatically search for motifs in unaligned sequences—indicated the presence of potential regulatory elements for a subset of key early and early-late genes *(7)*.

The ability to rapidly perform parallel gene-expression analysis at the whole viral genome level is also beginning to reveal new aspects of viral biology. For example, a previously unidentified class of viral transcripts, termed virion RNAs, has been discovered using HCMV microarrays *(10)*. These specific transcripts are packaged within virions, and allow for viral genes to be expressed within an infected cell immediately after virus entry. The role of this new class of transcripts is unknown. In other studies, fabricated microarrays of viral genomes are helping to reveal new relationships between lytic and latent gene-expression classes *(9)*. In the future, viral DNA microarrays will play an important role in defining classes of virus transcription activity in latency. It is noteworthy that the patterns (signature) of viral gene expression are influenced either directly or indirectly by the expression of cellular proteins, and as a result, quantitative and qualitative differences in the profile of viral gene expression have been shown to vary, depending on host-cell background *(8)*. With this connection, a better understanding of a virus transcription-replication cycle can be appreciated by future studies, which aim to integrate host-cell expression with viral gene expression.

Viral Chips for Diagnostics, Pharmacogenomics, and Drug Discovery

Naturally occurring viral mutants in infected patients have important implications for therapy. Thus, viral genotyping methods for detecting the prevalence of drug-resistant mutations/polymorphisms or virulent strains/isolates from patients are of high priority. For this reason, some of the first applications of viral DNA microarrays have been to rapidly identify sequence variation (genotype) among different virus strains/isolates. In the last few years, a wide variety of microarray technology platforms have been applied to viral genotyping. These include DNA microarrays for human immunodeficiency virus, hepatitis C virus, poliovirus, and influenza viruses *(11–16)*. Generally, these studies clearly show that viral DNA microarray technology provides a useful supplement—and, in the future, an alternative—to PCR-based diagnostic methods. Moreover, the global diagnostic microarray approach is likely to disclose many key clinical features that may help tailor drug regimes. For example, in DNA microarray sequence studies of HIV, it was found that sequence changes known to contribute to drug resistance occurred as natural polymorphisms in isolates from some patients who were naive to inhibitors *(12)*. In such cases, an alternative drug combination may be recommended, as well as the incorporation of resistance testing as a standard of care for treatment.

Viral DNA microarray analysis of gene expression has also been shown to provide a fingerprint for the mode of action of antiviral drugs that target viral gene products *(7)*. Therefore, viral-expression profiles of drug inhibition can be used to select for inhibitory drugs with a different profile. The variation in signature profiles would be indicative of a different mechanism of action for new lead compounds. The viral target for these compounds would be identified by the generation, in the laboratory, of a mutant strain resistant to inhibition by the lead compound and by gene-expression profiling of the mutant. A corollary from this is that a viral mutant which renders the putative target gene defective should have an expression signature that matches the drug-inhibition expression profile. Thus, drug inhibition of an essential viral gene will result in a restricted gene-expression profile that should be identical in profile to that obtained from a genetic knockout of the gene. A precedent for this has been established in studies comparing knockout mutants and drug-inhibition profiles in yeast *(17)*. In the future, it may be possible to perform such experiments *in silico* by performing cluster analyses of expression profiles from drug-inhibition studies with those obtained from a database of gene-expression profiles from a library of virus mutants.

As discussed in the previous section, antiviral drugs may also target host-encoded gene products that play a vital role (directly or indirectly) in the viral life cycle. Again, viral microarrays provide an efficient method to assess the interaction of the host regulatory pathway in the virus transcription-replication cycle. This approach, combined with the strategies outlined here, will help to identify novel antiviral therapeutics. In addition, specialized viral databases will dramatically enhance comparative analysis of antiviral strategies and help to identify broad-spectrum and virus-specific antiviral drugs.

Finally, the combination of viral transcript profiling with genotype analysis is beginning to open pathways for a more rigorous pharmacogenomics approach to viral biology. Currently, there are some technical limitations regarding marker generation, genotyping, and biostatistical analysis, which must be overcome before this becomes a reality. Nevertheless, viral DNA microarrays used for phenotypic assays and virus genotyping could become a standard in drug development as well as for infectious disease treatment.

USING MICROARRAYS TO STUDY CHANGES IN THE HOST-CELL GENE-EXPRESSION PATTERN

Examples for Host-Cell Pathways Important for Viral Infection

Viruses are entirely dependent on host factors for their survival, and are therefore vulnerable to inhibition of host-cell biochemical pathways. Since each step of the viral life cycle is dependent on host-cell proteins, inhibiting any of these essential functions should prevent virus growth. Therefore, it can be assumed that these host-encoded proteins represent a treasure trove of potential drug targets. Since many of the virus/host interactions are currently unknown, we are just beginning to discover such targets, and it is likely that the currently known examples are the mere tip of a vast iceberg. One example for a host-cell function found to be essential for HCMV replication is the stress-induced kinase complex *p38*. Inhibitors of *p38* that block the MAP-kinase signaling pathway prevent HCMV replication *(18)*. However, the exact role of this host-cell pathway for HCMV growth is unknown. Moreover, KSHV-infected cells undergo apoptosis upon inhibition of the transcriptional activator, NfkappaB *(19)*. Indeed, microarray experiments show a strong induction of the NfkappaB-dependent pro-inflammatory pathway (Luukkonen M., Bell Y., Moses A. and K. Früh, *unpublished results*). These results show that intracellular signaling events are essential for herpesvirus replication and can be targeted for intervention. It is very likely that many more such signaling cascades will be revealed by DNA microarray analysis. Another area of potential intervention is viral cell-cycle control. For instance, HCMV arrests infected cells in the G1 phase of the cell cycle, and this block is accompanied by an increase in the cell-cycle-dependent kinase 2 (cdk2)/cyclin E complex. Accordingly, roscovitine—an inhibitor of cdk-1, 2, and 5, but not cdk-4 and 6—inhibited HCMV replication, whereas other cell-cycle inhibitors had no effect *(20)*. Moreover, HSV 1 and 2 were also inhibited by roscovitine as well as olomoucine, another cdk-inhibitor *(21)*. Thus, different viruses may depend on the same cellular pathway, suggesting that certain compounds may inhibit different or unrelated viruses. This concept is strongly supported by recent observations that budding of the retroviruses HIV and Rous sarcoma virus as well as the unrelated Ebolavirus, the filovirus, seems to require the same or similar intracellular pathways *(22–25)*. The gag proteins of these viruses are linked to ubiquitin via their so-called L domains. Ubiquitination of gag was shown to be essential for virus release because inhibition of the proteasome, which reduces the intracellular concentration of ubiquitin, resulted in accumulation of virus particles at the plasma membrane. However, viral particles were not released. Another cellular target is the Golgi-protease furin. A protein inhibitor of furin was found to decrease the release of infectious HCMV, probably because furin is required for the processing of the HCMV glycoprotein B, one of the essential proteins *(26)*. Whether or not furin inhibitors prevent the release of other viruses remains to be established. These examples clearly demonstrate that inhibiting various host-cell pathways can prevent virus growth.

Common Host-Cell Pathways Affected by Different Viruses

Whereas different virus species may have learned to employ similar cellular pathways to their own advantage, the infected cell has developed antiviral countermeasures that can be activated by various viral species. DNA microarray analysis of host-cell gene expression from different cell types infected with various viruses revealed such common patterns. One of the most commonly observed patterns of transcriptional activation upon viral infection is the induction of interferon-stimulated genes (ISG). To date, DNA microarray analysis has revealed the activation of ISG expression by the following viruses or viral proteins: HCMV, whole virus *(27,28)* or isolated glycoprotein B *(29);* HSV, UV-treated or VP16-mutant *(30);* KSHV, whole virus (Luukkonen M., Bell Y., Moses A. and K. Früh, *unpublished result*), or transfected major latency transcript LANA *(31);* Marek's disease virus (a virus that infects chicken) *(32).* Thus, a representative of each herpesviral class, alpha (HSV, MDV), beta (HCMV), and gamma (KSHV), was shown to induce ISGs. The triggers of this response are currently unknown, but are most likely complex. For instance, HCMV does not seem to activate ISGs by induction of the interferon (IFN) gene and subsequent IFN production in the infected cell. Instead, HCMV induces ISGs directly as soon as the major ligand, glycoprotein B, binds to its unknown cellular receptor, which is distinct from the IFN receptor *(29* and references therein). By contrast, DNA microarray analysis of the other viruses influenza *(33);* HIV-1 *(34),* Coxsackievirus B3 *(35),* rabies virus *(36),* or hepatitis C virus *(37)* did not reveal ISG induction. In fact, expression profiling of cells infected with the tumorigenic human papillomavirus (HPV) *(38)* or transfected with the HPV-encoded oncogenes E6 and E7 *(39)* showed a suppressed interferon response and were found to be unresponsive to exogenous interferon. Since many of the interferon-stimulated genes perform antiviral functions *(40),* these data may suggest that infected cells are particularly immune against herpesviral assault. However, herpesviruses have developed whole arsenals of viral proteins that thwart the antiviral response of the host. Different from mutant HSV, wild-type HSV does not induce the interferon-response *(30),* suggesting that some of its viral functions are able to prevent their expression. HCMV is also known to interfere with signaling from the interferon-receptor *(41,42).* Moreover, one of the KSHV-encoded genes shows high homology to interferon response factor (IRF), a transactivator required for ISG induction, and the viral IRF is known to interfere with ISG induction *(43).* Thus, one of the general themes emerging from expression profiling of cells infected with herpesviruses seems to be their induction and the subsequent subversion of the interferon response. The molecular mechanisms by which herpesviruses counteract the antiviral action of these host-cell gene products may represent novel targets for therapeutic intervention.

Virus-Specific Host-Cell Pathways

Aside from activation of the innate cellular antiviral-response pathways, viruses induce host-cell genes that seem to be specific for certain viruses. For example, tumorigenic viruses are responsible for dramatic changes in the cellular transcriptional program during transformation. Among the herpesviruses, the gamma-herpesviruses Epstein-Barr Virus (EBV) and KSHV are able to transform cells. These transformation events can be evaluated with functional genomics tools. We have begun a systematic analysis of KSHV-infected and transformed cells by DNA microarrays (Luukkonen M., Bell Y., Moses A. and K. Früh, *unpublished results*). Changes in the gene-expression profile of KSHV-infected endothelial cells revealed the upregulation of proteins characteristic of precursors of the endothelial-cell lineage, consistent with a KSHV-induced de-differentiation of endothelial cells.

A comparison of the gene-expression profiles in chronic viral hepatitis tissues from different donors also revealed a clear distinction between hepatitis caused by HCV vs hepatitis caused by HBV *(44)*. Thus, the gene-expression profile was specific for either virus with HBV, inducing the expression of pro-inflammatory genes but HCV inducing anti-inflammatory genes. The ultimate cause of these transcriptional changes is unknown, but it can be assumed that they are the end product of a gene-expression cascade triggered by the expression of viral genes. The dissection of host-cell gene expression triggered by individual viral proteins is therefore an important step in unraveling the molecular mechanisms that lead to disease. However, in the case of HCV, DNA-microarray analysis of cells transfected with a partial genome encoding the nonstructural genes revealed few changes *(37)*. Further analysis is needed to clarify the role of HCV nonstructural proteins in host-cell gene expression. Structural proteins may also be involved in regulating host-cell gene expression. Such a role was clearly demonstrated in the case of the HCMV glycoprotein B *(29)*. Moreover, heat-inactivated or UV-inactivated influenza virus was found to induce host-cell genes, which may have been triggered by structural components of the virus *(33)*.

Most of the currently available microarray experiments with virally infected cells are based on a small number of arrays that are usually restricted to one strain of virus and one particular cell type (reviewed in *45*). However, the unequivocal identification of host genes specifically induced by viruses requires the analysis of multiple strains in various cell types. We have begun such an analysis using murine cytomegalovirus infection of various mouse cell lines. Preliminary data analysis suggests that although the cellular changes induced by this virus differ from cell type to cell type for the majority of host genes, there are also host gene groups that are consistently induced in different cell types (S. Kurz, S. Olek, P. Ghazal and K. Früh, *unpublished results*). If some of the genes required for viral replication are already expressed in a particular cell type prior to infection, it is also possible that the virus does not need to or is unable to further induce these genes. Such host genes can be found by comparing the expression levels rather than the induction ratios between different cell types infected by the same virus. An additional layer of complexity is added when the host-cell expression profiles are analyzed for different strains or different lab-generated mutants of a particular virus species. Here it is important to combine the characterization of viral gene-expression patterns, using viral chips and the host-cell gene-expression pattern. Tracking, storing, and comparing such data will require the generation of dedicated databases. However, as discussed in the next section, even the relatively simple bioinformatics tools available today have allowed the identification of previously unknown host-cell pathways that are crucial for viral replication or for virus-induced host-cell transformation.

FUNCTION OF VIRALLY INDUCED CELLULAR TRANSCRIPTS

To validate the importance of viral host gene induction or repression detected by DNA microarrays, it is necessary to disturb the function or expression of these genes and to evaluate the effect in the context of viral infection. Depending on the viral system used, this validation step may monitor viral replication or virally induced morphological changes such as transformation or cell migration.

Using KSHV-infected endothelial cells as a test system, we have performed such a systematic analysis. In this cell system, KSHV remains latent and transforms the endothelial cells to become spindle cells *(46)*. However, KSHV enters the lytic replication cycle upon induction with phorbolesters. We have examined the function of host-cell proteins that are specifically upregulated during the lytic cycle of replication. A group of approximately 20 human genes with known function or known regulation was selected on the basis of specific upregulation during lytic infection. We examined a series of compounds known to inhibit the respective protein function or gene induction, for their ability to prevent KSHV replication. Interestingly, two of these compounds specifically inhibited KSHV replication (Luukkonen M., Bell Y., Moses A., and K Früh, *unpublished observation*). These preliminary observations suggest that a systematic, data-driven approach to microarray-based target identification in viral systems is possible. In addition to these systematic approaches, we evaluated the role of selected gene products specifically induced by latent KSHV for their importance for KSHV-induced transformation. One of the gene products upregulated in KSHV-infected endothelial cells was the stem-cell growth factor receptor c-kit (Luukkonen M., Bell Y., Moses A., and K Früh, *unpublished observation*). When c-kit signaling was inhibited either through small molecules or by transfecting dominant-negative variants of c-kit, a reversal of the KSHV-induced morphological changes, such as spindle-cell phenotypes, was observed (Moses, A., *unpublished results*). Thus, it is possible that inhibitors of c-kit signaling may be able to interfere with KSHV-induced tumor formation. Since receptor tyrosine-kinase inhibitors that also inhibit c-kit signaling *(47)* are already in use for the treatment of chronic myelogenic leukemia *(48),* such compounds can be evaluated for the treatment of Kaposi's sarcoma.

As another example, the role of individual genes that were found to be upregulated during HCMV-infection has been examined by T. Shenk and colleagues. Zhu et al. noted that genes, such as cyclooxygenase 2 (cox-2), upregulated in HCMV-infected cells, are involved in the regulation of prostaglandin synthesis *(27)*. Accordingly, it was found that HCMV-infected cells showed an increased release of prostaglandin E2. Most importantly, blocking cox-2 activity inhibited HCMV growth in tissue culture (J-P. Cong, H. Zhu, W. Bresnahan, and T. Shenk, *personal communication*). Moreover, exogenous addition of prostaglandins restored HCMV growth, suggesting an important role of this pathway for HCMV to complete its replicative cycle. Thus, although most published results of DNA microarray analysis of virally infected cells are rather descriptive and quite preliminary, often lacking replicates or independent confirmation, these first functional data should encourage a more systematic approach to using functional genomics tools to combat viral infection.

ACKNOWLEDGMENTS

We acknowledge the helpful discussions and the sharing of unpublished results by the following colleagues and collaborators: Thomas Shenk, Ashlee Moses, Jay Nelson, Sabine Kurz, Kenny Simmen, Yolanda Bell, and Mattias Luukkonen.

REFERENCES

1. Human genome sequencing consortium. Initial sequencing and analysis of the human genome. Nature 2001; 409:860–921.
2. Venter et al. The sequence of the human genome. Science 2001; 291:1304–1351.
3. Ideker T, Thorsson V, Ranish JA, Christmas R, Buhler J, Eng JK, et al. Integrated genomic and proteomic analyses of a systematically perturbed metabolic network. Science 2001; 292:929–934.
4. DeRisi JL, Iyer VR, Brown PO. Exploring the metabolic and genetic control of gene expression on a genomic scale. Science 1997; 278:680–686.
5. Chee M, Yang R, Hubbell E, Berno A, Huang XC, Stern D, et al. Accessing genetic information with high-density DNA arrays. Science 1996; 274:610–614.
6. Manger ID, Relman DA. How the host "sees" pathogens: global gene expression responses to infection. Curr Opin Immunol 2000; 12:215–218.
7. Chambers J, Angulo A, Amaratunga D, Guo H, Jiang Y, Wan JS, et al. DNA microarrays of the complex human cytomegalovirus genome: profiling kinetic class with drug sensitivity of viral gene expression. J Virol 1999; 73:5757–5766.
8. Stingley SW, Ramirez JJG, Aguilar SA, Simmen K, Sandri-Goldin RM, Ghazal PH, et al. Global Analysis of HSV type 1 transcription using an oligonucleotide-based DNA microarray. J Virol 2000; 74:9916–9927ss.
9. Jenner RG, Alba MM, Boshoff C, Kellam P. Kaposi's sarcoma-associated herpesvirus latent and lytic gene expression as revealed by DNA arrays. J Virol 2001; 75:891–902.
10. Bresnahan WA, Shenk T. A subset of viral transcripts packaged within human cytomegalovirus particles. Science 2000; 288:2373–2376.
11. Li J, Chen S, Evans DH. Typing and subtyping influenza virus using DNA microarrays and multiplex reverse transcriptase PCR J Clin Microbiol 2001; 39:696–704.
12. Kozal MJ, Shah N, Shen N, Yang R, Fucini R, Merigan TC, et al. Extensive polymorphisms observed in HIV-1 clade B protease gene using high-density oligonucleotide arrays. Nat Med 1996; 2:753–759.
13. Livache T, Fouque B, Roget A, Marchand J, Bidan G, Teoule R, et al. Polypyrrole DNA chip on a silicon device: example of hepatitis C virus genotyping. Anal Biochem 1998; 255:188–194.
14. Bean P, Wilson J. HIV genotyping by chip technology. Am Clin Lab 2000; 19:16–17.
15. Wilson JW, Bean P, Robins T, Graziano F, Persing DH. Comparative evaluation of three human immunodeficiency virus genotyping systems: the HIV-GenotypR method, the HIV PRT GeneChip assay, and the HIV-1 RT line probe assay. J Clin Microbiol 2000; 38:3022–3028.
16. Proudnikov D, Kirillov E, Chumakov K, Donlon J, Rezapkin G, Mirzabekov A. Analysis of mutations in oral poliovirus vaccine by hybridization with generic oligonucleotide microchips. Biologicals 2000; 28:57–66.
17. Hughes TR, Marton MJ, Jones AR, Roberts CJ, Stoughton R, Armour CD, et al. Functional discovery via a compendium of expression profiles. Cell 2000; 102:109–126.
18. Johnson RA, Huong SM, Huang ES. Inhibitory effect of 4-(4-fluorophenyl)-2-(4-hydroxyphenyl)-5-(4-pyridyl) 1H-imidazole on HCMV DNA replication and permissive infection. Antivir Res 1999; 41:101–111.
19. Keller SA, Schattner EJ, Cesarman E. Inhibition of NF-kappaB induces apoptosis of KSHV-infected primary effusion lymphoma cells. Blood 2000; 96:2537–2542.
20. Bresnahan WA, Boldogh I, Chi P, Thompson EA, Albrecht T. Inhibition of cellular Cdk2 activity blocks human cytomegalovirus replication. Virology 1997; 231:239–247.
21. Schang LM, Phillips J, Schaffer PA. Requirement for cellular cyclin-dependent kinases in herpes simplex virus replication and transcription. J Virol 1998; 72:5626–5637.

22. Harty RN, Brown ME, Wang G, Huibregtse J, Hayes FP. A PPxY motif within the VP40 protein of Ebola virus interacts physically and functionally with a ubiquitin ligase: implications for filovirus budding. Proc Natl Acad Sci USA 2000; 97:13,871–13,876.

23. Patnaik A, Chau V, Wills JW. Ubiquitin is part of the retrovirus budding machinery. Proc Natl Acad Sci USA 2000; 97:13,069–13,074.

24. Schubert U, Ott DE, Chertova EN, Welker R, Tessmer U. Princiotta MF, et al. Proteasome inhibition interferes with gag polyprotein processing, release, and maturation of HIV-1 and HIV-2. Proc Natl Acad Sci USA 2000; 97:13,057–13,062.

25. Strack B, Calistri A, Accola MA, Palu G, Gottlinger HG. A role for ubiquitin ligase recruitment in retrovirus release. Proc Natl Acad Sci USA 2000; 97:13,063–13,068.

26. Jean F, Thomas L, Molloy SS, Liu G, Jarvis MA, Nelson JA, et al. A protein-based therapeutic for human cytomegalovirus infection. Proc Natl Acad Sci USA 2000; 97:2864–2869.

27. Zhu H, Cong J-P, Mamtora G, Gingeras T, Shenk T. Cellular gene expression altered by human cytomegalovirus: global monitoring with oligonucleotide arrays. Proc Natl Acad Sci USA 1998; 95:14,470–14,475.

28. Zhu H, Cong J-P, Shenk T. Use of differential display analysis to assess the effect of human cytomegalovirus infection on the accumulation of cellular RNAs: induction of interferon-responsive RNAs. Proc Natl Acad Sci USA 1997; 94:13,985–13,990.

29. Simmen KA, Singh J, Luukkonen BGM, Lopper M, Bittner A, Miller NE, et al. Global modulation of cellular transcription by human cytomegalovirus is initiated by viral glycoprotein B. Proc Natl Acad Sci USA 2001; 98:7140–7145.

30. Mossman KL, Macgregor PF, Rozmus JJ, Goryachev AB, Edwards AM, Smiley JR. Herpes simplex virus triggers and then disarms a host antiviral response. J Virol 2001; 75:750–758.

31. Renne R, Barry C, Dittmer D, Compitello N, Brown PO, Ganem D. Modulation of cellular and viral gene expression by the latency-associated nuclear antigen of Kaposi's sarcoma-associated herpesvirus. J Virol 2001; 75:458–468.

32. Morgan RW, Sofer L, Anderson AS, Bernberg EL, Cui J, Burnside J. Induction of host gene expression following infection of chicken embryo fibroblasts with oncogenic Marek's disease virus. J Virol 2001; 75:533–539.

33. Geiss GK, MC, An Bumgarner RE, Hammersmark E, Cunningham D, Katze MG. Global impact of influenza virus on cellular pathways is mediated by both replication-dependent and -independent events. J Virol 2001; 75:4321–4331.

34. Geiss GK, Bumgarner RE, An MC, Agy MB, van't Wout AB, Hammersmark E, et al. Large-scale monitoring of host cell gene expression during HIV-1 infection using cDNA microarrays. Virology 2000; 266:8–16.

35. Taylor LA, Carthy CM, Yang D, Saad K, Wong D, Schreiner G, et al. Host gene regulation during coxsackievirus B3 infection in mice: assessment by microarrays. Circ Res 2000; 87:328–334.

36. Prosniak M, Hooper DC, Dietzschold B, Koprowski H. Effect of rabies virus infection on gene expression in mouse brain. Proc Natl Acad Sci USA 2001; 98:2758–2763.

37. Huang Y, Uchiyama Y, Fujimura T, Kanamori H, Doi T, Takamizawa A, et al. A human hepatoma cell line expressing hepatitis C virus nonstructural proteins tightly regulated by tetracycline. Biochem Biophys Res Commun 2001; 281:732–740.

38. Chang YE, Laimins LA. Microarray analysis identifies interferon-inducible genes and Stat-1 as major transcriptional targets of human papillomavirus type 31. J Virol 2000; 74:4174–4182.

39. Nees M, Geoghegan JM, Hyman T, Frank S, Miller L, Woodworth CD. Papillomavirus type 16 oncogenes downregulate expression of interferon-responsive genes and upregulate proliferation-associated and NF-kappaB-responsive genes in cervical keratinocytes. J Virol 2001; 75:4283–4296.

40. Boehm U, Klamp T, Groot M, Howard JC. Cellular responses to interferon-gamma. Annu Rev Immunol. 1997; 15:749–795.

41. Miller DM, Rahill BM, Boss JM, Lairmore MD, Durbin JE, Waldman JW, et al. Human cytomegalovirus inhibits major histocompatibility complex class II expression by disruption of the Jak/Stat pathway. J Exp Med 1998; 187:675–683.

42. Miller DM, Zhang Y, Rahill BM, Waldman WJ, and Sedmak DD. Human cytomegalovirus inhibits IFN-alpha-stimulated antiviral and immunoregulatory responses by blocking multiple levels of IFN-alpha signal transduction. J Immunol 1999; 162:6107–6113.

43. Gao SJ, Boshoff C, Jayachandra S, Weiss RA, Chang Y, Moore PS. KSHV ORF K9 (vIRF) is an oncogene which inhibits the interferon signaling pathway. Oncogene 1997; 15:1979–1985.

44. Honda M, Kaneko S, Kawai H, Shirota Y, Kobayashi K. differential gene expression between chronic hepatitis B and C hepatic lesion. Gastroenterology 2001; 120:955–966.

45. Früh K, Simmen K, Luukkonen BGM, Bell YC, Ghazal P. Virogenomics: a novel approach to antiviral drug discovery. Drug Discovery Today 2001; 6:601–608.

46. Moses AV, Fish KN, Ruhl R, Smith PP, Strussenberg JG, Zhu D, et al. Long-term infection and transformation of dermal microvascular endothelial cells by human herpesvirus 8 J Virol 1999; 73:6892–6902.

47. Heinrich MC, Griffith DJ, Druker BJ, Wait CL, Ott KA, Zigler AJ. Inhibition of c-kit receptor tyrosine kinase activity by STI 571, a selective tyrosine kinase inhibitor Blood 2000; 96:925–932.

48. Druker BJ, Lydon NB. Lessons learned from the development of an Abl tyrosine kinase inhibitor for chronic myelogenous leukemia J Clin Investing 2000; 105:3–7.

2

Chipping Away at HIV Pathogenesis

Steffney Elise Rought, Roman Sasik, Davey Mitchell Smith, and Jacques Corbeil

THE NEW AND IMPROVED GENETIC CODE

Completion of the Human Genome Project *(1,2)* has spawned a new set of questions aimed at discovering its meaning. With 2.91 billion basepairs (bp), characterizing this is no easy task. Traditionally, investigators have been confined to mining the human genome a few genes at a time. Fortunately, recent technology has allowed investigators to study it in a comprehensive manner, with the aim of translating genetic sequence information into physiologic relevance. Methodologies such as microarray (cDNA and oligonucleotide) and high-density oligonucleotide array (GeneChips from Affymetrix) analysis allow the interrogation of thousands of genes simultaneously, revealing their expression patterns and the subsequent cellular pathways associated with a particular perturbation. This is particularly useful in studying the effects of microbes on their hosts, which allows both genomes to be investigated simultaneously.

GENECHIP TECHNOLOGY IN GENOMICS RESEARCH

Differential expression data can provide a clearer understanding of cellular pathways triggered by specific stimuli. GeneChip expression probe arrays assist in genomics research by quantitatively and simultaneously monitoring the expression of thousands of genes *(3,4)*. For example, the U95Av2 Chip has a platform of over 12000 gene-specific oligonucleotides anchored to a glass substrate. GeneChip probe arrays identify mRNA expression level changes of greater than twofold between experiments, and are able to detect mRNA transcripts from the level of only a few copies per cell to more than several hundred thousand copies. In contrast to spotting methods, in which a single clone is used to analyze each mRNA, GeneChip expression arrays use approximately 16 pairs of specific oligonucleotide probes to interrogate each transcript with specificity. GeneChip expression arrays are capable of specifically detecting individual gene transcripts and splice variants and can even differentiate among closely related members of gene families. Each GeneChip expression array contains probes that correspond to a number of reference and control genes. Data from different experiments can be normalized and scaled to compare

From: *Pathogen Genomics: Impact on Human Health*
Edited by: K. J. Shaw © Humana Press Inc., Totowa, NJ

multiple experiments quantitatively. These results are typically validated by quantitative real-time RT-PCR.

GeneChip technology has broad applications. Since 1998, the number of publications involving expression monitoring using high-density oligonucleotide probe arrays has increased by approximately sevenfold (see http://www.affymetrix.com/resources/papers.shtml for a complete list). The fields of cancer (5–23), toxicology (24–26), cardiology (27–28), nutrition and aging (29–34), bacteriology (35–38) and mycology (39–45) have all benefited from this technology. Surprisingly, there are only a few publications describing Human Immunodeficiency Virus (HIV)-induced changes in host-gene-expression patterns (46–48) and in identifying HIV-associated mutations using the HIV PRT probe array (49–52).

OVERVIEW OF HIV PATHOGENESIS

Since the presentation of HIV in the early 1980s, billions of dollars have been devoted to its eradication. As of December 2000, 21.8 million people have died globally from acquired immunodeficiency syndrome (AIDS). In addition, 5.3 million people were newly infected in the year 2000 *(53)*. These statistics clearly demonstrate the need for more resources to further the investigation into HIV pathogenesis. Although great progress has been made, the effect on host target cells has not been fully characterized. The inability to directly examine HIV as an intracellular pathogen on a comprehensive level has been a limiting factor. Several aspects of HIV pathogenesis are targets for study by GeneChip probe arrays. At each stage of the infection process, probe arrays could identify changes in gene-expression target and bystander immune cells. The following is a brief overview of potential areas of investigation.

Host Entry

HIV invades the human host through mucosa and blood. There, it has access to its target cells, CD4+ T lymphocytes and monocyte/macrophages. Attachment of the virion is mediated by the interaction of viral-envelope glycoproteins (gp120-gp41) with host cellular-receptor CD4. A conformational change in gp120 allows gp41 to bind to coreceptors such as CXCR4 or CCR5, facilitating cell-viral membrane fusion. The initial contact between HIV and its target cell may be enough to alter host-cell gene expression, as HIV carries host-encoded proteins such as CD80 and CD86 on its surface *(54–56)*.

Manifestation of Disease

Clinically, HIV infection can be defined in three stages: (1) primary, (2) asymptomatic, and *(3)* symptomatic disease progression. During acute infection, within the initial 6 mo, viral replication is intense, as are both humoral and cellular factors that act to control it *(57)*. In this early stage, flu-like symptoms—which appear in some but not all people—probably reflect the humoral and cellular changes that are occurring. The next phase of HIV progression is the aymptomatic period, which can last for several years. This stage is reflected by relatively low levels of HIV antigens and a high turnover of virus. CD4+ cells also turnover rapidly, but their numbers remain relatively steady because of the balance between replenishment and death. Finally, AIDS develops,

CD4+ levels decline, opportunistic infections arise, and death ensues. Each of these stages involves different systems of viral replication and immune response; GeneChip analysis may be an ideal method to evaluate these differences.

Target-Cell Depletion and Apoptosis

One of the hallmarks of HIV progression is CD4+ T-cell depletion. The decline in cell number results from a complex mixture of infected and bystander-cell apoptosis and direct killing by HIV. As CD4 cell numbers decline, viral load increases, directly contributing to pathogenesis. It has been reported the HIV gp120 crosslinking to CD4 receptor enhances susceptibility to apoptosis *(58,59)*. Other HIV proteins implicated in target-cell apoptosis include nef, tat, protease, and vpr (60–63). It is clear that this battle between the immune system and the virus could be explored more finitely using probe-array technology. This would aid in the discovery of apoptosis inhibitors, which could boost the immune response to infection.

BIOINFORMATIC ANALYSIS OF HIV EFFECTS

The utility of gene-array experimental data has been limited by the paradoxical occurrence of too much and too little data. The number of mRNA copies detected for thousands of gene loci represents too much data to be comprehended by unaided human cognition. This scientific problem has been likened to "trying to drink from a fire hose." At the same time, the paucity of semantic information—the *meaning* of gene activation patterns—derives from the fact that GeneChip and gene-array analyzers output only signal-strength information about individual loci, and is accompanied by minimal identifying information such as a GenBank accession number and a short description associated with that accession number. Bioinformatics, the science of developing methodologies for interpretation of biological research, has become an essential tool for understanding genomics. This field of computer science was precipitated by the Human Genome Project as a means of managing the vast amount of information now at our disposal. Organizing gene-expression data into clusters (for example, see Fig. 1) points to co-regulated genes and indicates potential pathways as a consequence of the experimental conditions. The bottleneck of interpreting results from new technologies such as GeneChip is aided by bioinformatic analysis.

Recently, we published data *(46)* on the HIV-1/host-cell relationship over a 72-h time period. Using HuFL GeneChips, we monitored 6800 human genes in a CEM-GFP lymphoblastoid cell line infected by HIV_{LAI} (0.5 MOI). In our paper, we reported these responses to infection: (1) after 72 h, one-third of the total transcripts present in the host cells represented HIV transcripts; (2) mitochondrial and DNA-repair gene expression was decreased, (3) *p53* and the *p53*-induced product Bax were upregulated, and (4) caspases 2, 3, and 9 were activated. HIV-1 transcription resulted in the repression of a large portion of cellular RNA expression and was associated with the induction of apoptosis only in infected cells but not bystander cells. The CEM-GFP host gene responses imply that the subversion of the cell transcriptional machinery for the purpose of HIV-1 replication is similar to that observed in genotoxic stress. This process may play a role in HIV-induced apoptosis, ultimately leading to CD4+ T-cell loss and immunosuppression.

A

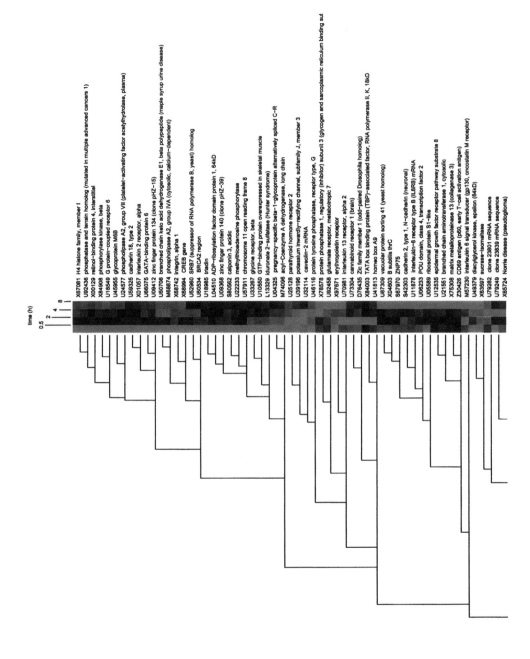

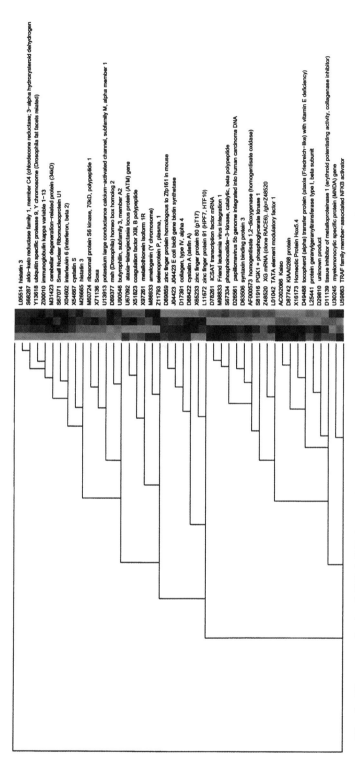

Fig. 1. Cluster analysis of CEM-GFP host-cell genes modulated by HIV within 8 h post-infection (A). (*Continued*)

17

B

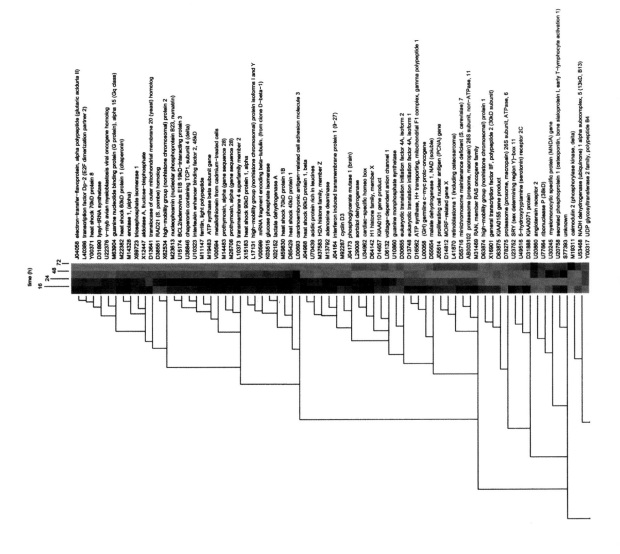

18

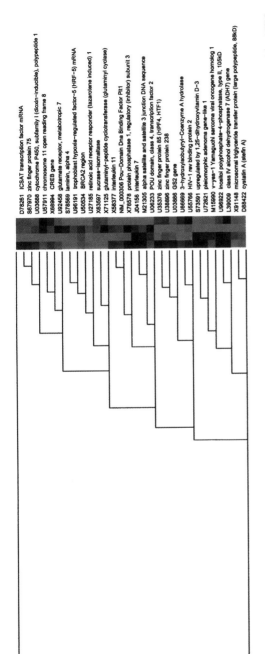

Fig. 1. (*Continued*). and 16-72 hrs (**B**) post-infection. Green = downregulated in HIV, red = upregulated in HIV.

19

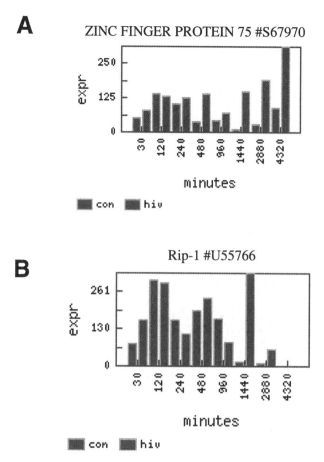

Fig. 2. Expression of zinc-finger protein 75 (**A**) and rev-binding protein (**B**) in uninfected (con) and HIV$_{LAI}$ infected CEM-GFP cells over a 72-h time-course.

Further examination of the GeneChip data revealed some interesting results. Specifically, a number of zinc finger (ZNF) proteins all belonging to the Kruppel group were significantly modulated during HIV infection, such as ZNF 75 (Fig. 2A). The human genome is estimated to contain 300–700 ZNF genes. ZNFs, which bind nucleic acids, perform many key functions; the most important is regulating transcription. The C2H2 ZNF family is characterized by repeated ZNF motifs of approximately 28 amino acids, which chelate a zinc ion using 2 cysteine and 2 histidine residues. The vast majority of these ZNFs are classified as Kruppel-like because they contain conserved 6-amino acid H/C links—regions that connect successive finger repeats. About one-third of Kruppel-like ZNFs contain a conserved motif of approximately 75 amino acids, called the Kruppel-associated box (KRAB), in their N-terminal nonfinger region *(64)*.

Another gene previously associated with HIV was highly upregulated in our experiments. This gene, HIV-1 rev-binding protein 2, (also know as rev-interacting protein (Rip-1) accession number U55766) was highly expressed at 24 h and 48 h after infection (see Fig. 2B). The functional relevance of such an upregulation is under investigation.

FUTURE OF GENOMICS

Discovery-driven approaches in genomics using high-density gene-expression microarrays have led to the establishment of new avenues of research. They have also enabled the identification of pathways and signal-transduction events pertinent to the process of HIV-1 infection. High-density microarray interrogation of gene expression represents a powerful tool to explore the relationships between an infectious agent and its host. The magnitude of knowledge gained by the global survey of effects of pathogens such as HIV on its host will provide a solid foundation for future studies. The study of proteins in a global context may also play an equally important role in the analysis of differential expression of human genomic sequence information.

REFERENCES

1. Venter JC et al. The sequence of the human genome. Science 2001;91:1304–1351.
2. The Genome International Sequencing Consortium. Initial sequencing and analysis of the human genome. Nature 2001;409:860–921.
3. Lockhart DJ, Dong H, Byrne MC, Follettie MT, Gallo MV, Chee MS, et al. Expression monitoring by hybridization to high-density oligonucleotide arrays. Nat Biotechnol 1996;14:1675–1680.
4. Lipshutz RJ, Fodor SPA, Gingeras TR, Lockhart DJ. High density synthetic oligonucleotide arrays. Nat Genet 1999;21:20–24.
5. Virtaneva K, Wright FA, Tanner SM, Yuan B, Lemon WJ, Caligiuri MA, et al. Expression profiling reveals fundamental biological differences in acute myeloid leukemia with isolated trisomy 8 and normal cytogenetics. PNAS 2001;98:1124–1129.
6. Brem R, Certa U, Neeb M, Nair AP, Moroni C. Global analysis of differential gene expression after transformation with the v-H-ras oncogene in a murine tumor model. Oncogene 2001;20:2854–2858.
7. Certa U, Seiler M, Padovan E, Spagnoli GC. High density oligonucleotide array analysis of interferon- alpha 2a sensitivity and transcriptional response in melanoma cells. Br J Cancer 2001;85:107–114.
8. Graveel CR, Jatkoe T, Madore SJ, Holt AL, Farnham PJ. Expression profiling and identification of novel genes in hepatocellular carcinomas. Oncogene 2001;20:2704–2712.
9. Ladanyi M, Chan WC, Triche TJ, Gerald WL. Expression profiling of human tumors: the end of surgical pathology? J Mol Diagn 2001;3:92–97.
10. Luzzi V, Holtschlag V, Watson MA. Expression profiling of ductal carcinoma in situ by laser capture microdissection and high-density oligonucleotide arrays. Am J Pathol 2001;158:2005–2010.
11. Markert JM, Fuller C, Gillespie GY, Bubien JK, McLean LA, Hong RL, et al. Differential gene expression profiling in human brain tumors. Physiol Genomics 2001;5:21–33.
12. Nishizuka S, Winokur ST, Simon M, Martin J, Tsujimoto H, Stanbridge EJ. Oligonucleotide microarray expression analysis of genes whose expression is correlated with tumorigenic and non-tumorigenic phenotype of HeLa x human fibroblast hybrid cells. Cancer Lett 2001;165:201–209.
13. Notterman DA, Alon U, Sierk AJ, Levine AJ. Transcriptional gene expression profiles of colorectal adenoma, adenocarcinoma, and normal tissue examined by oligonucleotide arrays. Cancer Res 2001;61:3124–3130.
14. Schwirzke M, Evtimova V, Burtscher H, Jarsch M, Tarin D, Weidle UH. Identification of metastasis-associated genes by transcriptional profiling of a pair of metastatic versus non-metastatic human mammary carcinoma cell lines. Anticancer Res 2001;21:1771–1776.
15. Tackels-Horne D, Goodman MD, Williams AJ, Wilson DJ, Eskandari T, Vogt LM, et al. Identification of differentially expressed genes in hepatocellular carcinoma and metastatic liver tumors by oligonucleotide expression profiling. Cancer 2001;92:395–405.

16. Thykjaer T, Workman C, Kruhoffer M, Demtroder K, Wolf H, Andersen LD, et al. Identification of gene expression patterns in superficial and invasive human bladder cancer. Cancer Res 2001;61:2492–2499.

17. Welsh JB, Zarrinkar PP, Sapinoso LM, Kern SG, Behling CA, Monk BJ, et al. Analysis of gene expression profiles in normal and neoplastic ovarian tissue samples identifies candidate molecular markers of epithelial ovarian cancer. PNAS 2001;98:1176–1181.

18. Welsh JB, Sapinoso LM, Su AI, Kern SG, Wang-Rodriguez J, Moskaluk CA, et al. Analysis of gene expression identifies candidate markers and pharmacological targets in prostate cancer. Cancer Res 2001 Aug 15; 61(16):5974–5978.

19. Zhang H, Yu CY, Singer B, Xiong M. Recursive partitioning for tumor classification with gene expression microarray data. PNAS 2001;98:6730–6735.

20. Clark EA, Golub TR, Lander ES, Hynes RO. Genomic analysis of metastasis reveals an essential role for RhoC. Nature 2000;406:532–535.

21. Alon U, Barkai N, Notterman DA, Gish K, Ybarra S, Mack D, et al. Broad patterns of gene expression revealed by clustering analysis of tumor and normal colon tissues probed by oligonucleotide arrays. PNAS 1999;96:6745–6750.

22. Golub TR, Slonim DK, Tamayo P, Huard C, Gaasenbeek M, Mesirov JP, et al. Molecular classification of cancer: class discovery and class prediction by gene expression monitoring. Science 1999;286:531–537.

23. Lee SB, Huang K, Palmer R, Truong VB, Herzlinger D, Kolquist KA, et al. The Wilms Tumor Suppressor WT1 encodes a transcriptional activator of amphiregulin. Cell 1999;98:663–673.

24. Gerhold D, Lu M, Xu J, Austin C, Caskey CT, Rushmore T. Monitoring expression of genes involved in drug metabolism and toxicology using DNA microarrays. Physiol Genomics 2001;5:161–170.

25. He B, Munson AE, Meade BJ. Analysis of gene expression induced by irritant and sensitizing chemicals using oligonucleotide arrays. Int Immunopharmacol 2001;1:867–879.

26. Reilly TP, Bourdi M, Brady JN, Pise-Masison CA, Radonovich MF, George JW, et al. Expression profiling of acetaminophen liver toxicity in mice using microarray technology. Biochem Biophys Res Commun 2001;282:321–328.

27. Jin H, Yang R, Awad TA, Wang F, Li W, Williams SP, et al. Effects of early angiotensin-converting enzyme inhibition on cardiac gene expression after acute myocardial infarction. Circulation 2001;103:737–742.

28. Redfern CH, Degtyarev MY, Kwa AT, Salomonis N, Cotte N, Nanevicz T, et al. Conditional expression of a Gi-coupled receptor causes ventricular conduction delay and a lethal cardiomyopathy. PNAS 2000;97:4826–4831.

29. Jiang CH, Tsien JZ, Schult PG, Hu YH. The effects of aging on gene expression in the hypothalamus and cortex of mice. PNAS 2001;98:1930–1934.

30. Garcia CK, Mues G, Liao Y, Hyatt T, Patil N, Cohen JC, et al. Sequence diversity in genes of lipid metabolism. Genome Res 2001;11:1043–1052.

31. Kayo T, Allison DB, Weindruch R, Prolla TA. Influences of aging and caloric restriction on the transcriptional profile of skeletal muscle from rhesus monkeys. PNAS 2001;98:5093–5098.

32. Lee CK, Weindruch R, Prolla TA. Gene-expression profile of the aging brain in mice. Nat Genet 2000;25:294–297.

33. Ly DH, Lockhart DJ, Lerner RA, Schultz PG. Mitotic misregulation and human aging. Science 2000;287:2486–2492.

34. Lee CK, Klopp RG, Weindruch R, Prolla TA. Gene expression profile of aging and its retardation by caloric restriction. Science 1999;285:1390–1393.

35. Hooper LV, Wong MH, Thelin A, Hansson L, Falk PG, Gordon JI. Molecular analysis of commensal host-microbial relationships in the intestine. Science 2001;291:881–884.

36. Belcher CE, Drenkow J, Kehoe B, Gingeras TR, McNamara N, Lemjabbar H, et al. The transcriptional responses of respiratory epithelial cells to Bordetella pertussis reveal host defensive and pathogen counter-defensive strategies. PNAS 2000;97:13,847–13,852.

37. Gingeras TR, Rosenow C. Studying microbial genomes with high-density oligonucleotide arrays. ASM News 2000;66:463–469.

38. Selinger DW, Cheung KJ, Mei R, Johansson EM, Richmond CS, Blattner FR, et al. RNA expression analysis using a 30 base pair resolution Escherichia coli genome array. Nat Biotechnol 2000;18:1262–1268.

39. Jelinsky SA, Estep P, Church GM, Samson LD. Regulatory networks revealed by transcriptional profiling of damaged Saccharomyces cerevisiae cells: Rpn4 links base excision repair with proteasomes. Mol Cell Biol 2000;20:8157–8167.

40. Nau ME, Emerson LR, Martin RK, Kyle DE, Wirth DF, Vahey M. Technical assessment of the Affymetrix Yeast Expression GeneChip YE6100 Platform in a heterologous model of genes that confer resistance to antimalarial drugs in yeast. J Clin Microbiol 2000;38:1901–1908.

41. Primig M, Williams RM, Winzeler EA, Tevzadze GG, Conway AR, Hwang SY, et al. The core meiotic transcriptome in budding yeasts. Nat Genet 2000;26:415–423.

42. Lelivelt MJ, Culbertson MR. Yeast Upf proteins required for RNA surveillance affect global expression of the yeast transcriptome. Mol Cell Biol 1999;19:6710–6719.

43. Winzeler EA, Shoemaker DD, Astromoff A, Liang H, Anderson K, Andre B, et al. Functional characterization of the S. cerevisiae genome by gene deletion and parallel analysis. Science 1999;285:901–906.

44. Wyrick JJ, Holstege FCP, Jennings EG, Causton HC, Shore D, Grunstein M, et al. Chromosomal landscape of nucleosome-dependent gene expression and silencing in yeast. Nature 1999;402:418–421.

45. Wodicka L, Dong H, Mittmann M, Ho MH, Lockhart DJ. A genome-wide expression monitoring in Saccharomyces cerevisiae. Nat Biotechnol 1997;15:1359–1367.

46. Corbeil J, Sheeter DA, Genini D, Rought SE, Leoni L, Du P, et al. Temporal gene regulation during HIV-1 infection of human CD4+ T cells. Genome Res 2001;11:1198–1204.

47. Ryo A, Suzuki Y, Arai M, Kondoh N, Wakatsuki T, Hada A, et al. Identification and characterization of differentially expressed mRNAs in HIV type 1-infected human T cells. AIDS Res Hum Retrovir 2000;16:995–1005.

48. Ryo A, Suzuki Y, Ichiyama K, Wakatsuki T, Kondoh N, Hada A, et al. Serial analysis of gene expression in HIV-1-infected T cell lines. FEBS Lett 1999;462:182–186.

49. Kozal MJ, Shah N, Shen N, Yang R, Fucini R, Merigan TC, et al. Extensive polymorphisms observed in HIV-1 clade B protease gene using high-density oligonucleotide arrays. Nat Med 1996;2:753–759.

50. Wilson JW, Bean P, Robins T, Graziano F, Persing DH. Comparative evaluation of three human immunodeficiency virus genotyping systems: the HIV-GenotypR method, the HIV PRT GeneChip assay, and the HIV-1 RT line probe assay. J Clin Microbiol 2000;38:3022–3028.

51. Vahey M, Nau ME, Barrick S, Cooley JD, Sawyer R, Sleeker AA, et al. Performance of the Affymetrix GeneChip HIV PRT 440 platform for antiretroviral drug resistance genotyping of human immunodeficiency virus type 1 clades and viral isolates with length polymorphisms. J Clin Microbiol 1999;37:2533–2537.

52. Gunthard HF, Wong JK, Ignacio CC, Havlir DV, Richman DD. Comparative performance of high-density oligonucleotide sequencing and dideoxynucleotide sequencing of HIV type 1 pol from clinical samples. AIDS Res Hum Retrovir 1998;14:869–876.

53. UNAIDS. Report on the global HIV/AIDS epidemic: December 2000.

54. Tremblay MJ, Fortin JF, Cantin R. The acquisition of host-encoded proteins by nascent HIV-1. Immunol Today 1998;19:346–351.

55. Bounou S, Dumais N, Tremblay MJ. Attachment of human immunodeficiency virus-1 (HIV-1) particles bearing host-encoded B7-2 proteins leads to nuclear factor-kappaB- and nuclear factor of activated T cells-dependent activation of HIV-1 long terminal repeat transcription. J Biol Chem 2001;276:6359–6369.

56. Esser MT, Graham DR, Coren LV, Trubey CM, Bess JW Jr, Arthur LO, et al. Differential incorporation of CD45, CD80 (B7-1), CD86 (B7-2), and major histocompatibility complex class I and II molecules into human immunodeficiency virus type 1 virions and microvesicles: implications for viral pathogenesis and immune regulation. J Virol 2001 75:6173–6182.

57. Daar ES. Virology and immunology of acute HIV type 1 infection. AIDS Res Hum Retrovir 1998 Oct; 14 Suppl 3:S229–S234.

58. Banda NK, Bernier J, Kurahara DK, Kurrle R, Haigwood N, Sekaly RP, et al. Crosslinking CD4 by human immunodeficiency virus gp120 primes T cells for activation-induced apoptosis. J Exp Med 1992;176:1099–1106.

59. Oyaizu N, McCloskey TW, Coronesi M, Chirmule N, Kalyanaraman VS, Pahwa S. Accelerated apoptosis in peripheral blood mononuclear cells (PBMCs) from human immunodeficiency virus type-1 infected patients and in CD4 cross-linked PBMCs from normal individuals. Blood 82:3392–3400.

60. Rasola A, Gramaglia D, Boccaccio C, Comoglio PM. Apoptosis enhancement by the HIV-1 Nef protein. J Immunol 2001;166:81–88.

61. Purvis SF, Jacobberger JW, Sramkoski RM, Patki AH, Lederman MM. HIV type 1 Tat protein induces apoptosis and death in Jurkat cells. AIDS Res Hum Retrovir 1995;11:443–450.

62. Strack PR, Frey MW, Rizzo CJ, Cordova B, George HJ, Meade R, et al. Apoptosis mediated by HIV protease is preceded by cleavage of Bcl-2. PNAS 1996;93:9571–9576.

63. Stewart SA, Poon B, Jowett JB, Chen IS. Human immunodeficiency virus type 1 Vpr induces apoptosis following cell cycle arrest. J Virol 1997;71:5579–5592.

64. Bellefroid EJ, Poncelet DA, Lecocq PJ, Revelant O, Martial JA. The evolutionarily conserved Kruppel-associated box domain defines a subfamily of eukaryotic multifingered proteins. PNAS 1991;88:3608–3612.

Microarray Analysis of Human Papillomavirus Pathogenesis

Yijan Elaine Chang and Laimonis A. Laimins

OVERVIEW

Human papillomaviruses (HPVs) have a complex life cycle, which is associated with the differentiation state of the host cell. Over eighty-five different types have been identified to date, and each exhibits strict tissue specificity. The genome of HPV is relatively small, and the majority of necessary enzymatic activities are provided by the host cells. Thus, the regulation of viral life cycle and the control of cellular activities are intimately intertwined. The advancement of new analytical technologies, combined with the wealth of information on human genome that has recently become available have paved the way for new developments in HPV research in the coming years.

PATHOGENESIS OF HPV

Classification of HPVs and Related Symptoms

HPVs are a group of small DNA viruses that cause hyperproliferation of infected epithelial cells. About one-half of the HPV types identified to date infect cutaneous epithelia and induce hyperproliferative benign warts *(1,2)*. Common lesions associated with low-risk HPV infections include plantar warts on the soles of feet (verruca plantaris) caused by HPV 1 infection, and common hand warts (verruca vulgaris) resulting from HPV 2 infection. A subset of cutaneous types HPVs (including HPV 5 and 8) infects patients with a rare genetic skin disease, epidermodysplasia verruciformis (EV), and in combination with ultraviolet (UV) exposure, can lead to the development of carcinomas *(2)*. In addition, HPV has been shown to be involved in the development of approximately 20% of oropharyngeal cancers, in conjunction with environmental carcinogenic factors *(3)*. Approximately one-half of the HPV types infect the anogenital mucosa. This group of HPV can be further categorized into the low-risk types, such as HPV 6 and 11, which cause benign lesions, or the high-risk type, such as HPV 16, 18, 31, 33, 45 and 54, which are the etiological agent of cancers of the anogenital region *(4)*. Genital infection by HPVs is the most common viral sexually transmitted disease in the United States, with approximately 24–40 million individuals infected. The initial stages of infection are asymptomatic, and the lesions usually resolve without treatment *(5)*. Infection by the high-risk HPV types in the anogenital tract is the primary risk fac-

From: *Pathogen Genomics: Impact on Human Health*
Edited by: K. J. Shaw © Humana Press Inc., Totowa, NJ

tor for the development of cancers of the cervix, vagina, vulva, and penis *(2)*. Cancer of the cervix is the second most common cancer worldwide, and HPV infection is associated with over 95% of these cases *(4)*. The number of individuals who develop cervical cancer in the United States and other developed countries has dropped dramatically in the past 40 years because of the widespread usage of the Papanicolau (Pap) smear. The Pap smear detects precancerous cells that are indicative of cervical intra-epithelial neoplasia (CIN), or dysplasia induced by HPV infection. Although low-grade CIN frequently resolves within a short period of time, on occasion, low-grade CIN may develop into high-grade CIN, which is the precursor of cancer. Typically, HPV-induced lesions resolve within 2 yr following infection, and the failure to clear these infections is a major risk factor for the development of genital malignancy *(2)*.

The HPV Genome and Functions of Individual Viral Genes

The genome of all HPV types consists of double-stranded DNA of approx 8 kb in length. The genome organization is highly conserved among all HPV types *(1)* (Fig.1). HPVs infect epithelial cells in the basal layer through open wounds, and establish persistent infection in these cells. During this persistent infection, the viral genome is maintained as extrachromosomal episomes whose replication coincides with cellular DNA replication. In these infected cells, the viral genome copy number is maintained constant at approximately 20–100 copies per cell *(4)*.

The viral genes can be roughly divided into early (E) and late (L) units based on the timing of expression. Messages encoding early proteins are transcribed from the early promoter located upstream of the E6 open reading frame (ORF). Early transcripts are heterogeneous, and each transcript has the potential to encode a subset of early genes (E1,E2,E4,E5,E6, and E7), depending on the particular splicing pattern. The late viral promoter is located within the E7 ORF and directs the expression of the E1^E4 fusion protein, E5 as well as the L1 and L2 genes encoding the capsid proteins. Upon epithelial differentiation, the productive stage of the viral life cycle is initiated, and the late promoter is dramatically activated. In addition, viral genomes are amplified to thousands of copies per cell, late proteins are synthesized, and infectious virions are assembled and released.

The E1 and E2 proteins encode the replication factors of the virus *(6,7)*. E1 recognizes and binds to the viral replication origin located in the upstream regulatory region (URR) and recruits cellular replication proteins *(7,8)*. In addition, E1 functions as a helicase during viral replication in a manner similar to the Simian virus 40 (SV40) T-antigen *(9)*. E2 plays a dual role in the viral life cycle. E2 forms a complex with E1 and enhances viral genome replication by facilitating E1 binding to the viral origin of replication *(10,11)*. In bovine papillomavirus 1 (BPV1), E2 transactivates the viral early promoter *(12,13)*. However, E2 appears to primarily play a negative role in viral gene transcription in the human viral types, and may act to autoregulate its own expression *(14,15)*. This autoregulation is likely to contribute to copy-number control in infected basal cells.

E4 is the most abundantly expressed viral protein, but its function still remains unclear. E4 is translated from a spliced transcript that forms a fusion between the first four amino acids of E1 and the E4 ORF. The E4 protein may potentially be translated from some of the early transcripts, but its expression is greatly elevated upon differen-

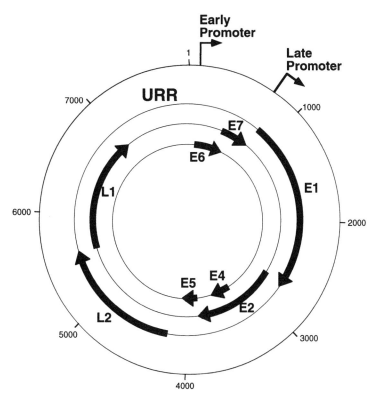

Fig. 1. Circular map of HPV genome. Viral early (E) or late (L) ORFs are indicated as bold arrow. Function of each ORF is described in the text. Nucleotide number is indicated on top of the outermost circle. Early and late promoters are labeled with the direction of transcription. URR, upstream regulatory region

tiation. When expressed in transformed keratinocytes, E4 interacts with cytokeratin intermediate filaments, and in some HPVs induces the collapse of the cytokeratin network *(16)*. However, it is likely that E4 has other uncharacterized functions in the viral life cycle. The HPV E5 protein is expressed from the same transcripts as the E1^E4 fusion protein. In BPV1, E5 is the major transforming protein of the virus; however, its role in HPVs remains elusive. The E5 protein by itself has weak transforming activity, and may augment the transformation activities of the major transforming proteins, E6 and E7 *(17)*. E5 is believed to alter the acidification of endosome, which results in deregulation of epithelial growth-factor receptor (EGFR) turnover. The prolonged presence of EGFR on the cell surface may sustain the proliferating effect of EGF signaling *(18,19)*.

The major transforming proteins in high-risk HPVs are E6 and E7, and significant efforts have been focused on the study of these two proteins. E6 and E7 are both small proteins (149 to 158 amino acids, and 97 to 110 amino acids in length, respectively), with versatile functions. Numerous cellular proteins are targeted by E6 and E7 at either the transcriptional or post-transcriptional level. E6 binds to p53 through its association with the cellular ubiquitin ligase E6AP *(20,21),* resulting in the rapid turnover of p53[22].

E6 has also been shown to activate expression of the catalytic subunit of telomerase, resulting in high-level telomerase activity in cells containing high-risk HPVs *(23,24)*. Furthermore, the E6 protein has a broad spectrum of effects on cellular activities, such as abrogation of G1/S checkpoint and G2/M checkpoint, prevention of apoptosis, resistance to differentiation, and alteration of interferon signaling *(25–28)*. These effects may result from interactions of E6 with a variety of cellular proteins, including p53, E6AP, MCM7, CEBP/p300, hDLG, E6TP1, E6BP, paxillin, clathrin-adaptor protein 1 (AP-1), IRF3, and Tyk2 *(20,21,29–36)*. It is surprising that a protein expressed at such a low level in cells can have such broad effects.

The E7 protein also has a wide variety of cellular binding partners. E7 binds to the retinoblastoma (Rb) protein pRB, and other members of the pocket protein family, p107 and p130 *(36,37)*. Other E7 binding partners include cyclin A and E cyclin-dependent kinase (cdk) inhibitors (CKI) p21 and p27, and histone deacetylase *(39–41)*. In normal cells, pRB regulates the G1/S and G2/M checkpoints *(42)*. Hypophosphory-lated Rb binds to E2F and prevents activation of S-phase specific genes. Upon stimulation by a mitogenic signal, cyclin D/cdk 4 phosphorylates Rb, which results in the release of E2F1 and activation of S-phase-specific genes. E7 abrogates the G1/S checkpoint directly by binding and sequestering Rb, resulting in activation of E2F proteins *(26,43)*. The association of E7 with Rb family members also plays an important role in blocking the exit from the cell cycle of epithelial cells during differentiation. This process allows for the productive phase of the viral life cycle in differentiated suprabasal cells *(44,45)*. E7 has also been shown to interact with p48 (ISGF3γ) and the tumor-suppressor protein IRF1 *(45–47)*.

Mechanism of HPV Transformation and Tumorigenesis

Expression of the E6 and E7 proteins of high-risk HPVs is sufficient to immortalize primary keratinocytes *(1,2)*. Activation of telomerase activity by E6 and inactivation of the Rb/p16 pathway by E7 are the major factors in mediating immortalization *(49)*. In addition, inactivation of p53 leads to the loss of checkpoint control, which increases the frequency of mutations in the host genome *(50)*. The degradation of p53 facilitated by E6 may therefore be the most important factor for oncogenesis. E6 may also affect cell-cycle regulation via p53-independent pathways by interacting with other tumor-suppressor proteins *(30)*. The ability to bypass cell-cycle checkpoints through the action of E6 and E7 proteins clearly gives infected cells a growth advantage.

Hyperproliferative lesions induced by HPVs usually regress after a period of time because of the activation of the host's immune response to viral infection. The failure to mount an adequate immune response results in persistent infection of the HPV. Persistent HPV infection can be sustained for several decades, resulting in increased level of genomic instability and the accumulation of chromosomal mutations *(51)*. One of the consequences of genomic instability may also be the integration of HPV DNA into a host genome, as a high percentage of HPV-induced cancers contain integrated copies of HPV DNA *(1)*. This integration usually results in interruption of E2 gene expression, and consequently, in altered regulation of E6 and E7 expression. The latently infected virus depends on terminal differentiation of keratinocytes to amplify the genome. Conversely, the normal differentiation program of the cells is altered to sustain the growth of the virus, and may lead to hyperproliferation and the development of warts. All of these factors may also facilitate the onset and maintenance of a tumorigenic state.

Current Treatment for High- and Low-Risk HPVs

Although there is no cure for HPV infection, various treatments are available to relieve symptoms. The prognosis varies considerably depending on the type of HPV, the course of infection, and the patient's genetic background. The types of treatments commonly used include surgical removal, cytotoxic agents, and immunomodulating therapy *(52)*. Warts are usually removed by surgical excision, electrosurgery, cryotherapy, or laser surgery. The problem with surgical removal is that the chance for recurrence of disease is high. It is difficult to identify and remove all the abnormal tissues, and it is possible that HPV DNA is harbored in a latent state in cells with a normal appearance. Cytotoxic agents used to treat HPV lesions include podophyllin, podophyllotoxin, colchicine, trichloroacetic acid, and 5-fluorouracil *(51)*. All of those agents may achieve varying degrees of clearance of infection, and consequently may result in a varying recurrence rate of the disease.

The host immune system, especially cellular immunity, plays an important role in the determining the course of HPV infection *(53)*. Immune-suppressed patients, such as those undergoing organ transplantation, often develop extensive and persistent warts. In addition, AIDS patients often develop extensive HPV-induced lesions and are at high risk for the development of cervical cancer *(53,54)*. Immunomodulation therapies and the development of prophylactic or therapeutic HPV vaccines are two areas that are currently under active study *(54,56)*. The prophylactic vaccines use viral-like particles (VLPs), which consist of L1 and L2 proteins expressed from heterologous systems *(56)*. In addition, type I interferon (IFN α, β) and type II interferon (IFN γ) have been used in clinical trials with varying degree of success. Although treatment of low-risk HPV-associated hyperproliferation with IFN remains promising, some of the initial success reported with high-risk HPV-associated neoplasia could not be reproduced in controlled trials *(57,58)*. The effectiveness of treatment of high-risk HPV infection with interferon has not yet been shown to be effective. Although interferon has been shown in BPV1-transformed cells to diminish the replication of BPV1 genome *(59)*, neoplasia induced from integrated HPV genomes may be resistant to the effects of interferon, as demonstrated with transformed cells with integrated SV40 genomes *(60)*.

APPLICATION OF MICROARRAY TECHNOLOGY IN UNDERSTANDING HPV PATHOGENESIS

Although the HPV viral life cycle is tightly regulated by cellular differentiation, viral proteins in turn modify many cellular activities. These changes include the altered expression of cellular genes. Several studies have used differential display and other transcription profiling approaches to examine the changes in cellular transcription caused by HPV infection. The application of microarray technology to the study of HPV infection is still at an early stage, and this area promises to yield useful information on virus-cell interactions. Here we describe published and ongoing studies using microarray and other global approaches to understand the effect of HPV on the host cells.

Tissue-Culture Systems for Studying HPV

As mentioned previously, the course of HPV infection can be divided into two stages: persistent infection in basal cells and productive infection in differentiated cells. In the case of high-risk HPV, there may be another level of host-virus interaction—malignant transformation. To study HPV infection in vitro, a model system that closely resembles the first two stages of infection is needed. The failure to find a good in vitro tissue-culture system has been the major obstacle in the study of HPV biology. In the past, expression systems have been extensively used in which one or two HPV gene products were expressed under a heterologous promoter independent of other viral genes. Although these methods have been informative, they may not accurately reflect what occurs when the gene products are expressed at physiological levels, or when the gene is expressed in the context of the viral genome. In addition, cells used for these heterologous expression studies were often not the natural host of HPV—i.e., keratinocyte, in order to achieve high transfection efficiency. The interpretation of results derived from cells that are not the natural host of HPV is difficult, considering the strict cell-type specificity of HPVs. The use of retroviral vectors is a more advantageous alternative system, which allows the study of a more uniform population of cells expressing the target protein at a near-physiological level *(45)*. However, for a true representation of the effects of HPV viral activities on host cells during infection, the presence of the entire viral genome is crucial *(61)*.

In recent years, several model systems have been developed that have made a genetic analysis of HPV functions during the productive life cycle possible *(62–64)*. Cell lines derived form biopsy or normal keratinocytes stably transfected with either high- or low-risk HPV genomes can be maintained in culture for various periods of time. These growth conditions reflect the latent infection state, as evidenced by the stable maintenance of a low copy number of HPV genomes and the expression of early genes. The productive infection requires the induction of terminal differentiation of epithelial cells—a result that has been achieved in several systems. A xenograft model has been successfully used to induce hyperproliferation caused by several HPVs by implanting HPV-infected human keratinocytes under the renal capsule of athymic mice *(65)*. One highly effective system for in vitro differentiation is the organotypic culture system, which triggers stratification of keratinocytes and gives rise to differentiated epidermal tissue closely resembling normal or infected tissue in vivo *(66)*. Differentiation induced by a high concentration of calcium in the media or by suspending cells in semisolid media are more cost-effective models which show promise *(67–69)*. These latter two systems allow RNA to be harvested at different times and subjected to microarray analysis. Because cells differentiate at a fairly uniform rate in these systems, it is possible to obtain a homogenous population of differentiated cells.

Another approach to the study of changes in cellular gene expression induced by HPVs is to use RNA isolated from biopsy samples of cervical neoplasia at various stages of disease progression. One concern with the use of biopsy samples for analyzing changes in global gene expression is that the cell types may be very heterogeneous. With recent advances in the use of laser-capture microdissection technique (LCM) *(70,71)*, it is now possible to isolate uniform cell types from tissues. The sensitivity of microarray analysis makes it possible to examine small amounts of RNA through an amplification process. The use of these methodologies allows for a detailed analysis of HPV effects on cellular gene expression during various phases of the viral life cycle.

Alteration of Cellular Gene Expression During Latent Infection by HPV

Prior to the introduction of microarray technology, numerous studies were conducted using other global transcriptional profiling methods such as differential display. These studies focused primarily on the effects of the E6 and E7 oncoproteins. In high-risk HPV-immortalized human keratinocytes, or cells transfected with only the E6 and E7 genes, the expression of several cellular genes were found to be altered *(72–80)*. These changes were likely the result of modulation of p53 and Rb, and thus indirectly the E2F activities. These studies using differential display have provided an initial analysis of the spectrum of cellular genes targeted by HPV oncoproteins. However, the information is fragmented, and the relevance of the cell lines chosen from these studies often makes interpretation difficult.

Microarray analysis allows a nonbiased and more vigorous examination of changes in the cellular transcriptional pattern during various stages of HPV infection. If a large representation of human genes is present on the array, groups of genes that carry out similar activities or participate in the same pathways can be easily identified. Recently, several studies have described the use of this technique to examine changes induced during HPV infection. One of these studies specifically examines the changes in cellular gene transcription during persistent HPV infection in undifferentiated cells *(81)*. Normal human keratinocytes from foreskin tissue was transfected and subsequently immortalized with the complete genome of the high-risk HPV type 31. This HPV31-positive cell line was propagated in monolayer culture, and represents a latent infection with HPV31.

Microarray analysis was performed using RNAs isolated from HPV31-positive cells, and these were compared to normal keratinocytes isolated from the same donor and grown under the same conditions. Among 7075 genes expressed sequence tags (ESTs) examined, only a small portion (4.6%) of genes were identified with an expression level altered by at least twofold. The genes whose expression was altered could be classified into three classes; genes that are involved in regulating cell growth, genes that are structural components and/or specific in keratinocytes, and genes that are important in the interferon pathway. Since normal keratinocytes have a limited life-span in culture, the process of immortalization itself undoubtedly alters normal cell-cycle regulation and thus cellular gene expression. Consistent with this activity, positive cell-proliferation regulators, such as myc, and negative regulators, such as p21 and Mad, were found to be up- or downregulated in HPV31 cells, respectively *(82,83)*. The second class of genes whose expression was found to be altered by HPV includes genes that encode keratinocyte-specific proteins such as SPRK and SprII, which are small, proline-rich proteins induced by UV irradiation *(84)* Downregulation of this type of genes in HPV31-positive cells may suggest an altered response to external stress in HPV31-positive cells. In addition, downregulation of desmoplakin and desmocollin was observed, and the alteration of expression of these cell-cell junction proteins may alter the mobility of HPV-positive cells *(84)*.

The most dramatic change observed was the suppression of the basal level of type I interferon-responsive genes in HPV-positive cells. As a result, HPV31-positive cells exhibit a delayed response to interferon (IFN) stimulation. HPV may actively suppress IFN response to evade host immune surveillance, and thus to maintain a latent infection. One of the major regulators in the IFN pathway, Stat-1 (Signal Transducer and Activator of Transcription 1) was also found to be suppressed in HPV31-positive cells *(86)*. Stat-1 belongs to a family of proteins which play vital roles in signal transduction, stimulated by a variety of cytokines and growth factors. This class of proteins usually resides in the cytoplasm in its hypophosphorylated and inactive form. Upon stimulation by binding of cell-surface receptors and ligands, Stat proteins are phosphorylated on tyrosine residues, translocated into the nucleus, and target gene expression. The best-studied stimulation of Stat-1 protein is with the type I type II interferons. Upon the stimulation of type I interferon, Stat-1 and Stat-2 are phosphorylated, heterodimerized, and complex with p48 to form the nuclear transactivation complex ISGF3. Type II interferon stimulation leads to the formation of Stat-1 homodimer *(87)*. This suppression of the basal level of Stat-1 in HPV31-positive cells occurs at both the transcriptional and post-transcriptional levels (Chang and Laimins, *unpublished data*). It is possible that the delayed response and reduced basal level of IFN-responsive genes in HPV31 cells could be a result of long-term suppression of Stat-1. Thomas et al. used a similar approach to examine cellular changes during latent infection with low-risk HPV type 11 *(88)*. Interestingly, no reduction was observed in the expression of type I IFN-responsive genes, and a slight activation of these genes by HPV11 was observed. This differential ability of low- and high-risk HPV to modulate host immune response may have important clinical implications. This difference is consistent with the difficulty reported in applying interferon therapy to high-risk HPV patients. *(54)*.

Alteration of Cellular Gene Expression by Viral Gene Products During Keratinocyte Differentiation

In addition to studies of changes induced by HPV in undifferentiated cells, studies have been initiated to examine altered cellular gene expression in differentiated cells.

Two types of experiments were conducted to address the question. Nees et al. examined the effects of HPV16 E6/E7 on keratinocytes during differentiation using human ectocervical keratinocytes that expressed E6 and E7 proteins *(89,90)*. These cells were treated with high concentrations of calcium to induce differentiation, and then analyzed for changes in cellular gene expression. RNAs from E6/E7 retroviral-infected cells and vector-infected cells were isolated and then processed for comparison on a cDNA array. From these studies, the authors identified several groups of genes with altered expression. First, genes involved in DNA replication, nucleotide metabolism, and cell-cycle progression were upregulated. Secondly, differentiation-induced TGF-β2 responses and proapoptotic genes were found to be downregulated. Consistent with studies with HPV31, interferon-responsive genes were found to be downregulated *(81)*. Finally, proliferation-related NF-κB-responsive genes were upregulated in E6/E7 cells during calcium-induced differentiation of cervical keratinocytes.

The regulation of TGF-β is complex and the function of TGF-β is pleotropic, as it regulates epithelial-cell remolding and blocks cell-cycle progression *(91)*. Furthermore, TGF-β acts as a tumor suppressor as it inhibits tumor progression in the animal model.

E6 and E7 proteins suppress the effect of TGF-β induced either by differentiation or other cytokines in a p53- and Rb-dependent fashion. Interestingly, expression of Stat-1 RNA was not affected by E6 and E7, but the total amount—and especially nuclear Stat-1 protein—was dramatically reduced in the cells that expressed E6 and E7. Nuclear Stat-1 activity was found to be decreased, as demonstrated by gel-shift assay. This effect was the result of the activity of E6 protein, and is only partially dependent on its ability to degrade p53 *(90)*. The authors also determined that the activation of NF-κB activity could be a result of an increased amount of CBP/p300 caused by the degradation of p53 by E6. NF-κB has been shown to protect keratinocytes from apoptosis, and elevated activity has been observed during mouse-skin carcinogenesis *(92)*.

Chang and Laimins have also examined cellular changes in HPV 31-immortalized foreskin keratinocytes differentiated in semisolid medium, and observed similar changes (Chang and Laimins, *manuscript in preparation*). In this study, genes involved in DNA synthesis and chromosome maintenance were upregulated. In addition, it appeared that the normal differentiation program was delayed based on the altered patterns of expression of specific types of keratin, and the reduced response to TGF-β. Since expression of only the E6 and E7 proteins of high-risk HPV has been shown to alter cellular differentiation, revive cellular DNA replication machinery, and stimulate cell-cycle progression, these findings are not unexpected *(44,93,94)*. In fact, it is possible that E6 and E7 are the main players in HPV-induced alteration of keratinocyte differentiation in the productive viral life cycle, and the contribution of other viral genes in this process is minimal.

The use of microarrays to analyze effects on cellular gene expression is valuable because it provides a nonbiased global view of all the alterations at the transcriptional level. As further information on the human genome becomes available, more surprises may appear as the interaction between HPV and the host cell is revealed. Much of the hyperproliferation and tumorigenic effects of HPVs can be understood by analysis of parallel studies using other relevant systems, such as, global gene profiling of an E2F-inducible cell line, specific types of cancer cells, and immortalized vs transformed cells *(95–97)*. In the future, HPV research will take advantage of microarray technologies to answer the important questions regarding the differences between low-risk and high-risk HPVs, cellular changes induced during the progression from a hyperproliferative state to cervical neoplasia, and the effects of specific mutations introduced into the viral genome. The fuller understanding of the effects of cellular gene expression by HPVs revealed by microarray analysis may help the interpretation of results from clinical trials, and suggest new directions for treatment and new targets for novel therapeutic drug development.

REFERENCES

1. Howley PM. Papillomavirinae: The verses and Their Replication. In: Fields BN, Knipe DM, Howley PM (eds.) Fundamental Virology. New York: Raven Press, 1996, pp. 947–978.
2. zur Hausen H, de Villiers EM. Human papillomaviruses (Review). Annu Rev Microbiol 1994; 48:427–447.
3. Syrjanen SM. Human papillomavirus infections in the oral cavity. In: Syrjanen K, Gissmann L, G. KL (eds.) Papillomaviruses and Human Disease. Heidelberg: Springer- Verlag, 1987, pp. 104–137.

4. Laimins LA. The biology of human papillomaviruses: from warts to cancer. Infectious Agents and Diseases 1993; 2:74–86.

5. Ho M. Interferon for the treatment of infections. Anna Rev Med 1987; 38:51–59.

6. Frattini MG, Laimins LA. The role of the E1 and E2 proteins in the replication of human papillomavirus type 31b. Virology 1994; 204:799–804.

7. Ustav M, Ustav E, Szymanski P, Stenlund A. Identification of the origin of replication of bovine papillomavirus and characterization of the viral origin recognition factor E1. EMBO J 1991; 10:4321–4329.

8. Kuo SR, Liu JS, Broker TR, Chow LT. Cell-free replication of the human papillomavirus DNA with homologous viral E1 and E2 proteins and human cell extracts. J Biol Chem 1994; 269:24,058–24,065.

9. Hughes FJ, Romanos MA. E1 protein of human papillomavirus is a DNA helicase/ATPase. Nucleic Acids Res 1993; 21:5817–5823.

10. Frattini MG, Laimins LA. Binding of the human papillomavirus E1 origin-recognition protein is regulated through complex formation with the E2 enhancer-binding protein. Proc Natl Acad Sci USA 1994; 91:12,398–12,402.

11. Mohr IJ, Clark R, Sun S, Androphy EJ, MacPherson P, Botchan MR. Targeting the E1 replication protein to the papillomavirus origin of replication by complex formation with the E2 transactivator. Science 1990; 250:1694–1699.

12. Yang L, Li R, Mohr IJ, Clark R, Botchan MR. Activation of BPV-1 replication in vitro by the transcription factor E2. Nature 1991; 353:628–632.

13. Spalholz BA, Yang YC, Howley PM. Transactivation of a bovine papilloma virus transcriptional regulatory element by the E2 gene product. Cell 1985; 42:183–191.

14. Bouvard V, Storey A, Pim D, Banks L. Characterization of the human papillomavirus E2 protein: evidence of trans-activation and trans-repression in cervical keratinocytes. EMBO J 1994; 13:5451–5459.

15. McBride AA, Romanczuk H, Howley PM. The papillomavirus E2 regulatory proteins. J Biol Chem 1991; 266:18,411–18,414.

16. Doorbar J, Ely S, Sterling J, McLean C, Crawford L. Specific interaction between HPV-16 E1-E4 and cytokeratins results in collapse of the epithelial cell intermediate filament network. Nature 1991; 352:824–827.

17. Bouvard V, Matlashewski G, Gu ZM, Storey A, Banks L. The human papillomavirus type 16 E5 gene cooperates with the E7 gene to stimulate proliferation of primary cells and increases viral gene expression. Virology 1994; 203:73–80.

18. Straight SW, Herman B, McCance DJ. The E5 oncoprotein of human papillomavirus type 16 inhibits the acidification of endosomes in human keratinocytes. J Virol 1995; 69:3185–3192.

19. Leechanachai P, Banks L, Moreau F, Matlashewski G. The E5 gene from human papillomavirus type 16 is an oncogene which enhances growth factor-mediated signal transduction to the nucleus. Oncogene 1992; 7:19–25.

20. Werness BA, Levine AJ, Howley PM. Association of human papillomavirus types 16 and 18 E6 proteins with p53. Science 1990; 248:76–79.

21. Scheffner M, Huibregtse JM, Vierstra RD, Howley PM. The HPV-16 E6 and E6-AP complex functions as a ubiquitin-protein ligase in the ubiquitination of p53. Cell 1993; 75:495–505.

22. Scheffner M, Werness BA, Huibregtse JM, Levine AJ, Howley PM. The E6 oncoprotein encoded by human papillomavirus types 16 and 18 promotes the degradation of p53. Cell 1990; 63:1129–1136.

23. Oh ST, Kyo S, Laimins LA. Telomerase activation by human papillomavirus type 16 E6 protein: induction of human telomerase reverse transcriptase expression through myc and GC-rich spl binding sites. J Virol 2001; 75:5559–66.

24. Klingelhutz AJ, Foster SA, McDougall JK. Telomerase activation by the E6 gene product of human papillomavirus type 16. Nature 1996; 380:79–82.

25. Livingstone LR, White A, Sprouse J, Livanos E, Jacks T, Tlsty TD. Altered cell cycle arrest and gene amplification potential accompany loss of wild-type p53. Cell 1992; 70:923–935.

26. Thomas JT, Laimins LA. Human papillomavirus oncoproteins E6 and E7 independently abrogate the mitotic spindle checkpoint. J Virol 1998; 72:1131–1137.

27. Pan H, Griep AE. Temporally distinct patterns of p53-dependent and p53-independent apoptosis during mouse lens development. Genes Dev 1995; 9:2157–2169.

28. Thomas M, Banks L. Inhibition of Bak-induced apoptosis by HPV18-E6. Oncogene 1998; 17:2943–2954.

29. Tong X, Howley PM. The bovine papillomavirus E6 oncoprotein interacts with paxillin and disrupts the actin cytoskeleton. Proc Natl Acad Sci USA 1997; 94:4412–4417.

30. Kiyono T, Hiraiwa A, Fujita M, Hayashi Y, Akiyama T, Ishibashi M. Binding of high-risk human papillomavirus E6 oncoproteins to the human homologue of the Drosophila disc large tumor suppressor protein. Proc Natl Acad Sci USA 1997; 94:11,612–11,616.

31. Chen JJ, Reid CE, Band V, Androphy EJ. Interaction of papillomavirus E6 oncoproteins with a putative calcium-binding protein. Science 1995; 269:529–531.

32. Ronco LV, Karpova AY, Vidal M, Howley PM. Human papillomavirus 16 E6 oncoprotein binds to interferon regulatory factor-3 and inhibits its transcriptional activity. Genes Dev 1998; 12:2061–2072.

33. Tong X, Boll W, Kirchhausen T, Howley PM. Interaction of bovine papillomavirus E6 protein with the clathrin adaptor complex AP-1. J Virol 1998; 72:476–482.

34. Li S, Labrecque S, Gauzzi MC, et al. The human papilloma virus (HPV)-18 E6 oncoprotein physically associates with Tyk2 and impairs Jak-STAT activation by interferon-alpha. Oncogene 1999; 18:5727–5737.

35. Gao Q, Srinivasan S, Boyer SN, Wazer DE, Band V. The E6 oncoproteins of high-risk papillomaviruses bind to a novel putative GAP protein, E6TP1, and target it for degradation. Mol Cell Biol 1999; 19:733–744.

36. Patel D, Huang SM, Baglia LA, McCance DJ. The E6 protein of human papillomavirus type 16 binds to and inhibits co-activation by CBP and p300. EMBO J 1999; 18:5061–5072.

37. Dyson N, Howley PM, Munger K, Harlow E. The human papillomavirus-16 E7 oncoprotein is able to bind to the retinoblastoma gene product. Science 1989; 243:934–937.

38. Munger K, Werness BA, Dyson N, Phelps WC, Harlow E, Howley PM. Complex formation of human papillomavirus E7 proteins with the retinoblastoma tumor suppressor gene product. EMBO J 1989; 8:4099–4105.

39. Brehm A, Nielsen SJ, Miska EA, et al. The E7 oncoprotein associates with Mi2 and histone deacetylase activity to promote cell growth. EMBO J 1999; 18:2449–2458.

40. Funk JO, Waga S, Harry JB, Espling E, Stillman B, Galloway DA. Inhibition of CDK activity and PCNA-dependent DNA replication by p21 is blocked by interaction with the HPV-16 E7 ocoprotein. Genes Dev 1997; 11:2090–2100.

41. Martin LG, Demers GW, Galloway DA. Disruption of the G1/S transition in human papillomavirus type 16 E7-expressing human cells is associated with altered regulation of cyclin E. J Virol 1998; 72:975–985.

42. Chellappan SP, Hiebert S, Mudryj M, Horowitz JM, Nevins JR. The E2F transcription factor is a cellular target for the RB protein. Cell 1991; 65:1053–1061.

43. Chellappan S, Kraus VB, Kroger B, et al. Adenovirus E1A, simian virus 40 tumor antigen, and human papillomavirus E7 protein share the capacity to disrupt the interaction between transcription factor E2F and the retinoblastoma gene product. Proc Natl Acad Sci USA 1992; 89:4549–4553.

44. Cheng S, Schmidt GD, Murant T, Broker TR, Chow LT. Differentiation-dependent up-regulation of the human papillomavirus E7 gene reactivates cellular DNA replication in suprabasal differentiated keratinocytes. Genes Dev 1995; 9:2335–2349.

45. Halbert CL, Demers GW, Galloway DA. The E7 gene of human papillomavirus type 16 is sufficient for immortalization of human epithelial cells. J Virol 1991; 65:473–478.

46. Barnard P, McMillan NAJ. The human papillomavirus E7 oncoprotein abrogates signaling mediated by interferon-α. Virology 1999; 259:305–313.

47. Park JS, Kim EJ, Kwon HJ, Hwang ES, Namkoong SE, Um SJ. Inactivation of interferon regulatory factor-1 tumor suppressor protein by HPV E7 oncoprotein. Implication for the E7-mediated immune evasion mechanism in cervical carcinogenesis. J Biol Chem 2000; 275:6764–6769.

48. Tanaka N, Ishihara M, Lamphier MS, et al. Cooperation of the tumour suppressors IRF-1 and p53 in response to DNA damage. Nature 1996; 382:816–818.

49. Kiyono T, Foster SA, Koop JI, McDougall JK, Galloway DA, Klingelhutz AJ. Both Rb/p16INK4a inactivation and telomerase activity are required to immortalize human epithelial cells. Nature 1998; 396:84–88.

50. Kemp CJ, Donehower LA, Bradley A, Balmain A. Reduction of p53 gene dosage does not increase initiation or promotion but enhances malignant progression of chemically induced skin tumors. Cell 1993; 74:813–822.

51. Kessis TD, Slebos RJ, Nelson WG, et al. Human papillomavirus 16 E6 expression disrupts the p53-mediated cellular response to DNA damage. Proc Natl Acad Sci USA 1993; 90:3988–3992.

52. von Krogh G. Treatment of human papillomavirus-induced lesions of the skin and anogenital region. In: Syrjanen K, Gissmann L, Koss LG (eds.). Papillomaviruses and Human Disease. Berlin, Germany: Springer-Verlag, 1987, pp. 296–333.

53. Tindle RW, Frazer IH. Immune response to human papillomaviruses and the prospects for human papillomavirus-specific immunisation. (Review). Curr Top Microbiol Immunol 1994; 186:217–253.

54. Gross G. Treatment of human papillomavirus infection. In: Mindel A (ed.). Genital warts, human papillomavirus infection. London, UK: St. Edmundsbury Press, 1995, pp. 198–236.

55. Frisch M, Biggar RJ, Goedert JJ. Human papillomavirus-associated cancers in patients with human immunodeficiency virus infection and acquired immunodeficiency syndrome. J Natl Cancer Inst 2000; 92:1500–1510.

56. Tindle R. Immunomodulation of HPV infection and disease: an overview. In: Tindle R (ed.). Vaccines for human papillomavirus infection and anogenital disease. Georgetown, TX: Landes Company, 1999, pp. 1–12.

57. De Palo G, Stefanon B, Rilke F, Pilotti S, Ghione M. Human fibroblast interferon in cervical and vulvar intraepithelial neoplasia associated with viral cytopathic effects. J Reprod Med 1985; 30:404–408.

58. Frost L, Skajaa K, Hvidman LE, Fay SJ, Larsen PM. No effect of intralesional injection of interferon on moderate cervical intraepithelial neoplasia. Br J Obstet Gynaecol 1990; 97:626–630.

59. Turek LP, Byrne JC, Lowy DR, Dvoretzky I, Friedman RM, Howley PM. Interferon induces morphologic reversion with elimination of extrachromosomal viral genomes in bovine papillomavirus-transformed mouse cells. Proc Natl Acad Sci USA 1982; 79:7914–7918.

60. Garcia-Blanco MA, Ghosh PK, Jayaram BM, Ivory S, Lebowitz P, Lengyel P. Selectivity of interferon action in simian virus 40-transformed cells superinfected with simian virus 40. J Virol 1985; 53:893–898.

61. Thomas JT, Hubert WG, Ruesch MN, Laimins LA. Human papillomavirus type 31 oncoproteins E6 and E7 are required for the maintenance of episomes during the viral life cycle in normal human keratinocytes. Proc Natl Acad Sci USA 1999; 96:8449–8454.

62. Frattini MG, Lim HB, Laimins LA. In vitro synthesis of oncogenic human papillomaviruses requires episomal genomes for differentiation-dependent late expression. Proc Natl Acad Sci USA 1996; 93:3062–3067.

63. Meyers C, Mayer TJ, Ozbun MA. Synthesis of infectious human papillomavirus type 18 in differentiating epithelium transfected with viral DNA. J Virol 1997; 71:7381–7386.

64. Dollard SC, Wilson JL, Demeter LM, et al. Production of human papillomavirus and modulation of the infectious program in epithelial raft cultures. Genes Dev 1992; 6:1131–1142.

65. Kreider JW, Howett MK, Lill NL, et al. In vivo transformation of human skin with human papillomavirus type 11 from condylomata acuminata. J Virol 1986; 59:369–376.

66. Meyers C, Frattini MG, Hudson JB, Laimins LA. Biosynthesis of human papillomavirus from a continuous cell line upon epithelial differentiation. Science 1992; 257:971–973.

67. Boyce ST, Ham R. Calcium-regulated differentiation of normal human epidermal keratinocytes in chemically defined clonal culture and serum-free serial culture. J Investing Dermatol 1983; 81:33s–40s.

68. Ruesch MN, Stubenrauch F, Laimins LA. Activation of papillomavirus late gene transcription and genome amplification upon differentiation in semisolid medium is coincident with expression of involucrin and transglutaminase but not keratin-10. J Virol 1998; 72:5016–5024.

69. Breitburd FV. Cell culture systems for the study of papillomaviruses. In: Syrjanen K, Gissmann L, Koss LG (eds). Papillomaviruses and human disease. Berlin, Germany: Springer-Verlag, 1987, pp. 371–392.

70. Simone NL, Bonner RF, Gillespie JW, Emmert-Buck MR, Liotta LA. Laser-capture microdissection: opening the microscopic frontier to molecular analysis. Trends Genet 1998; 14:272–276.

71. Jin L, Tsumanuma I, Ruebel KH, Bayliss JM, Lloyd RV. Analysis of homogeneous populations of anterior pituitary folliculostellate cells by laser capture microdissection and reverse transcription-polymerase chain reaction. Endocrinology 2001; 142:1703–1709.

72. Nees M, van Wijngaarden E, Bakos E, Schneider A, Durst M. Identification of novel molecular markers which correlate with HPV-induced tumor progression. Oncogene 1998; 16:2447–2458.

73. Steinmann KE, Pei XF, Stoppler H, Schlegel R. Elevated expression and activity of mitotic regulatory proteins in human papillomavirus-immortalized keratinocytes. Oncogene 1994; 9:387–394.

74. Rey O, Lee S, Park NH. Human papillomavirus type 16 E7 oncoprotein represses transcription of human fibronectin. J Virol 2000; 74:4912–4918.

75. Shino Y, Shirasawa H, Kinoshita T, Simizu B. Human papillomavirus type 16 E6 protein transcriptionally modulates fibronectin gene expression by induction of protein complexes binding to the cyclic AMP response element. J Virol 1997; 71:4310–4318.

76. Vogt B, Zerfass-Thome K, Schulze A, Botz JW, Zwerschke W, Jansen-Durr P. Regulation of cyclin E gene expression by the human papillomavirus type 16 E7 oncoprotein. J Gen Virol 1999; 80:2103–2113.

77. Lam EW, Morris JD, Davies R, Crook T, Watson RJ, Vousden KH. HPV16 E7 oncoprotein deregulates B-myb expression: correlation with targeting of p107/E2F complexes. EMBO J 1994; 13:871–878.

78. Hellung Schonning B, Bevort M, Mikkelsen S, et al. Human papillomavirus type 16 E7-regulated genes: regulation of S100P and ADP/ATP carrier protein genes identified by differential-display technology. J Gen Virol 2000; 81 Pt 4:1009–1115.

79. Yang X, Nakao Y, Pater MM, Pater A. Identification of two novel cellular genes associated with multistage carcinogenesis of human endocervical cells by mRNA differential display. Carcinogenesis 1996; 17:563–567.

80. Sheibani N, Rhim JS, Allen HB. Malignant human papillomavirus type16-transformed human keratinocytes exhibit altered expression of extracellular matrix glycoproteins. Cancer Res 1991; 51:5967–5975.

81. Chang YE, Laimins LA. Microarray analysis identifies interferon-inducible genes and Stat-1 as major transcriptional targets of human papillomavirus type 31. J Virol 2000; 74:4147–4182.

82. Macleod KF, Sherry N, Hannon G, et al. p53-dependent and independent expression of p21 during cell growth, differentiation, and DNA damage. Genes Dev 1995; 9:935–944.

83. Ayer DE, Kretzner L, Eisenman RN. Mad: a heterodimeric partner for Max that antagonizes Myc transcriptional activity. Cell 1993; 72:211–222.

84. Kartasova T, Van De Putte P. Isolation, characterization, and UV-stimulated expression of two families of genes encoding polypeptides of related structure in human epidermal keratinocytes. Mol Cell Biol 1988; 8:2195–2203.

85. Tselepis C, Chidgey M, North A, Garrod D. Desmosomal adhesion inhibits invasive behavior. Proc Natl Acad Sci USA 1998; 95:8064–8069.

86. Darnell JEJ, Kerr IM, Stark GR. Jak-STAT pathways and transcriptional activation in response to IFNs and other extracellular signaling proteins. Science 1994; 264:1415–1421.

87. Horvath CM, Darnell JEJ. The state of the STATs: recent developments in the study of signal transduction to the nucleus. Curr Opin Cell Biol 1997; 9:233–239.

88. Thomas JT, Oh ST, Terhune SS, Laimins LA. Cellular changes induced by low-risk human papillomavirus type 11 in keratinocytes that stably maintain viral episomes. J Virol 2001; 75:7564–7571.

89. Nees M, Geoghegan JM, Munson P, et al. Human papillomavirus type 16 E6 and E7 proteins inhibit differentiation-dependent expression of transforming growth factor-beta2 in cervical keratinocytes. Cancer Res 2000; 60:4289–98.

90. Nees M, Geoghegan JM, Hyman T, Frank S, Miller L, Woodworth CD. Papillomavirus type 16 oncogenes downregulate expression of interferon-responsive genes and upregulate proliferation associated and nf-kappab-responsive genes in cervical keratinocytes. J Virol 2001; 75:4283–4296.

91. Massague J, Cheifetz S, Laiho M, Ralph DA, Weis FM, Zentella A. Transforming growth factor-beta. Cancer Surv 1992; 12:81–103.

92. Budunova IV, Perez P, Vaden VR, Spiegelman VS, Slaga TJ, Jorcano JL. Increased expression of p50-NF-kappaB and constitutive activation of NF-kappaB transcription factors during mouse skin carcinogenesis. Oncogene 1999; 18:7423–7431.

93. Sherman L, Schlegel R. Serum- and calcium-induced differentiation of human keratinocytes is inhibited by the E6 oncoprotein of human papillomavirus type 16. J Virol 1996; 70:3269–3279.

94. Woodworth CD, Cheng S, Simpson S, et al. Recombinant retroviruses encoding human papillomavirus type 18 E6 and E7 genes stimulate proliferation and delay differentiation of human keratinocytes early after infection. Oncogene 1992; 7:619–626.

95. Muller H, Bracken AP, Vernell R, et al. E2Fs regulate the expression of genes involved in differentiation, development, proliferation, and apoptosis. Genes Dev 2001; 15:267–285.

96. Clark EA, Golub TR, Lander ES, Hynes RO. Genomic analysis of metastasis reveals an essential role for RhoC. Nature 2000; 406:532–535.

97. Perou CM, Sorlie T, Eisen MB, et al. Molecular portraits of human breast tumours. Nature 2000; 406:747–752.

4

Ribozymes as Gene Therapeutic Agents for HIV/AIDS

A Potential Paradigm Shift

Gregory C. Fanning, Janet L. Macpherson, and Geoff Symonds

INTRODUCTION

The study of Human Immunodeficiency Virus/Acquired Immune Deficiency (HIV/AIDS) remains at the forefront of medical research because of the urgent need to supplement current anti-retroviral drugs. At present, anti-retroviral treatment (ART) consists of a combination of drugs, usually two non-nucleoside reverse-transcriptase inhibitors (NNRTI) and one nucleoside reverse-transcriptase inhibitor (NRTI) or two NNRTI and one protease inhibitor (PI), to reduce plasma viral load to less than detectable levels *(1–5)*. Since their relatively recent inception, these drug regimens have had a major impact on AIDS patient care, reducing both morbidity and mortality. However, the emergence of escape-mutants *(6,7)*, the existence of anatomical barriers, the presence of cellular viral reservoirs which are highly impervious to ART *(8,9)*, and side effects that can be severe all limit the efficacy of existing treatments. Thus, the quest for new drugs and improved strategies remains a priority for the treatment of HIV/AIDS. The rational design of gene therapeutics for HIV-1 has been facilitated by the widespread availability of sequence data of viral subtypes and escape-mutants. This chapter addresses the potential use of the new modality of gene therapy to suppress viral gene expression and viral replication and to impact on T-lymphocyte survival and disease progression. Anti-sense *(10)*, intracellular antibodies *(11,12)*, RNA decoys *(13,14)*, mutant HIV genes *(15–18)*, and ribozymes *(19–26)* are all examples of gene therapies that have been used to suppress the replication of HIV-1 in vitro. However, the more complex issue of in vivo utility is only now being addressed by clinical studies of the feasibility of gene introduction and the safety of the expression of the gene constructs within the patient. This chapter highlights the overall anti-HIV gene-therapy approach and examines aspects of Clinical Trials aimed at introducing a specific hammerhead ribozyme (Rz2) into either CD4+ lymphocytes or CD34+ mobilized hematopoietic stem cells.

From: *Pathogen Genomics: Impact on Human Health*
Edited by: K. J. Shaw © Humana Press Inc., Totowa, NJ

HIV PATHOGENESIS AND ANTI-RETROVIRAL THERAPY

HIV infection generally occurs via the mucosal epithelium or skin; from this point of entry the HIV virions are transported to lymphoid tissue via the innate trafficking of specific immune cells. HIV can bind to receptors such as DC-SIGN on the surface of dendritic cells and be transported to the lymphoid tissue on the dendritic-cell surface *(27)*, or can infect cells such as macrophages and be transported intracellularly. This trafficking exposes CD4+ T-lymphocytes, the primary target for HIV, to infection by the virus. If HIV replication proceeds unchecked, an inexorable decline in the CD4+ T lymphocyte population ensues, resulting in an AIDS-related complex and a life-threatening susceptibility to opportunistic infections.

Clinical trials and current therapeutic practice have demonstrated the efficacy of ART in terms of (1) reducing viral load to levels in plasma that are undetectable by polymerase chain reaction (PCR) (<50 copies/mL) and (2) stabilizing CD4+T-lymphocyte counts *(1–5)*. Initial excitement at the ability of this treatment to control infection gave way (based on the existence of latent reservoirs) to estimates that 10–60 y of ART would be required to eliminate HIV-1 completely from such reservoirs *(8,9)*. This is viewed as an impractical proposition, given the often pronounced side effects, the adherence issues associated with this treatment strategy, and the evolution of drug-resistant mutant HIV strains. Progress has been made on adherence issues through the introduction of single-tablet combination drugs, thus reducing the pill burden and improving compliance. Yet side effects, viral reservoirs, and drug-resistant mutants that facilitate disease progression still remain issues. Latently infected CD4+ T-lymphocytes are believed to be one source of continued viral replication during ART *(28–31)*, and clinical trials aimed at supplementing ART with interleukin-2 (IL2) to stimulate proliferation of these reservoirs and thereby make them susceptible to ART have had some success *(30,32)*. However, it is now apparent that there are other reservoirs of HIV-1, such as macrophages, which do not respond to these strategies *(33–35)*. Despite these limitations, it is clear that the introduction of ART, particularly the use of protease inhibitors, has revolutionized AIDS patient care by stabilizing the patient for a period of time and thus reducing the morbidity and mortality associated with HIV-1 infection. However, for the reasons cited above here—lack of adherence to drug regimes, viral breakthrough, and side effects—other new treatment modalities are required.

RIBOZYME DESIGN AND IN VITRO EFFICACY

We and others *(14–18,20,22–25,36–39)* have sought to address the limitations of conventional ART by investigating alternative approaches to the treatment of HIV-1 infection. Many of these approaches have been based on the known sequence of HIV-1—approaches that have been collectively termed intracellular vaccination, a process to make the individual cell resistant to HIV infection *(40)*. Such gene therapeutics include anti-sense RNA *(10)*, intracellular antibodies *(11,12)*, RNA decoys *(13,14)*, mutant HIV genes or transdominant proteins *(15–18)*, and ribozymes *(19–26)*. These approaches share the requirement for cellular expression of the gene construct, and aim to suppress viral replication by preventing viral genome integration and/or suppression of viral gene expression. We have focused on the use of ribozymes catalytic RNA molecules, which can be targeted to specific regions of the HIV-1 genome. There are five major types of ribozymes defined by their catalytic core: the hairpin *(41,42)*, hammerhead *(43)*, group I intron *(44)*, ribonuclease P *(45)*, and hepatitis delta virus ribozyme *(46)*. The hammerhead ribozyme has been the most extensively studied as a means to target known genes, partly because of the short sequence requirement of the hammerhead ribozyme. It has three basic components: a 22-nucleotide-catalytic domain; a recognition sequence NUX, for which N is any nucleotide and X is A, C, or U *(19)*; and basepairing hybridizing arms flanking the susceptible 3′,5′-phosphodiester bond. Enzymatic cleavage involves the binding of the flanking sequences to the target; this is Mg^{2+}-dependent *(47)* and occurs 3′ to the recognition sequence. Such cleavage results in the formation of a terminus containing a 2′3′-cyclic phosphodiester and a 5′-hydroxyl terminus on the 3′ fragment. The reaction is catalytic, with multiple turnover of the ribozyme. The on-off rates are determined by both the length of the hybridizing arms and substrate homology *(20,22,48,49)*.

Specific ribozyme design starts with the identification of potential cleavage sites within the known RNA sequence of the target gene. There are a number of target nucleotide triplets that can result in cleavage by the hammerhead ribozyme, and comparative studies have shown that the cleavage rate decreases in the following order: AUC, GUC > GUA, AUA, CUC > AUU, UUC, UUA > GUU, GUA > UUU, CUU *(50–52)*. Several sites in the HIV-1 genome, including the 5′ leader region *(53,54)*, *gag* *(55)*, *tat (24,26,56)*, and the *psi*-packaging packaging site *(25)*, have been targeted by ribozymes. In our initial analysis, four suitable sites were identified in the *tat* gene, and corresponding ribozymes (Rz1, Rz2, Rz3, Rz4) were designed and tested (ref.*24*) and unpublished data).

In vitro cleavage of chemically synthesized targets is the first step in determining whether the particular ribozyme has cleavage activity *(19,22)*. In these experiments, labeled oligonucleotides containing RNA bases at or proximal to the cleavage site are synthesized, cleaved in the test tube, and then analyzed on an acrylamide gel. The efficiency of ribozyme cleavage can be assessed by analyzing relative amounts of cleaved and non-cleaved substrate over time. In these in vitro cleavage reactions, we have determined that one of the most efficient anti-HIV-1 ribozymes is a *tat*-targeted ribozyme termed Rz2 *(57)*. Cleavage is at a GUA site located at position 5842 within the HIV-1 genome (HIVHXB2 reference genome, accession number K03455), corresponding to the 4th codon of the *tat* gene and part of both codons 94 and 95 of the overlapping *vpr* gene (Fig. 1). Analysis of the large amount of sequence data available in databases such as the Los Alamos database, demonstrates the highly conserved nature of this target site *(unpublished data)*. Although there is marked genetic diversity of naturally occurring HIV-1 isolates of different subtypes or clades for other genes such as *env*, the Rz2 target site is highly conserved, suggesting that this sequence may be required for functional genes. This contention is further supported by preclinical experiments in T-cell lines that show no in vitro evolution of the target site during a 6-mo period of sequential HIV-1 challenge assays *(26)*. The potential for drug-resistant mutations is an important consideration in all therapies in HIV-1 (or other viral targets), and efforts to select highly conserved regions of the target genome are an important criterion for sequence-based gene therapies.

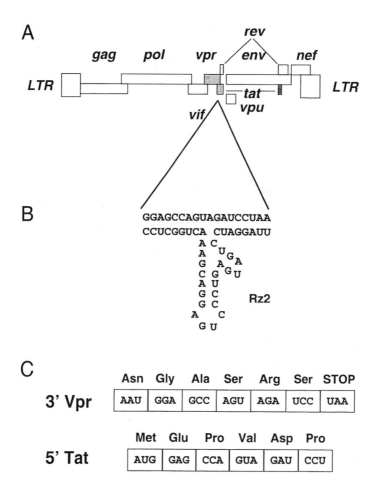

Fig. 1. (A) The HIV-1 reference genome (HXB2) is 9.7 kb in length, and the site targeted by Rz2 is located at position 5842 (Accession number: K03455). **(B)** The Rz2 sequence, showing a schematic of the hammerhead ribozyme catalytic core and flanking binding arms. **(C)** The cleavage at the RRz2 target site cuts the *tat* mRNA transcript at codon four, and the *vpr* mRNA transcript between codons 94 and 95.

Although in vitro cleavage experiments are a useful tool, they cannot predict how well a ribozyme will cleave intracellularly (Fig. 2). To address this, both a plasmid vector and a retroviral vector were engineered in which Rz2 was expressed as part of the 3′ untranslated region of the neomycin resistance (*neo*[R]) gene transcript *(24,25,57)*. In a series of experiments that assessed the activity of Rz2, the T-lymphocyte cell lines SupT1 (plasmid vector) and CEMT4, primary PBMC and CD8+ depleted lymphocytes (all transduced with a retroviral vector) were challenged with HIV-1. The ability of Rz2 to inhibit HIV-1 replication was determined by comparing the production of p24 (an HIV-1 viral protein) in cultured cells with and without Rz2. In these preclinical experiments, a rate of approximately 80% inhibition of HIV-1 replication by Rz2 containing cells was observed, as compared to cells that contained the *neo*[R] gene alone *(24–26,57)*.

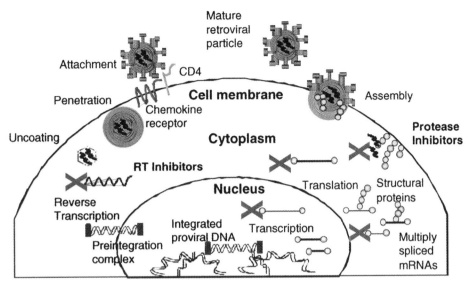

Fig. 2. The HIV-1 life cycle begins when a virion binds to receptors on the cell membrane and enters the cytoplasm. The HIV genomic RNA is uncoated and reverse-transcribed into DNA, combining with proteins to form the pre-integration complex. This complex enters the nucleus and is integrated into the host genome, where upon activation it is transcribed to produce new RNA and ultimately virus particles. Rz2, represented by scissors in this diagram, catalyzes the cleavage of RNA intermediates at various stages of the HIV-1 life cycle. These stages are: (1) after uncoating of the virus prior to reverse transcription, (2) at transcription of integrated HIV genome prior to and after RNA splicing and translation, and (3) during virion assembly.

IN VIVO EFFICACY-ANIMAL MODELS

There is an abundance of preclinical data demonstrating that cells lines which express a gene therapeutic can inhibit virus production *(14–18,20,22–25,36–39)*. In terms of animal-model data, Donahue et al. *(58)* demonstrated in vivo efficacy of gene therapy in a relevant animal model of HIV-1 infection. Rhesus macaques were infused with autologous CD4+ lymphocytes engineered to express a *tat/rev* anti-sense transcript. In earlier studies, this *tat/rev* anti-sense construct was shown to suppress Simian Immunodeficiency Virus (SIV) replication by 78% in tissue-culture experiments. In this animal study, three macaques were infused with engineered anti-HIV CD4+ T lymphocytes at doses that were equivalent to 9.6%, 7.8%, and 2.4% of the total CD4+ T lymphocyte population of each animal. Following infusion, each animal was infected with 100 Animal Infectious Units of SIV. Measurements of viral protein *(p27)* and lymph-node biopsy staining were performed to assess disease progression and the potential impact of this cell-delivered gene therapy. The study demonstrated that in animals with 7.8% or more engineered cells, viral replication could be attenuated and disease progression could be slowed in this animal model. The authors noted that the effective dose of engineered cells may be higher than 7.8%, and 9.8% was effectively higher if the target-cell population for SIV was considered to be the activated CD4+ lymphocytes. All the engineered cells were all activated, and only a small proportion of nonengineered cells were activated (infectable). It is clear from recent human disease data that cells other than CD4+ T lymphocytes, such as macrophages, are important in disease progression and maintenance of viral replication during ART. Therefore, the macrophage-cell population should also be considered. To the best of our knowledge, animal studies targeting these cell populations have not yet been reported.

GENE-THERAPY CLINICAL TRIALS

Gene therapy for HIV-1 is still in the transitional stage from the laboratory to the clinic. There have been several small Phase I studies demonstrating safety and feasibility, and to date the results of Phase II studies are not widely reported. There is little, if any, efficacy data. The clinical application of anti-HIV gene therapeutics can presently be divided into two procedure types, based on the target-cell population employed. As in the animal model described here, the first group of studies have utilized the HIV-1 susceptible CD4+ cells as the means of gene delivery to the patient. These studies include the anti-HIV ribozymes of Immusol and GeneShears *(59)* (Fig. 3A), transdominant Rev, and more recently, a combined anti-sense/transdominant protein approach at The National Human Genome Research Institute. In this Phase I/II study of 8 patients, the survival of transduced cells was reported. The largest study to date is a controlled Phase II study from Cell Genesys, where patients were treated with T-cell receptor modified CD4+ and CD8+ lymphocytes. The 40 patients who received the therapeutic T-cells were reported to show a reduction in the amount of virus cultured from blood (mean 0.4 log decrease) and rectal tissue (mean 0.5 log decrease) at 6 mo. Marked cells could be detected at 0.2–0.8% of total white blood cells for up to 6 mo.

The other type of study is based on the introduction of gene therapeutic agents into CD34+ hematopoietic stem cells (Fig. 3B). Cells are infused into the patient, travel to the bone marrow and engraft, and can then potentially contribute to all the lineages in the blood, including the CD4+ T- lymphocytes. Enzo Biochem continues to report early results for its anti-sense therapy HGTV43 (3 anti-sense genes) at large meetings including the 8th Conference on Retroviruses and Opportunistic Infections (Chicago). The five-patient trial was designed to test for safety and for engraftment and differentiation of the transduced cells. This study and others, including our own, have demonstrated that anti-HIV genes can be introduced successfully into CD34+ stem cells, and that the stem cells survive and contribute to the peripheral blood CD4+ cells, the cells that are susceptible to HIV infection. Other studies in this area usually report low numbers of marked cells detected in the peripheral blood for 12 mo.

DRUG RESISTANCE AND GENE THERAPY

HIV-1 evolves rapidly in response to environmental pressure. In terms of treatment, the effect of the selective pressure is the relatively rapid emergence of HIV-1 strains that are not inhibited by that anti-retroviral drug; these are the so-called drug-resistant mutants. Drug resistance was documented in the early days of anti-retroviral (Zidovudine) treatment *(6,7),* and such resistance has subsequently been shown to new drugs, including the emergence of multi-drug resistance *(60–62).* If there is emergence of a drug-resistant HIV mutants in a patient, this requires administration of a new combination of anti-retroviral drugs in order to control the ensuing rise in viral replication and HIV-1 plasma levels. The choice of drug combinations is limited by side effects and by the number of drug-resistant strains an individual has encountered or harbors as a result of drug-driven mutation. When this is addressed on a population basis, one may envision epidemics of infection by drug-resistant mutants, limiting the choice of drug combinations available to newly infected individuals. In support of this theory, reports from North America and Europe indicate that up to 14% of newly infected individuals carry drug resistant strains of HIV-1 (63–66). The use of a combination of drugs to treat AIDS addresses this problem in part, but the continually diminishing drug choices will eventually limit the effectiveness of therapy. The key question is: will new types of therapies be subject to this same problem? The rapid mutation of HIV-1 implies that if there is a protein or gene sequence that can elude therapy and significantly maintain function, then it will evolve. Although this theory remains untested in the area of gene therapy, there is the potential emergence of drug resistance. This probably means that pretreatment screening of clinical isolates by sequencing and follow-up monitoring (for emergence of drug-resistant isolates) will become an important part of any new HIV/AIDS therapy *(67)*.

HIV GENE THERAPY IN THE CLINIC

In its current form, gene therapy would most likely be carried out in the context of a bone-marrow transplant unit. In this model, the gene therapeutic would be supplied as a traditional pharmaceutical (in a bottle) with cell manipulation and transduction protocols provided. The steps in the process are as outlined in the CD34+ Clinical protocol (Fig. 3b). (1) CD34+ cell mobilization and apheresis, (2) Cell transduction, (3). Ex vivo expansion of genetically modified cells, (4). Infusion of cells, (5). Post-treatment monitoring and dose assessment.

At least conceptually, there are no adherence issues related to such treatment, and the most important parameter to be considered at time of treatment is the number and type of modified cells required to impact on disease as well as the surrogate markers used for assessment. Without further clinical trials, it is difficult to determine the level of gene-therapeutic expression in the different cell lineages required to impact on disease, resulting in a reduced viral load and/or increased CD4+ count.

SUMMARY—FROM SEQUENCE TO PRODUCT

Since the identification of HIV-1 as the cause of AIDS, this virus has been a major focus for research groups around the world, and has itself become a paradigm for viral pathology and viral disease. Despite this intense effort, there is a need for additional treatments, vaccines, and ultimately cures. The sequencing of HIV-1 subtypes and drug-resistant mutants has provided valuable information to enhance understanding of the limitations of current treatments and to provide valuable insights into the origin and spread of the disease. Our study and others have used this sequence knowledge as a basis for the rational design of gene therapies (Fig. 4). Knowledge of the sequence of the target pathogen is a significant fact, yet it represents a small step toward the development of an effective therapy. The next key step for HIV-1 research is to develop an understanding of the mechanism by which HIV-1 has evolved into

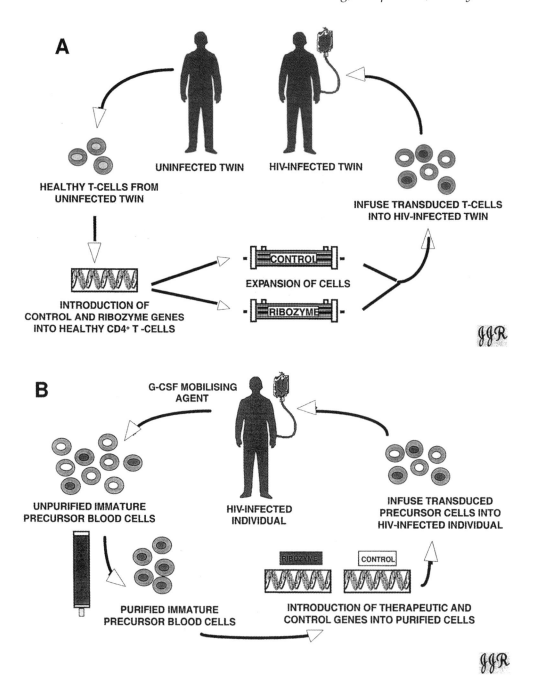

Fig. 3. (A) Flow diagram of the CD4+ Phase I Clinical Trial protocol. The trial involves pairs of identical twins discordant for HIV-1 infection. Healthy T-lymphocytes from the HIV negative twin were transduced with ribozyme-containing and control retrovirus vectors, expanded ex vivo, and then infused into the corresponding HIV positive sibling. **(B)** Flow diagram of the CD34+ Phase I Clinical Trial protocol. Autologous pluripotent CD34+ stem cells are collected from HIV-positive individuals following G-CSF mobilization, further purified, and then transduced with ribozyme containing and control retroviral vectors before reinfusion. The transduced CD34+ cells engraft into the bone marrow, where they begin to differentiate into the component cells of the hematopoietic system.

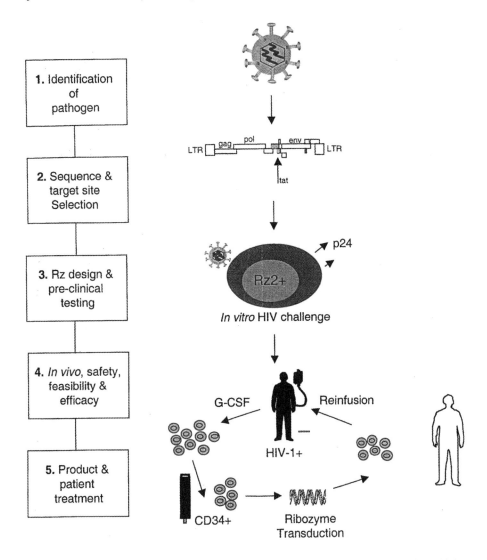

Fig. 4. From sequence to therapy a summary flow diagram of the process of identifying and sequencing HIV-1 to the development of a gene therapy treatment for AIDS patients.

such a successful virus, and to allow for the design of effective strategies to apply sequence specific gene therapies to AIDS. As part of this process, gene therapy will be clinically tested.

REFERENCES

1. Wong JK, Günthard HF, Havlir DV, et al. Reduction of HIV-1 in blood and lymph nodes following potent antiretroviral therapy and the virologic correlates of treatment failure. Proc Natl Acad Sci USA 1997; 94:12,574–12,579.
2. Cavert W, Notermans DW, Staskus K, et al. Kinetics of response in lymphoid tissues to antiretroviral therapy of HIV-1 infection. Science 1997; 276:960–964.

3. Carpenter CC, Fischl MA, Hammer SM, et al. Antiretroviral therapy for HIV infection in 1997. Updated recommendations of the International AIDS Society-USA panel. JAMA 1997; 277:1962–1969.

4. Gulick RM, Mellors JW, Havlir D, et al. Treatment with indinavir, zidovudine, and lamivudine in adults with human immunodeficiency virus infection and prior antiretroviral therapy. N Engl J Med 1997; 337:734–739.

5. Hammer SM, Katzenstein DA, Hughes MD, et al. A trial comparing nucleoside monotherapy with combination therapy in HIV-infected adults with CD4 cell counts from 200 to 500 per cubic millimeter. AIDS Clinical Trials Group Study 175 Study Team. N Engl J Med 1996; 335:1081–1090.

6. Larder BA, Darby G, Richman DD. HIV with reduced sensitivity to zidovudine (AZT) isolated during prolonged therapy. Science 1989; 243:1731–1734.

7. D'Aquila RT, Johnson VA, Welles SL, et al. Zidovudine resistance and HIV-1 disease progression during antiretroviral therapy. AIDS Clinical Trials Group Protocol 116B/117 Team and the Virology Committee Resistance Working Group. Ann Intern Med 1995; 122:401–408.

8. Zhang L, Ramratnam B, Tenner-Racz K, et al. Quantifying residual HIV-1 replication in patients receiving combination antiretroviral therapy. N Engl J Med 1999; 340:1605–1613.

9. Saag MS, Kilby JM. HIV-1 and HAART: a time to cure, a time to kill [news; comment]. Nat Med 1999; 5:609–611.

10. Smythe JA, Symonds G. Gene therapeutic agents: the use of ribozymes, antisense, and RNA decoys for HIV-1 infection. Inflamm Res 1995; 44:11–15.

11. Shaheen F, Duan L, Zhu M, Bagasra O, Pomerantz RJ. Targeting human immunodeficiency virus type 1 reverse transcriptase by intracellular expression of single-chain variable fragments to inhibit early stages of the viral life cycle. J Virol 1996; 70:3392–400.

12. Maciejewski JP, Weichold FF, Young NS, et al. Intracellular expression of antibody fragments directed against HIV reverse transcriptase prevents HIV infection in vitro. Nat Med 1995; 1:667–673.

13. Lee SW, Gallardo HF, Gilboa E, Smith C. Inhibition of human immunodeficiency virus type 1 in human T cells by a potent Rev response element decoy consisting of the 13-nucleotide minimal Rev-binding domain. J Virol 1994; 68:8254–8264.

14. Lisziewicz J, Rappaport J, Dhar R. Tat-regulated production of multimerized TAR RNA inhibits HIV-1 gene expression. New Biol 1991; 3:82–89.

15. Escaich S, Kalfoglou C, Plavec I, Kaushal S, Mosca JD, Böhnlein E. RevM10-mediated inhibition of HIV-1 replication in chronically infected T cells. Hum Gene Ther 1995; 6:625–634.

16. Aguilar-Cordova E, Chinen J, Donehower LA, et al. Inhibition of HIV-1 by a double transdominant fusion gene. Gene Ther 1995; 2:181–186.

17. Woffendin C, Ranga U, Yang Z-Y, Xu L, Nabel GJ. Expression of a protective gene prolongs survival of T-cells in human immunodeficiency virus-infected patients. Proc Natl Acad Sci USA 1996; 93:2889–2894.

18. Caputo A, Grossi MP, Bozzini R, et al. Inhibition of HIV-1 replication and reactivation from latency by tat transdominant negative mutants in the cysteine rich region. Gene Ther 1996; 3:235–245.

19. Haseloff J, Gerlach WL. Simple RNA enzymes with new and highly specific endoribonuclease activities. Nature 1988; 334:585–591.

20. Heidenreich O, Eckstein F. Hammerhead ribozyme-mediated cleavage of the long terminal repeat RNA of human immunodeficiency virus type 1. J Biol Chem 1992; 267:1904–1909.

21. Rossi JJ, Sarver N. Catalytic antisense RNA (ribozymes): their potential and use as anti-HIV-1 therapeutic agents. Adv Exp Med Biol 1992; 312:95–109.

22. Crisell P, Thompson S, James W. Inhibition of HIV-1 replication by ribozymes that show poor activity in vitro. Nucleic Acids Res 1993; 21:5251–5255.

23. Homann M, Tzortzakaki S, Rittner K, Sczakiel G, Tabler M. Incorporation of the catalytic domain of a hammerhead ribozyme into antisense RNA enhances its inhibitory effect on the replication of human immunodeficiency virus type 1. Nucleic Acids Res 1993; 21:2809–2814.

24. Sun LQ, Wang L, Gerlach WL, Symonds G. Target sequence-specific inhibition of HIV-1 replication by ribozymes directed to tat RNA. Nucleic Acids Res 1995; 23:2909–2913.

25. Sun LQ, Warrilow D, Wang L, Witherington C, Macpherson J, Symonds G. Ribozyme-mediated suppression of Moloney murine leukemia virus and human immunodeficiency virus type I replication in permissive cell lines. Proc Natl Acad Sci USA 1994; 91:9715–9719.

26. Wang L, Witherington C, King A, et al. Preclinical characterization of an anti-tat ribozyme for therapeutic application. Hum Gene Ther 1998; 9:1283–1291.

27. Geijtenbeek TB, Kwon DS, Torensma R, et al. DC-SIGN, a dendritic cell-specific HIV-1-binding protein that enhances trans-infection of T cells [see comments]. Cell 2000; 100:587–597.

28. Chun TW, Engel D, Berrey MM, Shea T, Corey L, Fauci AS. Early establishment of a pool of latently infected, resting CD4+ T cells during primary HIV-1 infection. Proc Natl Acad Sci USA 1998; 95:8869–8873.

29. Finzi D, Hermankova M, Pierson T, et al. Identification of a reservoir for HIV-1 in patients on highly active antiretroviral therapy. Science 1997; 278:1295–1300.

30. Finzi D, Blankson J, Siliciano JD, et al. Latent infection of CD4+ T cells provides a mechanism for lifelong persistence of HIV-1, even in patients on effective combination therapy [see comments]. Nat Med 1999; 5:512–517.

31. Wong JK, Hezareh M, Gunthard HF, et al. Recovery of replication-competent HIV despite prolonged suppression of plasma viremia. Science 1997; 278:1291–1295.

32. Chun TW, Engel D, Mizell SB, et al. Effect of interleukin-2 on the pool of latently infected, resting CD4+ T cells in HIV-1-infected patients receiving highly active antiretroviral therapy. Nat Med 1999; 5:651–655.

33. Chun TW, Carruth L, Finzi D, et al. Quantification of latent tissue reservoirs and total body viral load in HIV-1 infection [see comments]. Nature 1997; 387:183–188.

34. Brodie SJ. Nonlymphoid reservoirs of HIV replication in children with chronic-progressive disease. J Leukoc Biol 2000; 68:351–359.

35. Crowe SM, Sonza S. HIV-1 can be recovered from a variety of cells including peripheral blood monocytes of patients receiving highly active antiretroviral therapy: a further obstacle to eradication. J Leukoc Biol 2000; 68:345–350.

36. Lisziewicz J, Sun D, Metelev V, Zamecnik P, Gallo RC, Agrawal S. Long-term treatment of Human Immunodeficiency Virus-infected cells with antisense oligonucleotide phosphorothioates. Proc Natl Acad Sci USA 1993; 90:3860–3864.

37. Lisziewicz J, Sun D, Lisziewicz A, Gallo RC. Antitat gene therapy: a candidate for late-stage AIDS patients. Gene Ther 1995; 2:218–222.

38. Rossi JJ, Castanotto D, Krishnan A, et al. A human gene therapy trail of ribozyme gene transduced CD34+ hematopoietic cells. Am GTSoc Meeting 1999; 2nd meeting.

39. Rossi JJ, Elkins D, Zaia JA, Sullivan S. Ribozymes as anti-HIV-1 therapeutic agents: principles, applications, and problems. AIDS Res Hum Retrovir 1992; 8:183–189.

40. Baltimore D. Gene therapy. Intracellular immunization. Nature 1988; 335:395–396.

41. Hampel A, Tritz R. RNA catalytic properties of the minimum (–)sTRSV sequence. Biochemistry 1989; 28:4929–4933.

42. Hampel A, Tritz R, Hicks M, Cruz P. 'Hairpin' catalytic RNA model: evidence for helices and sequence requirement for substrate RNA. Nucleic Acids Res 1990; 18:299–304.

43. Buzayan JM, Gerlach WL, Bruening GB. PNAS 1986; 83:8859–8862.

44. Cech TR, Zaug AJ, Grabowski PJ. In vitro splicing of the robosomal RNA precursor of Terahymena: involvement of guanosine nucleotide in the excision of the intervening sequence. Cell 1981; 27:487–496.

45. Guerrier-Takada C, Gardiner K, Marsh T, Pace N, Altman S. Cell 1983:849–957.
46. Macnaughton TB, Wang YJ, Lai MM. Replication of hepatitis delta virus RNA: effect of mutations of the autocatalytic cleavage sites. J Virol 1993; 67:2228–2234.
47. Dahm SC, Uhlenbeck OC. Role of divalent metal ions in the hammerhead RNA cleavage reaction. Biochemistry 1991; 30:9464–9469.
48. Sioud M. Effects of variations in length of hammerhead ribozyme antisense arms upon the cleavage of longer RNA substrates. Nucleic Acids Res 1997; 25:333–338.
49. Hertel KJ, Herschlag D, Uhlenbeck OC. Specificity of hammerhead ribozyme cleavage. EMBO J 1996; 15:3751–3757.
50. Zoumadakis M, Tabler M. Comparative analysis of cleavage rates after systematic permutation of the NUX consensus target motif for hammerhead ribozymes. Nucleic Acids Res 1995; 23:1192–1196.
51. Perriman R, Delves A, Gerlach WL. Extended target-site specificity for a hammerhead ribozyme. Gene 1992; 113:157–163.
52. Shimayama T, Nishikawa S, Taira K. Generality of the NUX rule: kinetic analysis of the results of systematic mutations in the trinucleotide at the cleavage site of hammerhead ribozymes. Biochemistry 1995; 34:3649–3654.
53. Weerasinghe M, Liem SE, Asad S, Read SE, Joshi S. Resistance to human immunodeficiency virus type 1 (HIV-1) infection in human CD4+ lymphocyte-derived cell lines conferred by using retroviral vectors expressing an HIV-1 RNA-specific ribozyme. J Virol 1991; 65:5531–5534.
54. Ojwang JO, Hampel A, Looney DJ, Wong-Staal F, Rappaport J. Inhibition of human immunodeficiency virus type 1 expression by a hairpin ribozyme. Proc Natl Acad Sci USA 1992; 89:10,802–10,806.
55. Sarver N, Cantin EM, Chang PS, et al. Ribozymes as potential anti-HIV-1 therapeutic agents. Science 1990; 247:1222–1225.
56. Lo KM, Biasolo MA, Dehni G, Palu G, Haseltine WA. Inhibition of replication of HIV-1 by retroviral vectors expressing tat-antisense and anti-tat ribozyme RNA. Virology 1992; 190:176–183.
57. Sun LQ, Pyati J, Smythe J, et al. Resistance to human immunodeficiency virus type 1 infection conferred by transduction of human peripheral blood lymphocytes with ribozyme, antisense or polymeric trans-activation response element constructs. Proc Natl Acad Sci USA 1995; 92:7272–7276.
58. Donahue RE, Bunnell BA, Zink MC, et al. Reduction in SIV replication in rhesus macaques infused with autologous lymphocytes engineered with antiviral genes. Nat Med 1998; 4:181–186.
59. Cooper D, Penny R, Symonds G, et al. A marker study of therapeutically transduced CD4+ peripheral blood lymphocytes in HIV discordant identical twins. Hum Gene Ther 1999; 10:1401–1421.
60. Miller V, Phillips A, Rottmann C, et al. Dual resistance to zidovudine and lamivudine in patients treated with zidovudine-lamivudine combination therapy: association with therapy failure. J Infect Dis 1998; 177:1521–1532.
61. Zolopa AR, Shafer RW, Warford A, et al. HIV-1 genotypic resistance patterns predict response to saquinavir-ritonavir therapy in patients in whom previous protease inhibitor therapy had failed. Ann Intern Med 1999; 131:813–821.
62. DeGruttola V, Dix L, D'Aquila R, et al. The relation between baseline HIV drug resistance and response to antiretroviral therapy: re-analysis of retrospective and prospective studies using a standardized data analysis plan. Antivir Ther 2000; 5:41–48.
63. Boden D, Hurley A, Zhang L, et al. HIV-1 drug resistance in newly infected individuals. JAMA 1999; 282:1135–1141.

64. Little SJ, Daar ES, D'Aquila RT, et al. Reduced antiretroviral drug susceptibility among patients with primary HIV infection. JAMA 1999; 282:1142–1149.
65. Yerly S, Kaiser L, Race E, Bru JP, Clavel F, Perrin L. Transmission of antiretroviral-drug-resistant HIV-1 variants. Lancet 1999; 354:729–733.
66. UK Collaborative Group on Monitoring the Transmission of HIV Drug Resistance. Analysis of prevalence of HIV-1 drug resistance in primary infections in the United Kingdom. Br Med J 2001; 322:1087–1088.
67. Hirsch MS, Brun-Vezinet F, D'Aquila RT, et al. Antiretroviral drug resistance testing in adult HIV-1 infection: recommendations of an International AIDS Society-USA Panel. JAMA 2000; 283:2417–2426.

II Bacteria

5
Genomics and New Technologies Applied to Antibacterial Drug Discovery

Donald T. Moir

INTRODUCTION

The goal of this chapter is to review recent progress in the use of genomic information for the discovery and validation of new targets in antibacterial drug discovery and for the identification of appropriate assays and screens. Several recent studies have discussed these or related topics *(1–5),* but discoveries in this field occur rapidly, and frequent review is useful. Although this chapter provides an overview of the entire process of developing targets and screens from genomic sequences, the main focus is on the latest methods and results, especially as applied to potential drug targets of unknown function.

UPDATE ON GENOMIC SEQUENCE AND ANALYSIS RESOURCES AVAILABLE

Genomic resources available on the World Wide Web for antimicrobial target selection continue to grow in both number and quality, and most are publicly accessible at no cost (Table 1). The Institute for Genomic Research (TIGR) maintains a summary Web page, which monitors which bacterial genomes are being sequenced or have been completely sequenced, and provides a link for access to the information. Several groups, including TIGR, the Sanger Center, the University of Oklahoma, and Stanford University, have active sequencing centers focused on bacterial and fungal genomes, and have deposited large numbers of microbial genomes in public databases. Continued success with sequencing random shotgun clones followed by whole-genome assembly and finishing has validated this approach for completing bacterial genomes. Combined with the availability of affordable automated fluorescence sequencers, the shotgun sequencing method has provided an abundance of complete bacterial genomic sequences. For example, the NCBI web site listed 47 complete bacterial genomes as of August 2001. Surprisingly, the sequence of the genomes of many prominent pathogens have not yet been determined to completion. (e.g., *Enterococcus faecium, Staphylococcus epidermidis, Acinetobacter baumanii, Bacteroides fragilis, Moraxella catarrhalis, Proteus mirabilis,* and *Clostridium difficile*). However, recent publications of the complete genomic sequence of two different strains of *Staphylococcus aureus (6)* and of a

From: *Pathogen Genomics: Impact on Human Health*
Edited by: K. J. Shaw © Humana Press Inc., Totowa, NJ

Table 1
Resources Available on the Internet

Site	Topic	Maintained by:
http://www.tigr.org/tdb/mdb/mdbcomplete.html http://www.tigr.org/tdb/mdb/mdbinprogress.html	Status of microbial genomic sequencing, both complete and in progress, with links to data and tools	The Institute for Genomic Research (TIGR)
http://www.ncbi.nlm.nih.gov:80/PMGifs/Genomes/micr.html	Complete microbial genome sequences and sequence similarity analysis tools	National Center for Biotechnology Information (NCBI), NIH
http://www.ncbi.nlm.nih.gov/COG/	Clusters of Orthologous Groups of proteins (COGs) were delineated by comparing protein sequences encoded in 44 complete genomes, representing 30 major phylogenetic lineages. Each COG consists of individual proteins or groups of paralogs from at least 3 lineages and thus corresponds to an ancient conserved domain	National Center for Biotechnology Information (NCBI), NIH
http://pedant.gsf.de/ http://pedant.mips.biochem.mpg.de/	"Protein Extraction, Description, and Analysis Tool"; computational analysis of complete genomic sequences	Munich Information Center for Protein Sequences (MIPS)
http://www.genome.ad.jp/kegg/	Analysis of gene features and function; pathway analysis; and comparative genomics; "computerize current knowledge of molecular and cellular biology in terms of the information pathways that consist of interacting molecules or genes"	Bioinformatics Center, Institute for Chemical Research, Kyoto University
http://www.ecocyc.org/	Up-to-date annotations of all *E. coli* genes, as well as the DNA sequence of each *E. coli* gene; describes all known pathways of *E. coli* small-molecule metabolism. Each pathway and its component reactions and enzymes are annotated in rich detail, with extensive references to the biomedical literature	DoubleTwist (URL doubletwist.com); funded by a grant from the Comparative Medicine program at the NIH National Center for Research Resources
http://www.tigr.org/tigr-scripts/CMR2/CMRHomePage.spl	The Comprehensive Microbial Resource (CMR) CMR is a tool that allows access to all of the bacterial genome sequences completed to date	The Institute for Genomic Research (TIGR), with DOE funding

virulent *Streptococcus pneumoniae* strain *(7)* fill a critical information gap in the sequences of Gram-positive pathogens. In addition, many unfinished genomes are available for sequence similarity searching, although with some risk of missing a significant match because of the incomplete status of the sequence. More complete versions of many of these pathogens are available for searching by payment of a fee and completing a license agreement (see, for example, Compugen Inc. "Lab-on-Web", at URL www.labonweb.com).

In addition to sequence resources, the Web provides several excellent analysis resources (Table 1). For example, the *Kyoto Encyclopedia of Genes and Genomes* and the EcoCyc database provide access to microbial sequences parsed into genes and pathways, and provide comparative views. Similarly, the PEDANT™ site provides precomputed analysis of microbial genomes, including results of motif and pattern searches. The NCBI microbial genome site provides an excellent contextual view of genes as well as links to clustering results known as "clusters of orthologous groups" (COGs) which are helpful for predicting the presence of orthologs in multiple species. Note that precomputed comparative genomics and contextual views of genes within genomes are available for a fee from a few commercial vendors, such as Genome Therapeutics Corporation's PathoGenome™ database and Incyte Genomics' PathoSeq™ database, now administered by Elitra Pharmaceuticals.

COMPARATIVE GENOMICS

The availability of sequence information for complete genomes of multiple species enables drug developers to search for potential targets with particular prevalence characteristics. This is useful for three main reasons. First, there are too many essential genes (e.g., about 10–15% of the genes) in a single bacterial species to pursue as drug targets, and prioritization is difficult because of the paucity of annotated features for many genes. Second, development of a drug against a single bacterial species is usually impractical from a commercial and clinical perspective because its spectrum of activity might be too narrow. Third, if gene products chosen as drug targets have likely orthologs encoded in the human genome, then drugs against those targets may lack selectivity. For these reasons, it is helpful to compare genomes and find potential drug targets which are shared by a clinically important range of microbial species and are absent from the human host.

Techniques for comparing the gene content of many genomes have been described *(8)*. They are practical, yet require considerable computing power. Genome vs genome protein queries may be run via the Internet at sites such as the Comprehensive Microbial Resource maintained by TIGR (Table 1) or for a fee by subscribing to commercial databases, as noted previously. The more genomes compared, the smaller the list of shared genes obtained. This filtering and prioritization of gene targets by predicted breadth of spectrum and selectivity of a resulting drug is a very practical approach. As additional genomes become available, it will become increasingly possible to search for narrower-spectrum drug targets, for example, focused on particular disease indications such as upper respiratory tract or gastrointestinal tract infections. However, at present, sequences for some key species are still missing. A key genome for exclusion—the human genome—is also incomplete at this time, but about 98% of the euchromatic portion of the human genome has been sequenced at least in draft form, with 47% in finished form (see http://www.ncbi.nlm.nih.gov/genome/seq/). Thus, the accuracy with which human homologs of potential antibacterial targets can be detected is increasing.

EVALUATING TARGET ESSENTIALITY

The essential nature of the gene encoding a putative antibacterial drug target remains an important step in validating the target. Although a gene which is nonessential for growth or viability may yet represent a useful drug target if it is required for a critical step in pathogenesis, this has not been established in the marketplace with successful drugs in this category. Therefore, this review deals primarily with essential targets, with only a brief discussion of potential nonessential targets.

The most direct approach to establishing the essentiality of a gene for growth or viability of the bacterium is a directed knockout by allele replacement. This may be accomplished readily in a number of pathogenic bacterial species including *E. coli, S. aureus,* and *S. pneumoniae (9–11)*. However, efficiencies vary widely by species, and the approach is too ineffective to be useful in certain species without additional development. Furthermore, even when it is effective for knockout of individual genes, the method may be impractical to apply to hundreds of putative targets. Fortunately, higher-throughput methods have been developed.

Most high-throughput methods of determining gene essentiality depend on the random generation of insertional knockouts, and the majority make use some type of transposon to accomplish this goal. All approaches share the following basic steps— generation of a population of random insertion mutants, outgrowth under specific conditions, and identification of those insertions which permit growth, and by implication, those which prohibit growth. Recent reviews describe numerous variations in application of these steps, allowing this general approach to be applied to a wide variety of bacterial species *(12,13)*.

Two recent studies illustrate the utility of these methods. First, Hare et al. *(14)* described adaptation of the "genetic footprinting" method to the bacterium *E. coli.* First applied to yeast, this approach uses random transposon mutagenesis performed within cells to generate a mutagenized population. A DNA sample of the population is collected while transposition is occurring, then further transposition is shut off and cells are grown in a selective condition—in this case, a nutrient-rich laboratory medium. Cells containing transposon insertions within genes essential for that growth condition will die out of the population. DNA is collected after the selective growth condition, and polymerase chain reaction (PCR) products are generated from the transposon to each gene of interest and are visualized on a sequencing gel. The absence of PCR products representing the gene of interest after selective growth, but not before, demonstrates the essentiality of that gene for growth or viability under the conditions examined. Thus, the entire collection of knockout mutants is initially made in one step using random transposon insertion; then, each gene is queried rapidly with a PCR followed by gel analysis. Although Hare et al. *(14)* have described application of this approach to the *E. coli* genome, it could be applied to other species with some development effort. Clearly, important issues are the degree of randomness achieved in the transposon insertions and the ability to adequately turn off further transposition during the outgrowth phase under selective conditions.

Second, this general approach has also been applied under conditions of outgrowth in an animal model. Known as "signature-tagged mutagenesis" (STM), this method was developed by David Holden and colleagues to identify genes that are essential for growth and survival in vivo *(15)*. STM has been used widely and modified extensively since its first description (see, for example, ref. *(13)*. Since the randomly mutagenized population must be grown in vitro in the laboratory prior to testing in an animal model in vivo, the method will not detect genes which are essential for growth and viability in vitro. Instead, its strength lies in identifying genes critical for virulence and pathogenicity in vivo in a host organism. For example, application of STM to *S. aureus* identified a cluster of 10 genes, which attenuate *S. aureus* growth in vivo when mutated *(16)*. Critical aspects of this approach include the randomness of the generation of mutants and the choice of animal host. The complexity of the pool of mutants introduced into the animal must be evaluated with respect to the cell number required to initiate infection in the model.

Since random transposon-based STM methods cannot establish the in vivo essentiality of an in vitro essential gene, various approaches are required to determine if an in vitro essential gene is also essential in vivo. Clearly, the ultimate goal is understanding pathogen gene essentiality in the human host environment. This has been addressed in two ways. First, researchers typically test essentiality on very nutrient-rich agar media, simulating the condition in a human tissue. Factors that are diffusible and may supplement the needs of a drug-inhibited bacterium may be present in the nutrient-rich laboratory medium. In this way, gene knockouts, which are merely auxotrophic defects, may be detected. Second, methods have been developed for testing essentiality directly in an animal model (see, for example, ref. *17*). This may be accomplished by engineering the bacterium to contain a regulatable promoter driving expression of the gene of interest. As long as the promoter inducer or repressor can be provided in an effective manner in the animal host, this method should provide a reliable answer. However, few bacterial promoters are completely shut off in the repressed or uninduced state, and this is the challenge for developing effective methods of this type and for interpreting the results. Tao et al. *(17)* and Blum et al. *(18)* have used upregulation of a promoter driving an inhibitor to demonstrate the essentiality of targets. In this way, it is not necessary to turn off expression from the promoter entirely, but merely to increase expression significantly, an experimentally more achievable goal. To apply this approach, it is necessary to first identify a strong peptide inhibitor of the target of interest. Although this can often be accomplished by using peptide phage display or yeast two-hybrid methods, success is not guaranteed. An alternate approach is to drive expression of an anti-sense transcript from an upregulatable promoter in vivo, and this has been configured using random shotgun clones to identify essential genes in a whole-genome survey *(19)*. Unfortunately, identification of a potent anti-sense sequence may not always be feasible. Nevertheless, the availability of several approaches ensures success for most potential gene targets.

POTENTIAL NEW TARGETS FROM GENOMIC APPROACHES

During the past three years, functions have been discovered for several genes that were previously of unknown function in many bacterial genomes. These genes do not necessarily encode appropriate targets for antibacterial drug development, because it is not yet clear whether they meet all of the criteria. For example, many are present in

Table 2
Functions recently identified for bacterial genes

Gene Names	Function	Method of Function Identification	Reference
kdtB (coaD)	CoA biosynthesis	N-terminal sequencing of purified protein; database search	*20*
yacE (coaE)	CoA biosynthesis	N-terminal sequencing of purified protein; database search	*21*
ybeN (nadD)	NAD biosynthesis	Mapping of mutations, motif and sensitive sequence homology searches between species	*22*
yaeM (dxr)	Isoprenoid biosynthesis	Sequencing of clones complementing methyl-erythritol (MER)-requiring mutants	*23*
ygbP	Isoprenoid biosynthesis	Purification of MER-phosphate converting activity, discovery of CTP utilization, similarity of CTP-utilizing *H. influenzae acs1* gene 5′ end to *ygbP* gene; codistribution of *ygbP* homologs among species known to use deoxyxylulose (or MEP) pathway for isoprenoids	*24*
ygbB	Isoprenoid biosynthesis	Genetic linkage to ygbP; codistribution as for *ygbP;* gene fusion to *ygbP* in some species	*25*
ychB	Isoprenoid biosynthesis	Codistribution in species with *dxr, dxs,* & *ygbP* in species known to utilize the MEP pathway	*26*
yaeS (uppS)	dolichol carrier	Protein purification, excised from PAGE, trypsin digested and MALDI-TOF identification by match to computer-predicted trypsin fragments of all *E. coli* proteins	*27*
yidC	Secretion/insertion of membrane proteins	Sequence similarity to mitochondrial gene *oxal,* required for insertion of some inner-membrane proteins into the mitochondrion	*28*

only a narrow spectrum of species. In addition, knockouts of some of these genes may generate auxotrophic strains, and thus, the genes may not be essential in an animal host. Nevertheless, it is worth reviewing how these functions were elucidated, because functional annotation of genomes is one of the central problems in genomics, and one of the main obstacles to conversion of genomic information into drug targets. Some of the genes that have been annotated recently for function are shown in Table 2, along with a summary of how the functions were discovered. Clearly, in all cases, the investigators benefited enormously from having access to the sequence of several bacterial genomes, and in some cases from having access to sequences of the yeast genome and of several higher eukaryotes for comparative purposes. The combination of classical biochemistry or mutational genetics with genome and predicted proteome information has driven rapid discovery of new functions. In some cases, investigators were able to purify the source of the catalytic activity and derive enough N-terminal amino-acid sequence to make an unambiguous match to the predicted proteome of the bacterial species of interest (e.g., identification of the function of the *kdtB, yacE,* and *yaeS* gene products, Table 2). In other cases, mutational genetic approaches provided strains that could be complemented with plasmid libraries of genomic fragments, followed by sequencing of the complementing fragment or mapping the mutations and identifying the corresponding gene in the genome (e.g., identification of the function of the *ybeN* and *yaeM* gene products, Table 2). Notably, in all cases, confirmation of the putative function was achieved by expressing the gene, purifying the product, and demonstrating that it catalyzed the predicted reaction effectively.

Perhaps one of the most surprising outcomes of these efforts was the discovery of genes encoding activities in an entirely new pathway of isoprenoid biosynthesis. Isoprenoids and derivatives play key roles in cellular pathways such as energy metabolism (ubiquinones) and cell-wall biosynthesis (dolichol). Until the mid-1990s, all bacteria were believed to produce isoprenoid compounds through the mevalonate pathway in a manner similar to that of eukaryotes. However, as early as 1981, biochemical and genetic evidence began building in support of an alternate pathway in some species of bacteria. Incorporation of labeled precursors into isoprenoid compounds in some bacterial species was not consistent with predictions from the mevalonate pathway (see review in ref. *29*). Studies with *E. coli* mutants confirmed that pyruvate and glyceraldehyde-3-phosphate are precursors in the synthesis of isoprenoids in that species, and a new hypothetical biosynthetic pathway was proposed *(30)*. This so-called "non-mevalonate pathway" or 2-methyl-erithrytol (MER) pathway has now been shown to function in many Gram-negative pathogenic bacteria, some Gram-positive bacteria, and most plastids in plants. Genes that encode the first two steps of this pathway in bacteria—dxs and dxr—were discovered in 1997 and 1998, and discovery of the biochemistry and genes involved in much of the rest of the pathway followed rapidly thereafter (see Table 2).

Much of this success has derived from computational evidence of functional linkage between genes. These methods have been reviewed recently by Eisenberg et al. *(31)* and include genetic linkage ("gene neighbor method"), codistribution of genes in species ("method of phylogenetic profiles"), and fusion patterns of protein domains ("Rosetta Stone sequences"). For example, bacteria frequently carry genes encoding steps in the same pathway in a linked manner and usually regulate and cotranscribe the entire linkage group as an operon. Therefore, tight linkage of a gene of unknown function with a gene known to play a role in the MER pathway is good evidence that the unknown gene may also encode an MER pathway enzyme. However, since cotranscribed genes do not always play roles in the same biochemical pathway, it is important to have additional supporting evidence before investing too much effort in confirmation attempts. Fortunately, the fact that some bacterial species utilize the mevalonate pathway and some use the MER pathway provides another useful bit of information, and this is evident in comparisons of the phylogenetic profiles of genes. Finally, the fact that the *ygbB* gene is fused to the *ygbP* gene in *H. pylori* and *T. pallidum* has implicated the *ygbB* gene in the MER pathway since the *ygbP* gene was demonstrated to play such a role *(25)*. In fact, the *ygbB* and *ychB* genes were hypothesized to encode enzymes catalyzing steps in the MER pathway by using at least one of these bits of information (Table 2). Since genes have not yet been identified for all of the MER pathway steps, these methods may help to elucidate the remainder of the pathway in the near future.

GENOMIC APPROACHES TO DISCOVERY OF FUNCTION— FUNCTIONAL GENOMICS

It is clear from the successes shown in Table 2 that a number of approaches have proven useful for elucidation of the functional role of various gene products in the cell. These include the computational methods described here, as well as experimental approaches such as isolating sufficient protein with the desired catalytic activity to permit amino-terminal-sequence determination for database matching or obtaining mutants for complementation with cloned fragments. However, these experimental methods may be extremely difficult to apply to very low-abundance proteins or to genes with a mutant phenotype that cannot be predicted. A discussion of methods based on predicting functional linkages between genes and proteins of unknown function with those of known function and the limitations of these approaches follows.

Genetic Linkage, Phylogenetic Linkage, and Protein Fusions

As Table 2 indicates, computational evidence of linkage between genes/proteins of unknown function with those of known function can be helpful. However, these methods must be interpreted with caution and ultimately supported with direct experimental evidence. For example, genetic linkage between the *kdtB* and *kdtA* genes in a number of species has suggested that the *kdtB* gene product likely played a role in the biosynthesis of lipopolysaccharide (LPS), as established for the *kdtA*-encoded protein. Surprisingly, the *kdtB* gene product was recently shown to catalyze a reaction in the biosynthesis of coenzyme A, a role only marginally related to LPS biosynthesis (ref. *20;* Table 2). Finally, it is important to point out that the "linkage" of a gene of unknown function with one of known function by fusion of genes in some species has not been widely useful for identification of potential antibacterial targets. This is primarily because fusion of genes and gene fragments encoding protein domains is much more common in eukaryotes, and preferred antibacterial targets are selected to lack eukaryotic homologs.

Gene-Expression Profiling

The notion that coregulated genes usually share a common functional role is based on substantial evidence. In fact, the use of genetic linkage in apparent operons to infer function is based on this principle. However, coregulation may frequently be achieved in the cell through unlinked clusters of genes which share a regulatory mechanism—a regulon. In extreme cases, eukaryotes which have no operons coordinately control multiple genes spread around the genome. Although genes encoding proteins with a variety of different functions may appear to be coregulated in a single experimental condition, the coregulation of genes under a variety of conditions provides stronger evidence of common function. The availability of microarrays provides a convenient method for assessing the transcriptome under a variety of experimental conditions, and thus building relationships between genes based on common expression patterns. For example, Peterson et al. *(32)* used microarrays representing a portion of the *S. pneumoniae* genome to identify eight loci that were not previously known to be induced by competence stimulating peptide. Clustering software enables rapid comparison of results from multiple experimental conditions. This is absolutely essential when using microarrays representing entire genomes, because of the large number of data points from even a single experiment.

In addition to suggesting function by detection of coregulation, gene-expression profiling offers two related benefits, one in the area of assay development and one in the area of determining the mode of action of an inhibitory compound. In yeast, experiments demonstrate that the gene-expression profile of cells grown in the presence of an inhibitory compound closely resembles that of cells engineered to underexpress the gene encoding the target of the compound *(33)*. Therefore, compounds inhibiting a particular gene product could, in principle, be discovered by screening for compounds which generate a gene-expression profile resembling that observed when the target gene is underexpressed. One method to convert this approach into a high-throughput screen would be to tag with reporters one or more of the genes whose expression is affected by underexpression of the target gene. Indeed, reporter assays of this type have been described previously. For example, Bianchi and Baneyx *(34)* describe *lacZ* fusions to promoters known to be induced in response to various cell stresses as a sensitive method of identifying compounds affecting critical cell pathways. Results from microarray experiments may provide an abundant source of potential reporter fusions for assay design.

The view of the entire cellular transcriptome provided by microarrays may reveal clues to the mode of action of a compound incubated with cells prior to RNA isolation and probe preparation. For example, Gmuender et al. *(35)* demonstrated that DNA gyrase inhibitors produce very different gene-expression profiles in *H. influenzae,* depending on whether they inhibit GyrA (e.g., Ciprofloxacin) or GyrB (e.g., Novobiocin). Similarly, Wilson et al. *(36)* used a microarray of *Mycobacteria tuberculosis* genes to demonstrate that incubation of cells with isoniazid induces transcription of several genes known to be related to the drug's mode of action, and a few genes with no obvious relationship to mycolic acid biosynthesis. As expected, another compound, which also inhibits mycolic acid synthesis, induced a very similar pattern of gene expression. However, compounds which inhibit growth by different mechanisms yielded highly distinct gene-expression profiles. These results argue that gene-expression profiles may be used as "fingerprints" to distinguish modes of action of different compounds, and possibly to identify the mode of action of a new compound. In some cases, the target gene of the inhibitory compound will be upregulated. In other cases, the effect may be dominated by classes of genes involved in SOS or heat-shock response, but even in those cases, the pattern of gene expression may be distinct for that particular compound. If the investigator has a library of expression profiles available in response to treatment with a variety of known drugs and/or downregulated expression of a variety of putative drug targets, then hierarchical clustering of the data will reveal which target or drug-associated pattern is most similar to that generated by the new compound.

Proteomics

Just as analysis of the entire transcriptome of bacterial cells by microarray has been useful for discovery and validation of potential drug targets, analysis of the entire proteome is also proving helpful. Although proteins in bacterial cells undergo fewer post-transcriptional modifications than proteins in mammalian cells and alternative splicing of messages is rare or nonexistent in bacteria, the bacterial proteome is not entirely predictable from its transcriptome. Indeed, the very short half-life of most bacterial messages (averaging approx 2.5 min.) means that the amount of a protein in the cell may bear little relationship to the amount of message detected in a microarray experiment. Methods for the analysis of the entire proteome of bacterial cells are still in development, and the problem is clearly much more difficult than that of analyzing the transcriptome because proteins vary considerably in their properties. Early methods utilizing 2-dimensional gel electrophoresis have been supplemented with mass spectrometric peptide fingerprinting (MALDI-TOF) for identification of proteins *(37)*. Key problems are adequate separation of the entire proteome, sensitivity, and quantitation of differences. A promising new method using isotope-coded affinity tags and tandem mass spectrometry offers solutions to two of these problems *(38)*. Proteins isolated from cells grown in two different conditions are labeled differentially with affinity-tagged, proton- or deuterium-labeled, thiol-reacting reagents. The proteins are then digested with trypsin and the labeled peptides are isolated by affinity chromatography. Finally, the peptides are analyzed by LC-MS (for quantitative comparison of the amounts of each protein in each condition) and by MS-MS scan to permit identification of the protein by its peptide sequence. Unfortunately, it is still not possible to analyze the entire proteome. For example, only about 25% of membrane proteins contain cysteine residues; so new labeling methods are needed to extend this method to include most of the proteome. Application of this method and microarray analysis to yeast cells grown in the presence and absence of galactose indicates that the correlation between the transcriptome and the proteome is significant, but weak ($r = 0.61$; $P < 13 \times 10^{-20}$; ref. *39*). The mRNA levels of many ribosomal genes, for example, increased significantly in the presence of galactose, but the protein levels remained quite steady. Clearly, proteome and transcriptome data are different, but it is also clear that they will be useful in complementary ways for drug-target discovery and validation.

ASSAYS/SCREENS FOR TARGETS OF UNKNOWN OR INTRACTABLE FUNCTION

As noted previously, methods to identify the cellular role played by gene products lacking significant sequence similarity to known gene products are critical elements of a genomics strategy for drug development. However, they are not always successful in the time frame required, and even if they are successful, it is not always possible to design tractable biochemical assays and screens based on those functions. For these reasons, it is helpful to develop complementary screening methods not based on biochemical assays. Fortunately, a wide variety of such methods are now available, and forthcoming results should validate many of these approaches. Current methods can be

Table 3
Screening methods for targets of unknown function

Category	Method	Reference
Cell-based approaches	Over-expression rescue	*40*
	Under-expression hypersusceptibility	*40*
	Conditional mutants at semi-permissive conditions	*42*
	Reporter assays	*34*
Direct Binding approaches	"Any two ligand affinity screen" (ATLAS)	*43*
	Intrinsic fluorescence	*44*
	Capillary electrophoresis	*45*
	Mass spectrometry	*46*
Indirect-Binding methods	Time-resolved fluorescence	*47*
	Electrochemiluminescence	*48*
	Scintillation proximity assay (SPA)	*49*

organized into three basic categories—cell-based assays, direct-binding assays, and indirect-binding assays based on the use of a surrogate ligand (Table 3).

Cell-Based Assays

Cell-based assays are typically based on the principle that the amount of gene product affects the sensitivity of the cell to drugs that inhibit that enzymatic function. In this manner, regulated underexpression of a gene is predicted to result in hypersusceptibility of the cell to drugs which inhibit that gene product, and overexpression of a gene is expected to result in cells which are relatively more resistant to drugs that inhibit that enzyme. These expectations have been validated for several gene-drug combinations in model systems in the laboratory *(40)*. In addition, overexpression of the gene encoding the target is one recognized mechanism of drug resistance encountered clinically (e.g., overexpression of the *murA* gene confers resistance to fosfomycin *(41)*. An alternate approach to generate hypersensitive cells for screening involves the use of cells with conditional lethal mutations in key target genes *(42)*. In this case, essential genes were identified by the isolation of temperature-sensitive mutations. The ts mutants validated the targets as essential under the particular laboratory conditions used, but also provided a screening approach. Temperature-sensitive cells were grown at a semi-permissive temperature and used to screen for compounds which were more potent against the ts cells than against normal control cells. These approaches may also be used to construct secondary assays for confirmation of the specificity of compounds that kill whole cells. Although they are convenient, these assays will not be effective for every target. For example, some targets may be lethal when overproduced, and others may be part of multisubunit complexes, requiring overproduction of every component.

Reporter assays represent another distinct type of cell-based assays. As described above, the results from microarray studies may be used to identify appropriate genes for reporter fusions. In principle, the approach is generally applicable to most targets. However, it suffers from a relative lack of specificity. Therefore, carefully designed secondary assays are essential for filtering the resulting hits.

Direct Binding Assays

The second category of assays for targets of unknown or intractable function is based directly on affinity of the target for compounds. The "any two ligand affinity screen" (ATLAS) was one of the first such methods to be used for drug screening *(43)*. Although it is generally applicable, it is cumbersome to set up because it is based primarily on changes in the proteolytic susceptibility of the protein target upon binding of a small molecule, and requires development of antibodies to the protein target of interest. A simpler but less universally applicable method relies on changes in the intrinsic properties (e.g., fluorescence) of the target protein upon binding of a compound *(44)*. Another method is based on detecting electrophoretic mobility changes in capillary gels of the target protein upon binding of a small molecule *(45)*. Finally, small molecules that bind to a target of interest may be identified by their mass on a mass spectrometer after removal of unbound compounds by rapid gel filtration *(46)*. Limitations to these methods involve lack of control over the affinity of the binding, and over whether the small molecule is binding at an active site or an alternate site on the target. Generally, the highest affinity sites are expected to be in the substrate-binding pocket; however, further published examples are needed to confirm this expectation.

Indirect Binding Assays

A third category of assays and screens for targets of unknown or intractable function is based on detection of affinity in an indirect manner. According to these methods, novel small-molecule binders are identified by their ability to displace or compete with a surrogate ligand that has been labeled in some manner. Identification of a suitable surrogate ligand requires screening of an initial diverse set of compounds. Although screening to find a suitable ligand for screening appears to be paradoxical, in fact, most efforts have focused on initially identifying a peptide surrogate ligand. Methods such as panning peptide phage display libraries lend themselves readily to this problem *(17,47)*. Once an appropriate surrogate ligand has been identified and labeled, measurement of competition by members of a diverse chemical library may be accomplished in a relatively high-throughput manner by using techniques such as fluorescence polarization or time-resolved fluorescence *(47)*, electrochemiluminescence *(48)*, scintillation proximity assays *(49)*, or capillary electrophoretic mobility shifts *(45)*.

CONSIDERATION OF NONESSENTIAL TARGETS

The main focus of this chapter is essential gene products, yet it is clear that genomic information and techniques can equally assist in the discovery of nonessential gene products for drug discovery. The most widely suggested nonessential targets have been those involved in pathogenicity and virulence. Drugs directed against such targets would reduce the ability of the bacterium to cause disease, and would not kill the infectious organism. However, a host of unanswered question surrounds these types of targets. For example, will the selective pressure for drug resistance be lower for such drug-target combinations? How large a reduction in infectivity in an animal model is necessary to gauge efficacy in a human patient? How will lead compounds be optimized without a convenient in vitro assay? Will the host immune system deal adequately with the residual nonpathogenic, but live organisms? Will diagnostic methods be sufficiently rapid and accurate to permit correct choice of narrow-spectrum drugs targeting nonessential gene products? Perhaps such drugs would be used in combination to cover a wide spectrum until accurate diagnostic results are available. Perhaps such drugs will be used prophylactically in situations of high risk *(50)* to reduce the likelihood of a productive infection. The answers to these questions may not be revealed until a drug of this class is actually developed and tested.

Since pathogenicity is remarkably variable among infectious organisms, it is likely that drugs directed against such factors would exhibit rather narrow spectra. However, two types of pathogenicity factors have drawn wide attention because the potential spectra of drugs acting against them could be wide enough to include most Gram-positive organisms or most Gram-negative organisms. For example, sortase is a gene product found in most Gram-positive pathogens. It functions in a bacterial-specific manner to process secreted proteins bound for the cell-wall outer surface. Initially expected to be an essential gene, it was shown to be nonessential after it was cloned and knocked-out by Schneewind and colleagues *(51)*. Nevertheless, such deletion strains exhibit a 100-fold reduction in virulence in both a mouse renal abscess and a lethal infection model *(52)*. This function may be sufficiently critical to warrant drug development. Suitable uses could be for prophylaxis (e.g., in intravenous (iv) lines, catheters, prostheses, presurgery, post-trauma), decolonization (e.g., eliminate nasal carriage of *S. aureus*), or for therapy, but probably only in combination with other drugs.

Second, type III secretion systems (TTSS) are found only in pathogenic, Gram-negative species *(53)*. These systems are typically found on pathogenicity islands, and encode over 20 gene products involved in building bacterial-specific secretion machinery resembling a syringe and used for delivery of toxins to host cells. Although the toxins vary considerably from species to species, many of the genes encoding the delivery machinery are fairly conserved. However, it is still unclear whether they are sufficiently conserved to expect that a drug directed against such a target in one species would also block TTSS in another species.

FUTURE DIRECTIONS/CHALLENGES FOR GENOMICS

The previous section has emphasized the strength of genomic data and molecular genetic tools for the discovery and validation of drug targets and the development of screens. However, there are clearly some limitations to what can be accomplished with these methods alone. Some drug discovery needs will never be met by genomics, but the following two aspects of target validation may yet benefit from genomic tools. First, in the future, genomics approaches are likely to be of more assistance in predicting the rate and mechanism of development of drug resistance. As models of cellular pathways based on the genome and proteome improve, it will become possible to predict the existence of bypass pathways which may allow the cell to escape death because of inhibition of a particular enzymatic step. In addition, improved knowledge of the substrate specificity of drug modification enzymes and efflux pumps will permit predictions of the development of drug resistance by those mechanisms. Second, proteomic methods will provide an accurate view of the amount of each protein in the cell under particular conditions. This data, combined with knowledge of the minimal amount of each protein required for cell viability, will reveal which steps are most critical for each pathway, and therefore, which are the key rate-limiting steps to be targeted by new drugs.

In the meantime, the growing resources of microbial genomes and genomic tools provide increasingly valuable assistance for target discovery, validation, and screen development. Even if these approaches do not accelerate the process of developing a drug, they should increase the number of different targets for screening and entry into the development pipeline.

ACKNOWLEDGMENT

I thank all of my colleagues at Genome Therapeutics Corporation who have helped make this chapter possible by providing helpful discussions and relevant literature references. In particular, I thank Lucy Ling, Tim Opperman, Gilles Carmel, Jianhua Wu, Yibin Xiang, and Veronique Damagnez.

REFERENCES

1. Trias J. Perspectives on genomics and antibiotic discovery. Curr Opinion Investigational Drugs 2001;2:742–744.
2. Black T, Hare R. Will genomics reolutionize antimicrobial drug discovery? Curr Opinion Microbiol 2000;3:522–527.
3. Fraser CM, Eisen JA, Salzberg SL. Microbial genome sequencing. Nature 2000;406:799–803.
4. Rosamond J, Allsop A. Harnessing the power of the genome in the search for new antibiotics. Science 2000;287:1973–1976.
5. Moir DT, Shaw KJ, Hare, RA, Vovis GF. Genomics and antimicrobial drug discovery. Antimicrob. Agents Chemother 1999;43:439–446.
6. Kuroda M, Ohta T, Uchiyama I, Baba T, Yuzawa H, Kobayashi I, et al. Whole genome sequencing of methicillin-resistant Staphylococcus aureus, the major hospital pathogen. Lancet 2001;357:1225–1240.
7. Tettelin H, Nelson KE, Paulsen IT, Eisen JA, Read TD, Peterson S, et al. Complete genome sequence of a virulent isolate of Streptococcus pneumoniae. Science 2001;293:498–506.
8. Galperin MY, Koonin EV. Comparative genome analysis. Methods Biochem Anal 2001;43:359–392.
9. Murphy KC. Use of bacteriophage lambda recombination functions to promote gene replacement in Escherichia coli. J Bacteriol 1998;180:2063–2071.
10. Niemeyer DM, Pucci MJ, Thanassi JA, Sharma VK, Archer GL. Role of mecA transcriptional regulation in the phenotypic expression of methicillin resistance in Staphylococcus aureus. J Bacteriol 1996;178:5464–5471.
11. Lee MS, Dougherty BA, Madeo AC, Morrison DA. Construction and analysis of a library for random insertional mutagenesis in Streptococcus pneumoniae: use for recovery of mutants defective in genetic transformation and for identification of essential genes. Appl Environ Microbiol 1999;65:1883–1890.
12. Judson N, Mekalanos JJ. Transposon-based approaches to identify essential bacterial genes. Trends Microbiol 2000;8:521–526.
13. Lehoux DE, Levesque RC. Detection of genes essential in specific niches by signature-tagged mutagenesis. Curr Opinion Biotechnol 2000;11:434–439.
14. Hare RS, Walker SS, Dorman TE, Greene JR, Guzman L-M, Kenney TJ, et al. Genetic footprinting in bacteria. J Bacteriol 2001;183:1694–1706.
15. Shea JE, Hensel M, Gleeson C, Holden DW. Identification of a virulence locus encoding a second type III secretion system in Salmonella typhimurium. Proc Natl Acad Sci USA 1996;93:2593–2597.

16. Coulter SN, Schwan WR, Ng EY, Langhorn MH, Ritchie HD, Wesbrock-Wadman S, et al. Staphylococcus aureus genetic loci impacting growth and survival in multiple infection environments. Mol Microbiol 1998;30:393–404.

17. Tao J, Wendler P, Connelly G, Lim A, Zhang J, King M, et al. Drug target validation: lethal infection blocked by inducible peptide. Proc Natl Acad Sci USA 2000;97:783–786.

18. Blum JH, Dove SL, Hochschild A, Mekalanos JJ. Isolation of peptide aptamers that inhibit intracellular processes. Proc Natl Acad Sci USA 2000;97:2241–2246.

19. Zyskind JW, Forsyth RA. Method for identifying microbial proliferation genes. US Patent 6,228,579. May 8, 2001.

20. Geerlof A, Lewendon A, Shaw WV. Purification and characterization of phosphopantetheine adenylyltransferase from Escherichia coli. J Biol Chem 1999;274:27,105–27,111.

21. Mishra PK, Park PK, Drueckhammer DG. Identification of yacE (coaE) as the structural gene for dephosphocoenzyme A kinase in Escherichia coli K12. J Bacteriol 2001;183:2774–2778.

22. Mehl RA, Kinsland C, Begley TP. Identification of the Escherichia coli nicotinic acid mononucleotide adenylyltransferase gene. J Bacteriol 2000;182:4372–4374.

23. Takahashi S, Kuzuyama T, Watanabe H, Seto H. A 1-deoxy-D-xylulose 5-phosphate reductoisomerase catalyzing the formation of 2-C-methyl-D-erythritol 4-phosphate in an alternative non-mevalonate pathway for terpenoid biosynthesis. Proc Natl Acad Sci USA 1998;95:9879–9884.

24. Rohdich F, Wungsintaweekul J, Fellermeier M, Sagner S, Herz S, Kis K, et al. Cytidine 5′-triphosphate-dependent biosynthesis of isoprenoids: YgbP protein of Escherichia coli catalyzes the formation of 4-diphosphocytidyl-2-C-methylerythritol. Proc Natl Acad Sci USA 1999;96:11,758–11,763.

25. Herz S, Wungsintaweekul J, Schuhr CA, Hecht S, Luettgen H, Sagner S, et al. Biosynthesis of terpenoids: YgbB protein converts 4-diphosphocytidyl-2C-methyl-D-erythritol 2-phosphate to 2C-methyl-D-erythritol 2,4-cyclodiphosphate. Proc Natl Acad Sci USA 2000;97:2486–2490.

26. Luettgen H, Rohdich F, Herz S, Wungsintaweekul J, Hecht S, Schuhr CA, et al. Biosynthesis of terpenoids: YchB protein of Escherichia coli phosphorylates the 2-hydroxy group of 4-diphosphocytidyl-2C-methyl-D-erythritol. Proc Natl Acad Sci USA 2000;97:1062–1067.

27. Apfel CM, Takacs B, Fountoulakis M, Stieger M, Keck W. Use of genomics to identify bacterial undecaprenyl pyrophosphate synthetase: cloning, expression, and characterization of the essential uppS gene. J Bacteriol 1999;181:483–492.

28. Samuelson JC, Chen M, Jiang F, Moeller I, Wiedmann M, Kuhn A, et al. YidC mediates membrane protein insertion in bacteria. Nature 2000;406:637–641.

29. Rohmer M. Isoprenoid biosynthesis via the mevalonate-independent route, a novel target for antibacterial drugs? Prog Drug Res 1998;50:137–154.

30. Rohmer M, Seemann M, Horbach S, Bringer-Meyer S, Sahm H. Glyceraldehyde 3-phosphate and pyruvate as precursors of isoprenic units in an alternative non-mevalonate pathway for terpenoid biosynthesis. J Am Chem Soc 1996;118:2564–2566.

31. Eisenberg D, Marcotte EM, Xenarios I, Yeates TO. Protein function in the post-genomic era. Nature 2000;405:823–826.

32. Peterson S, Cline RT, Tettelin H, Sharov V, Morrison DA. Gene expression analysis of the Streptococcus pneumoniae competence regulons by use of DNA microarrays. J Bacteriol 2000;182:6192–6202.

33. Marton MJ, DeRisi JL, Bennett HA, Iyer VR, Meyer MR, Roberts CJ, et al. Drug target validation and identification of secondary drug target effects using DNA microarrays. Nat Med 1998;11:1293–1301.

34. Bianchi A, Baneyx F. Stress Response as a tool to detect and characterize the mode of action of antibacterial agents. Applied Environ Microbiol 1999;65:5023–5027.

35. Gmuender H, Kuratli K, Padova KD, Gray CP, Keck W, Evers S. Gene expression changes triggered by exposure of Haemophilus influenzae to novobiocin or ciprofloxacin: combined transcription and translation analysis. Genome Res 2001;11:28–42.

36. Wilson M, DeRisi J, Kristensen HH, Imboden P, Rane S, Brown PO, et al. Exploring drug-induced alterations in gene expression in Mycobacterium tuberculosis by microarray hybridization. Proc Natl Acad Sci USA 1999;96:12833–12838.
37. Washburn MP, Yates JR. Analysis of the microbial proteome. Curr Opin Microbiol 2000;3:292–297.
38. Gygi SP, Rist B, Gerber SA, Turecek F, Gelb MH, Aebersold R. Quantitative analysis of complex protein mixtures using isotope-coded affinity tags. Nat Biotechnol 1999;17:994–999.
39. Ideker T, Thorsson V, Ranish JA, Christmas R, Buhler J, Eng JK, et al. Integrated genomic and proteomic analyses of a systematically perturbed metabolic network. Science 2001;292:929–934.
40. Trias J, Young D, Rosenow C. Regulated target expression for screening. PCT patent application WO 99/52926. Oct. 21, 1999.
41. Horii T, Kimura T, Sato K, Shibayama K, Ohta M. Emergence of fosfomycin-resistant isolates of Shiga-like toxin-producing Escherichia coli O26. Antimicrob Agents Chemother 1999;43:789–793.
42. Benton B, Lee VJ, Malouin F, Martin PK, Schmid MB, Sun D. Methods of screening for compounds active on Staphylococcus aureus target genes. US Patent 6,037,123. March 14, 2000.
43. Bowie JU, Pakula A. Screening method for identifying ligands for target proteins. US Patent 5,679,582. Oct. 21, 1997.
44. Pantoliano MW, Petrella E, Salemme FR, Springer BA. Method for determining conditions that stabilize proteins. US Patent 6,232,085. May 15, 2001.
45. Dunayevskiy YM, Hughes DE, Waters JL. Capillary electrophoretic methods to detect new biologically active compounds in complex biological material. PCT Patent application WO 99/31496. June 24, 1999.
46. Lenz GR, Nash HM, Jindal S. Chemical ligands, genomics and drug discovery. Drug Develop Technol 2000;5:145–156.
47. Hyde-DeRuyscher R, Paige LA, Christensen DJ, Hyde-DeRuyscher N, Lim A, Fredericks ZL, et al. Detection of small-molecule enzyme inhibitors with peptides isolated from phage-displayed combinatorial peptide libraries. Chem Biol 2000;7:17–25.
48. Liljestrand J, Zhang J, Gambrel DR, Ivanov S, Wohlstadter JN. Apparatus for carrying out electrochemiluminescence test measurements. US Patent 6,200,531. March 13, 2001.
49. Alouani S. Scintillation proximity binding assay. Methods Mol Biol 2000;138:135–141.
50. Alksne LE, Projan S. Bacterial virulence as a target for antimicrobial chemotherapy. Curr Opinion Biotechnol 2000;11:625–636.
51. Mazmanian SK, Liu G, Ton-That H, Schneewind O. Staphylococcus aureus sortase, an enzyme that anchors surface proteins to the cell wall. Science 1999;285:760–763.
52. Mazmanian SK, Liu G, Jensen ER, Lenoy E, Schneewind O. Staphylococcus aureus sortase mutants defective in the display of surface proteins and in the pathogenesis of animal infections. Proc Natl Acad Sci USA 2000;97:5510–5515.
53. Hueck CJ. Type III protein secretion systems in bacterial pathogens of animals and plants. Microbiol Mol Biol Rev 1998;62:379–433.

6

Genomics of the *Mycobacterium tuberculosis* Complex and BCG Vaccines

Marcel A. Behr and Stephen V. Gordon

BACKGROUND

Despite the existence of the *M. bovis* bacillus Calmette-Guerin (BCG) vaccine since the 1920's (BCG) and the availability of effective antimicrobial therapy since the 1950s, tuberculosis (TB) remains a pathogen of major importance. Current estimates indicate that one-third of the world's population is infected by *M. tuberculosis* with an estimated 8 million new cases and 1.9 million deaths attributable to tuberculosis each year *(1)*. Although antimicrobial therapy should theoretically convert this deadly disease into a treatable bacterial infection, programmatic limitations prevent many of the victims from obtaining effective therapy. In regions where drugs have been available, inappropriate use has led to the selection of drug-resistant bacilli *(2)*. Furthermore, the synergy between HIV/AIDS and TB and the added difficulties of treating both these diseases with complex multi-drug cocktails suggest that control of TB with antimicrobial agents alone may remain an elusive challenge. This paucity of chemotherapeutic options is compounded by the variable efficacy of the live attenuated *M. bovis* BCG vaccine strains in clinical settings *(3)*.

For many infectious diseases, the preventive option provided by vaccination has led either to elimination of the disease (e.g., smallpox) or the brink of elimination (e.g., measles, polio). For TB, a vaccine could help serve at two points in the cycle of transmission and disease development. A vaccine given prior to infection with *M. tuberculosis* could prime the immune system to prevent the spread of the pathogenic strain, much the way that BCG vaccination is anticipated to delay or retard disease upon subsequent exposure *(4)*. Another option would be to provide a post-exposure immunologic stimulus to the 1.7 billion people infected with *M. tuberculosis*. Here, the goal would be to prevent these individuals from progressing to active disease at a later date. Unfortunately, no human vaccine currently exists for this purpose, and animal models of immunotherapy to date have focused on better control of active disease rather than immunoprophylaxis of latent infection *(5)*.

Whatever the ultimate strategy is for the use of a new vaccine, it is likely that such a product will result from a better understanding of the pathogenesis of the infection, and the role of host, bacterial, and environmental factors. Environmental factors, such as co-infection with HIV/AIDS, may be difficult to factor into vaccine design, but it is

From: *Pathogen Genomics: Impact on Human Health*
Edited by: K. J. Shaw © Humana Press Inc., Totowa, NJ

Table 1
Mycobacterial sequencing projects completed or ongoing

Organism	Status, summer 2001	Website
M. tuberculosis H37Rv	Completed	http://www.sanger.ac.uk/Projects/ M_tuberculosis/
M. tuberculosis CDC1551	Completed	http://www.tigr.org/tigr-scripts/CMR2/ GenomePage3.spl?database=gmt
M. tuberculosis strain 210	Nearing completion	http://www.tigr.org/cgi-bin/ BlastSearch/ReleaseDate.cgi
M. bovis 2122/97	Nearing completion	http://www.sanger.ac.uk/Projects/ M_bovis/
M. microtti	Ongoing	n.a.
M. bovis BCG Pasteur	Ongoing	http://www.pasteur.fr/recherche/ unites/Lgmb/mycogenomics.html
M. leprae	Completed	http://www.sanger.ac.uk/Projects/ M_leprae/
M. smegmatis	Ongoing	http://www.tigr.org/cgi-bin/ BlastSearch/ReleaseDate.cgi
M. avium 104	Ongoing	http://www.tigr.org/cgi-bin/ BlastSearch/ReleaseDate.cgi
M. avium paratuberculosis	Ongoing	http://www.cbc.umn.edu/ ResearchProjects/AGAC/Mptb/ Mptbhome.html
M. ulcerans	Ongoing	http://www.pasteur.fr/recherche/ unites/Lgmb/mycogenomics.html

clear that the vaccine should not generally cause disease in immunocompromised persons. Other environmental factors, such as nutritional status and exposure to other Mycobacteria, which may interfere with the development of a protective immune response, should be considered to ensure that the vaccine is given to individuals who have a realistic possibility of mounting an effective immune response. Host factors have not traditionally played a significant role in vaccine design; however, data from both animal models and human populations indicate that host genetic variability plays a significant role in our ability to contain *M. tuberculosis (6,7)*. Significantly, only 10% of persons infected with *M. tuberculosis* are expected to develop disease. Therefore a vaccine to prevent 10 cases may need to be given to 100 individuals, if it is not possible to identify in advance the subset of persons who are not naturally immune. From this perspective, the goal of new research should be to exploit information on why 90% of infected individuals do not develop TB in order to produce a vaccine that will generate an appropriate response in the 10% who do not do so already.

Considering the complexity of host and environmental issues, study of the pathogen offers an attractive system to learn more about the biology of disease. The wealth of genomic information available for the Mycobacterial genus provides the basis for explorations of traits such as virulence, strain variability, and host tropism (see Table 1). Genomics of BCG vaccine strains should also finally reveal the nature of the mutations that attenuated the *M. bovis* progenitor, which are still unknown after more than 75 years of use. The opportunities for comparative genomics in Mycobacteria have therefore been considerable, both from in silico comparisons of sequence data and in vitro comparisons of strains using modern genomic tools such as BAC libraries, DNA microarrays, and Affymetrix Genechips.

INFORMATION FROM COMPLETE GENOME SEQUENCING

The cornerstone of Mycobacterial genomic analysis has been the complete genome sequence of *M. tuberculosis* H37Rv, published in 1998 *(8)*. H37Rv is a clinical isolate from 1905 that spent most of the 20th century in research labs, yet it has retained its virulence in model systems and is the best standardized strain for use in experimental settings. From our knowledge of the H37Rv genome, it is now possible to compare sequence data from other isolates of the genus. The first order of comparison is strain-to-strain variability within *M. tuberculosis,* as the complete genome sequence of a recent clinical isolate known as *M. tuberculosis* CDC1551 is also available on-line *(9)*. Variability between clinical strains in the community will provide information on antigenic variability, and suggest whether one vaccine will be sufficient against all strains or whether different type-specific vaccines will be needed, as observed for other pathogens such as Influenza and *Streptococcus pneumoniae.* The next order of comparison is the study of differences within the closely related members of the *M. tuberculosis* complex—specifically differences between *M. tuberculosis,* a human pathogen, and *M. bovis,* which is primarily a veterinary pathogen. Genomic variation between the bacilli may suggest differences in host-pathogen interactions, yet similarities may indicate potential livestock uses of a human vaccine, or vice versa. Within the group of organisms known as *M. bovis* are found the live attenuated vaccine strains, known as *M bovis* BCG, or Bacille Calmette-Guerin, named in honor of the microbiologists who developed these attenuated forms of an *M. bovis* isolate between 1908 and 1921 *(10)*. The most obvious phenotype for study is the fact that these vaccines, which are given to millions of infants each year, rarely cause disease. Thus, analysis of BCG should provide insights into bacterial virulence by highlighting genomic features that are missing or mutated compared to naturally virulent strains. Finally, genomic comparisons are possible between *M. tuberculosis* and other Mycobacteria sequenced or in the process of being sequenced. The massive scale of gene decay in *M. leprae,* the causative agent of leprosy, suggests a minimal gene set needed for survival as an obligate intracellular pathogen *(11)*. The larger genomes of environmental Mycobacteria, such as *M. avium* and *M. smegmatis,* may point to genomic factors associated with a more varied lifestyle.

STRAIN-TO-STRAIN VARIABILITY WITHIN *M. tuberculosis* SSP. *tuberculosis*

Human tuberculosis is generally caused by members of the subspecies *M. tuberculosis.* Therefore, a vaccine to prevent TB in humans should be designed to be effective against all strains of the *M. tuberculosis* complex. Preliminary indications about strain-to-strain variability suggest that clinical isolates share high degrees of sequence identity. For instance, sequence analyses of a limited number of genes across a large collection of *M. tuberculosis* isolates revealed that single-nucleotide polymorphisms (SNPs) are exceedingly rare—approx 1 in 10,000 basepairs (bp) *(12)*. If these observations are confirmed on a larger scale, such homogeneity among clinical isolates would provide a window of optimism for vaccine design, suggesting that one product may provide protection against all isolates of *M. tuberculosis*. Yet converse data come from molecular typing efforts, where a number of variable loci in the genome have been exploited to permit tracking of organisms in molecular epidemiologic studies. A number of variable loci, such as insertion sequences (IS), tandem repeats, and polymorphic GC-rich sequences have been revealed, indicating that *M. tuberculosis* isolates circulating in the community are genetically heterogeneous, at least in a limited number of loci. The challenge in the post-genomic design of a novel vaccine will be to exploit the regions of homogeneity to develop a vaccine that is protective against all strains, acknowledging that variable regions exist which may play a role in the ability of the pathogen to elude host defenses.

To date, data regarding strain-to-strain genome variability of *M. tuberculosis* isolates have come from informative analysis of three genome-sequencing projects and molecular epidemiologic studies of *M. tuberculosis* clinical isolates.

Genome sequencing has now been completed for the recent clinical isolate *M. tuberculosis* CDC1551. Sequencing of a second recent isolate, *M. tuberculosis* strain 210, is not yet complete. Thus, comparative genomic analysis was not possible at the time of writing (http://www.tigr.org/cgi-bin/BlastSearch/ReleaseDate.cgi). However, analyses of the two complete *M. tuberculosis* sequences (H37Rv and CDC1551) have identified a number of variable genetic loci between these strains. Comparisons between the CDC1551 and H37Rv genomes can be visualized using the Apropos genome alignment tool (http://www.cmmi.ic.ac.uk/apropos/index.php). The CDC1551 isolate has 4,033 predicted open reading frames (ORFs), about 109 more than the genome sequence of H37Rv. In silico comparison suggests a frequency of polymorphism between the two strains of approx 1 in 3,000 bp, with approximately one-half the differences observed in intergenic regions *(13)*. This is higher than the frequency reported by Musser and colleagues in a study that was restricted to selected genes across geographically distinct isolates *(12)*.

In addition to SNPs, there are numerous insertions and deletions (indels) and gene-duplication events between the two strains. For example, a locus encoding a phospholipase C is present in CDC1551 but absent from H37Rv (a locus designated RvD2) *(14)*. This locus appears to have been deleted from H37Rv by recombination between proximal IS*6110* elements, with resulting loss of the intervening sequence. Comparison of the sequence flanking the insertion sites of IS*6110* elsewhere in the H37Rv genome identified three other IS*6110*-mediated deletions from the genome of *M. tuberculosis* H37Rv. As IS*6110* is the most promiscuous insertion sequence in the *M. tuberculosis* complex, ranging from 0–26 copies, this suggests that IS-catalyzed genome rearrangements may be a major generator of plasticity. Indeed, examination of the RvD2 locus across a range of clinical isolates has identified it as a region prone to indels *(15)*.

An apparent gene duplication in CDC1551 is observed at the locus eoncoding homologs of the H37Rv ORFs Rv2543 and Rv2544. These two ORFs share >85% nucleotide identity in H37Rv, implying that they originally arose through gene duplication. However, in CDC1551 the corresponding region has three genes—MT2618, MT2619, and MT2620. The middle gene, MT2619, has significant sequence similarity with the flanking genes, but does not have a homolog in H37Rv, suggesting that it represents an additional duplication. These observations, from the comparison of just two isolates, suggest that although nucleotide polymorphisms may be rare, other sources of genetic variability such as indels, duplications, and rearrangements may provide a source for *M. tuberculosis* strain-to-strain variability.

To pursue observations on *M. tuberculosis* genomic variability across a broader collection of strains, a number of different approaches have been employed. The *M. tuberculosis* H37 strain was originally dissociated into clones that showed a stable virulent or attenuated phenotype in animal models. To address the genetic basis of this variation, Brosch et al. used pulsed-field gel electrophoresis (PFGE) to construct physical maps of the genomes of *M. tuberculosis* H37Rv and its attenuated derivative H37Ra *(14)*. They were able to identify an IS-mediated deletion from H37Rv and an extra insertion of IS*6110* near the origin of replication in H37Ra. The IS-mediated deletion was found to correspond to RvD2, so its loss apparently did not alter virulence. Furthermore, complementation of the insertion of IS*6110* near *oriC* in H37Ra with the wild-type locus from H37Rv did not restore virulence in a mouse model, suggesting that this genetic event was not causally associated with the attenuated phenotype. These observations illustrate that analysis of genomic alterations can suggest phenotypic variants, but also indicate that these efforts are hypothesis-generating and still require formal testing.

A second approach to studying strain variability between *M. tuberculosis* isolates has involved Affymetrix Genechip™-based interrogation of well-defined clinical isolates. In this study, clones from San Francisco that came with described clinical and epidemiological parameters were tested for deletions with respect to the *M. tuberculosis* H37Rv genome, in order to determine the frequency of deletions in natural populations and the types of genes deleted *(16)*. Unlike analysis by restriction digests, genome libraries, or whole-genome sequencing, use of one sequence as a basis for studying deletions in other strains forcibly restricts analysis to a unidirectional view. Thus, duplications in clinical strains and deletions from H37Rv with respect to clinical isolates could not be tested *(17)*. Nonetheless, data from this analysis provided exciting clues into the genomic variability of clinical isolates, causing infection and disease in a natural human population.

The simplest observation from this analysis was that clonal isolates as defined by restriction fragment-length polymorphism (RFLP)-based typing shared the same genomic deletions, suggesting that deletion analysis may be a valuable genotyping tool for understanding population genetics of the *M. tuberculosis* complex. The mean number of deleted regions per clone was 2.9, containing on average 17.2 ORFs, or about 0.3% of the genome. Of ORFs deleted from clinical isolates, insertion elements and phages were over-represented, and genes predicted to have a role in information pathways were not observed in deletions. Most intriguing was the observation that clones with the most deleted genes had the least propensity to manifest as cavitary disease on chest radiograph, suggesting that a clinical virulence phenotype may be inversely associated with genomic deletions *(16)*.

In summary, preliminary analysis from sequencing of *M. tuberculosis* isolates and chip-based study of deleted regions confirms that *M. tuberculosis* isolates share a high degree of genetic similarity. It is important to note that analysis of the proteome of CDC1551 and H37Rv has also revealed a striking degree of conservation, indicating that global protein-expression profiles, at least in vitro, are highly similar *(18)*. This finding provides hope for vaccine development if the nature of antigenicity is equally conserved, but further evaluation is needed. The possibility exists that the small subset of genes that show genetic heterogeneity may play an important role in the immunopathogenesis of disease.

GENOMIC VARIABILITY BETWEEN SUBSPECIES OF THE *M. tuberculosis* COMPLEX

The *M. tuberculosis* complex comprises seven related species, namely *M. tuberculosis, M. bovis, M. microti, M. africanum, M. caprae,* and *M. canetti.* The hallmark of these strains is that they show greater than 99% DNA identity at the gene level, yet present diverse phenotypes. Thus, although *M. tuberculosis, M. africanum,* and *M. canettii* can all cause disease in immunocompetent individuals, *M. microti* is attenuated for the human host. Similarly, *M. bovis* is not a common human pathogen, yet it is isolated from tuberculous lesions in a range of wild and domesticated animals. The solution to this paradox of genetic homogeneity with phenotypic diversity is undoubtedly encoded in the genomes of the bacilli. Comparative genomics across the complex therefore represents a powerful tool to dissect the molecular basis of host tropism, virulence, and pathogenesis.

As an initial step toward comparative genomics of the *M. tuberculosis* complex, bacterial artificial chromosome (BAC) array comparisons have been used to identify deletions from *M. bovis* and *M. bovis* BCG relative to *M. tuberculosis (19)*. This process identified a set of deletions, designated RD4-RD10, which affect a range of metabolic pathways and putative virulence factors. For example, *M. bovis* has lost an operon encoding one of the putative mycobacterial Mce (macrophage cell entry) invasins. Similarly, three genes encoding phospholipase C have been lost from the bovine bacillus. It is evident that these are deletions from *M. bovis,* rather than insertions in *M. tuberculosis,* since the ORF structure at the deletion junction points is clearly disrupted. However, the physiological impact of the loss of these loci from *M. bovis,* or conversely their presence in *M. tuberculosis,* is difficult to predict.

The genome sequence of *M. bovis* 2122/97, an isolate from a tuberculous cow, should be completed by the end of 2001 (see Table 1). This will provide the first opportunity for exquisitely detailed genetic comparison of two species of the *M. tuberculosis* complex. Initial analysis of this data suggests that there are no major genomic loci unique to the bovine bacillus. Furthermore, the genes showing the major differences are the PE and PPE proteins, a class of proteins encoded by GC-rich genes whose sequences have been shown to be highly variable among disease isolates. The incomplete nature of the data makes predictions of SNP frequencies difficult, but these are expected to be similar to those described for the CDC1551 and H37Rv comparison.

The apparent lack of any *M. bovis*-specific genes suggests that the major phenotypic differences between this and the other members of the *M. tuberculosis* complex may be caused by variation in expression. Indeed, it is already known that the major antigens of *M. bovis,* MPB83 and MPB70, are expressed by *M. tuberculosis* at much lower levels *(20)*. It also possible that the classic biochemical marker tests used to differentiate human and bovine bacilli, such as nitrate reduction or niacin secretion, will be linked to expression differences. Transcriptome analysis will therefore prove fundamental to describing the global-expression profiles of *M. tuberculosis* and *M. bovis,* and will ultimately enable us to identify differential gene expression in vivo. Gene products identified in this way should provide ideal candidates for subunit vaccines, as well as targets whose inactivation could lead to the development of improved, life and attenuated vaccine strains.

The genome of *M. microti,* the vole bacillus, is currently being determined, and should be completed in 2002 (S.T. Cole, *personal communication*). Apart from BCG, this is the only other tubercle strain that has been used as a live vaccine against tuberculosis, and notably, this strain provided considerable protection against TB in a clinical trial *(21).* Preliminary analysis suggests that deletions will again be the most obvious genomic difference between *M. microti* and *M. tuberculosis.* Because this strain is attenuated for humans, it will be of great interest to identify genetic lesions that are shared by *M. microti* and BCG, as this promises to reveal virulence factors necessary for successful infection.

The other members of the complex, *M. africanum, M. caprae,* and *M. canettii,* have been investigated to determine whether they share the deletions observed, in *M. microti* and *M. bovis.* Using polymerase chain reaction (PCR) to amplify deletion junction points, it was found that some strains of *M. africanum* are deleted for RD9, yet *M. canettii* apparently has all its loci intact (R. Brosch, *personal communication*). *M. caprae* is similar to bovine strains in terms of deletions, except that the RD4 locus is present. The main problem with this type of analysis is that it can only identify deletions relative to the sequenced strains. However, it does suggest a genealogy for the *M. tuberculosis* complex, with *M. tuberculosis* and *M. canettii* being the closest to the common progenitor, followed by *M. africanum, M. microti, M. caprae,* and *M. bovis.* Intriguingly, because BCG was derived from the most "degenerate" tubercle bacillus, yet can protect against disease caused by *M. tuberculosis,* it suggests that the deletions do not have a major impact on the ability of BCG to induce protection. This holds the promise that new subunit or live attenuated vaccines could protect against both human and animal disease.

GENOMIC ANALYSIS OF *M. bovis* BCG VACCINES

At a first step toward understanding the genomic basis of anti-TB vaccination, a number of groups have attempted to dissect the origins of the BCG vaccines currently in use. These vaccines are a family of closely related BCG strains that shared a common ancestor in 1921 before being propagated in various vaccine production facilities for much of the 20th century *(22).* Before lyophilization permitted the immortalization of the vaccines in the 1960s and 1970s, most of these vaccines were being propagated in vitro by passage on fresh media every 10–14 days. The vaccine numbers provided with strains indicate passage number, so that BCG Pasteur 1173 was passaged 1173 times over 53 years in the laboratory, and BCG Danish 1331 had a higher passage number because of a shorter interval between passages. Because the record of strain dissemination was largely known and some strains had been obtained indirectly through other vaccine houses, it has been possible to assemble a genealogic tree of BCG strains (see Fig. 1) *(23).* This record of strain dissemination can then be used as a framework to assemble genomic differences between strains

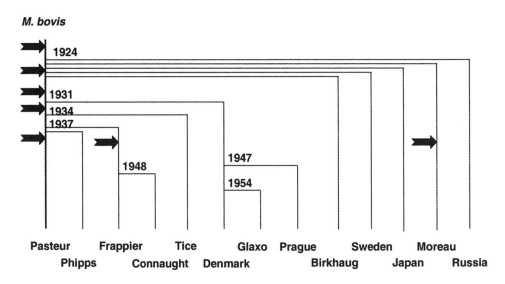

Fig. 1. Historical genealogy of BCG vaccine strains. The vertical axis scales to time, beginning with virulent *M. bovis* and ending at bottom with contemporary BCG vaccines. The horizontal axis represents different vaccine houses. Timing of deletions in the bacterial genome is illustrated with arrows.

and to validate a phylogenetic scenario for the evolution of BCG strains from virulent *M. bovis*.

Considering the wealth of information on BCG vaccines, it is important to highlight what is and is not known about them. Most importantly, the reasons for their attenuated virulence are unknown, and their ability to protect against TB is uncertain. That they are less virulent is the lesser virulence of BCG vaccines is undisputed, as disease following exposure to *M. tuberculosis* is estimated to occur in 10% of those infected, yet the rate of disease from BCG is estimated to be on the order of 1/1,000,000 *(24)*. Whether they protect against TB is less certain. Prevention of infantile forms of TB has been highly consistent, with most studies estimating over 80% less disease in vaccinated infants *(25)*. For this reason, BCG vaccination is likely to continue to be given to most children around the world. Unfortunately, protection against the contagious form of pulmonary TB has been widely inconsistent, with clinical trials demonstrating efficacy ranging from 80% to no difference compared to placebo. This may explain in part why the epidemic curves of countries which use BCG vaccinations are similar to those of countries that have never employed large-scale vaccination. Beyond the imprecise estimate of protection is the problem that when BCG vaccines have been successful, the mechanism of action has not been apparent. Therefore, it is not possible to simply extract the useful elements of BCG and assemble them into new vaccine. Some of the features that appear to predict whether BCG will protect are not bacterial factors. Age of the host at vaccination appears to be critical, as vaccination prior to exposure may provide protection against primary TB but vaccination later in life may be unable to protect against reactivation TB. Environmental factors also appear important, as pre-vaccination exposure to environmental Mycobacteria may interfere with the immune response of BCG.

Finally, vaccine factors have been the focus of recent attention, because of the known phenotypic and genetic differences between BCG strains.

Ongoing work on sequencing the type strain of BCG vaccines, known as BCG Pasteur 1173, is expected to provide some insights into the biological basis of attenuation. However, considering that BCG vaccines have been propagated in vitro for nearly a half century and have evolved into a family of closely related strains, it is expected that further comparisons between virulent strains of the *M. tuberculosis* complex and BCG vaccine strains will be required to reveal potential loci associated with reduced virulence. Although work on BCG Pasteur is awaiting completion, it is still possible to perform preliminary comparisons between *M. tuberculosis, M bovis,* and BCG strains, using both piecemeal analysis and in vitro comparative genomic techniques.

Studies in the latter half of the twentieth century had already identified phenotypic variations between BCG strains that suggested that they had evolved in vitro. These observations were confirmed in the 1990s, as analysis of specific genetic loci, such as insertion sequences *(26),* antigenic genes *(27),* and mycolic acid synthesis genes *(28)* demonstrated polymorphisms between BCG strains. Using analysis of these previously documented differences between BCG strains, it has been possible to compare these results to the framework suggested by historical records (see Fig. 1) *(23).* This exercise has provided a few discordant results that could be readily explained by ambiguous records, demonstrating that the genetic record of strain dissemination could be used to study the evolution of BCG Pasteur from 1908 to 1961.

The first genomic analysis of BCG strains to provide important insights into the biologic basis of attenuation employed subtractive hybridization to look for genomic regions of *M. bovis* that are absent from BCG vaccines. By comparing the Connaught strain of BCG with a virulent strain of *M. bovis,* Mahairas and colleagues were able to identify three polygenic regions absent from BCG Connaught *(29).* One of these regions, named RD1,was missing from all BCG strains, and appears to be present in all strains of *M. tuberculosis* and *M. bovis* tested. This deletion is specific for BCG strains, and therefore appeared to have occurred during the original derivation of BCG, between 1908 and 1921. A second region, RD2, was missing from BCG Connaught but present in BCG Moreau, a strain obtained from the Pasteur Institute in 1925, suggesting that the deletion occurred at the Pasteur Institute after 1925. A third deletion, RD3, is a prophage which is present variably in strains of *M. bovis,* and therefore may have been lost in the original attenuation of BCG or may have not been present in the ancestral strain which gave rise to BCG.

Further work on comparing BCG vaccines with virulent strains of the *M. tuberculosis* complex has made use of BAC libraries, whole-genome DNA microarrays, and Affymetrix Genechips. As noted previously, the BAC library approach allowed for analysis of deletions, and also detected two duplications in the BCG Pasteur genome *(30).* In contrast, genomic comparisons by microarrays and Genechips require only whole genomic DNA and are readily performed across a large number of isolates, including a collection of BCG strains *(31).* Genomic comparisons by microarrays and Genechips is biased toward detection of deletions, yet the ability to detect small deletions is enhanced with each technological advance. Thus, microarray-based comparisons revealed a deletion unique to BCG Pasteur not observed by BAC libraries (RD14). Genechip-based comparisons subsequently detected a smaller deletion not

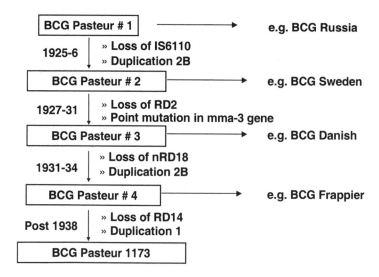

Fig. 2. Molecular events in the evolution of BCG strains from 1921 to 1961. RD=deletion, DU=duplication.

documented by microarray-based screening (n-RD18)*(17)*. Genetic events in the history of BCG vaccine propagation that have been reveated to date are shown in Fig. 2.

Analysis of deleted and duplicated genes provides a starting point for generating hypotheses as to the genetic basis of attenuation in BCG strains (see Table 2). The most striking observation is that ORFs predicted to have a role in regulatory pathways are over-represented in BCG deletions, providing a contrast to their strict conservation in clinical isolates from San Francisco. Analysis of BCG duplications is even more appealing. In BCG Pasteur, the entire region of the origin of replication is duplicated. Diploid genes include, among others, the chromosomal replication initiator *(dnaA),* DNA polymerase *(dnaN), recF,* DNA gyrase subunits a and b *(gyrA and gyrB), recF,* and a possible sigma factor *(sigM).* The other duplication, known as DU2, contains a second sigma factor, *sigH,* which is therefore diploid in most strains of BCG. Together, the presence of regulatory genes in deletions and duplications suggests that the BCG phenotype may result from differences in genetic expression. Preliminary data to this effect are provided by the differences in proteome between two strains of *M. tuberculosis* and two strains of BCG *(32).*

The linkage between genomic differences and altered phenotype is expected to provide important insights into the biology of BCG. To date, it is clear that BCG strains lack genes encoding certain antigenic proteins, such as ESAT-6 and Mpt64. Therefore, one can exploit the absence of these genes in developing specific diagnostic assays for wild-type *M. tuberculosis.* However, the impact of the absence of these genes on the immunogenicity of the vaccine product has not yet been determined. Recently, Horwitz and colleagues have demonstrated that overexpression of an antigenic protein already present in BCG strains translates into improved protection in a specific mouse model of TB[33]. These results demand an answer to whether replacement of an antigen missing from BCG may result in improved protection, and may therefore serve as the rational basis for developing a new BCG.

Table 2
Selected genes deleted or duplicated in the BCG vaccine strains

Class	Gene*	Deletion/Duplication¶	Description/Function
Metabolic functions	*aroA*	DU2	aromatic amino acid synthesis
	echA1	RD10	fatty acid synthesis
	ephA	RD8	degradation of epoxides
	cobL	RD9	cobalamin synthesis
	sseC	RD12	thiosulphate sulphurtransferase
Antigens	*esat6*	RD1	T-cell antigen
	cfp10	RD1	T-cell antigen
	mpt64	RD2	secreted antigen
Putative virulence factors	*plcABC*	RD5	phospholipase C enzymes
	mce3	RD7	putative invasin
Regulatory genes	*Rv1985c*	RD2	LysR-like regulator
	Rv1255c	RD13	AcrR-like regulator
	Rv1773c	RD16	IclR-like regulator
	sigM	DU1	sigma factor
	sigH	DU2	sigma factor
	whiB1	DU2	transcriptional regulator

* Gene designation taken from TubercuList (http://genolist.pasteur.fr/TubercuList)

¶ Nomenclature on deletions (RD) and duplications (DU) is available at: http://www.pasteur.fr/recherche/unites/Lgmb/

SUMMARY

In order to combat tuberculosis, there is a clear need for either a new vaccine or an improved version of BCG. Genomics of the *M. tuberculosis* complex will prove pivotal to the realization of either of these goals. Comparative genomics promises to reveal the virulence factors that make the tubercle bacilli such successful pathogens, exposing the genes and gene products we need to inactivate if we are to generate a new live, attenuated vaccine strain. Such analysis will also reveal targets for subunit vaccines, such as DNA vaccines or protein cocktails, which will not have the risks associated with using a live vaccine and that may also be used as an adjunct to BCG. Comparative genomics across the tubercle bacilli has revealed a remarkable degree of genetic homogeneity despite clear phenotypic distinctions between species. This gives real hope that one vaccine will elicit a protective response against all members of the *M. tuberculosis* complex and finally lessen the worldwide burden of tuberculosis.

REFERENCES

1. Dye C, Scheele S, Dolin P, Pathania V, Raviglione MC. Consensus statement. Global burden of tuberculosis: estimated incidence, prevalence, and mortality by country. WHO Global Surveillance and Monitoring Project. JAMA 1999;282(7):677–686.
2. Espinal MA, Laszlo A, Simonsen L, Boulahbal F, Kim SJ, Reniero A, et al. Global trends in resistance to antituberculosis drugs. World Health Organization-International Union against Tuberculosis and Lung Disease Working Group on Anti-Tuberculosis Drug Resistance Surveillance. N Engl J Med 2001;344(17):1294–1303.

3. Fine PE. Bacille Calmette-Guerin vaccines: a rough guide. Clin Infect Dis 1995;20(1):11–14.

4. Calmette A, Guérin C. Recherches expérimentales sur la défense de l'organisme contre l'infection tuberculeuse. Ann Inst Pasteur 1911;25:625–641.

5. Lowrie DB, Tascon RE, Bonato VL, Lima VM, Faccioli LH, Stavropoulos E, et al. Therapy of tuberculosis in mice by DNA vaccination. Nature 1999;400(6741):269–271.

6. Vidal SM, Malo D, Vogan K, Skamene E, Gros P. Natural resistance to infection with intracellular parasites: isolation of a candidate for BCG. Cell 1993;73(3):469–485.

7. Greenwood CM, Fujiwara TM, Boothroyd LJ, Miller MA, Frappier D, Fanning EA, et al. Linkage of tuberculosis to chromosome 2q35 loci, including NRAMP1, in a large aboriginal Canadian family. Am J Hum Genet 2000;67(2):405–416.

8. Cole ST, Brosch R, Parkhill J, Garnier T, Churcher C, Harris D, et al. Deciphering the biology of Mycobacterium tuberculosis from the complete genome sequence. Nature 1998;11;393(6685):537–544.

9. http://www.tigr.org/tigr-scripts/CMR2/GenomePage3.spl?database=gmt

10. Grange JM, Gibson J, Osborn TW, Collins CH, Yates MD. What is BCG? Tubercle 1983;64(2):129–139.

11. Cole ST, Eiglmeier K, Parkhill J, James KD, Thomson NR, Wheeler PR, et al. Massive gene decay in the leprosy bacillus. Nature 2001;22;409(6823):1007–1011.

12. Sreevatsan S, Pan X, Stockbauer KE, Connell ND, Kreiswirth BN, Whittam TS, et al. Restricted structural gene polymorphism in the Mycobacterium tuberculosis complex indicates evolutionarily recent global dissemination. Proc Natl Acad Sci USA 1997;94(18):9869–9874.

13. Fraser CM, Eisen J, Fleischmann RD, Ketchum KA, Peterson S. Comparative genomics and understanding of microbial biology. Emerg Infect Dis 2000;6(5):505–512.

14. Brosch R, Philipp WJ, Stavropoulos E, Colston MJ, Cole ST, Gordon SV. Genomic analysis reveals variation between Mycobacterium tuberculosis H37Rv and the attenuated M. tuberculosis H37Ra strain. Infect Immun 1999;67(11):5768–5774.

15. Ho TB, Robertson BD, Taylor GM, Shaw RJ, Young DB. Comparison of Mycobacterium tuberculosis genomes reveals frequent deletions in a 20 kb variable region in clinical isolates. Yeast 2000;17(4):272–282.

16. Kato-Maeda M, Rhee JT, Gingeras TR, Salamon H, Drenkow J, Smittipat N, et al. Comparing genomes within the species Mycobacterium tuberculosis. Genome Res 2001;11(4):547–554.

17. Salamon H, Kato-Maeda M, Small PM, Drenkow J, Gingeras TR. Detection of deleted genomic DNA using a semiautomated computational analysis of GeneChip data. Genome Res 2000;10(12):2044–2054.

18. Betts JC, Dodson P, Quan S, Lewis AP, Thomas PJ, Duncan K, et al. Comparison of the proteome of Mycobacterium tuberculosis strain H37Rv with clinical isolate CDC 1551. Microbiology 2000;146 Pt 12:3205–3216.

19. Gordon SV, Brosch R, Billault A, Garnier T, Eiglmeier K, Cole ST. Identification of variable regions in the genomes of tubercle bacilli using bacterial artificial chromosome arrays. Mol Microbiol 1999;32(3):643–655.

20. Hewinson RG, Michell SL, Russell WP, McAdam RA, Jacobs WR Jr. Molecular characterization of MPT83: a seroreactive antigen of Mycobacterium tuberculosis with homology to MPT70. Scand J Immunol 1996;43(5):490–499.

21. Hart PD, Sutherland I. BCG and vole bacillus vaccines in the prevention of tuberculosis in adolescence and early adult life. Br Med J 1977;2(6082):293–295.

22. Oettinger T, Jorgensen M, Ladefoged A, Haslov K, Andersen P. Development of the Mycobacterium bovis BCG vaccine: review of the historical and biochemical evidence for a genealogical tree. Tubercle Lung Dis 1999;79(4):243–250.

23. Behr MA, Small PM. A historical and molecular phylogeny of BCG strains. Vaccine 1999 Feb 26;17(7–8):915–922.

24. Casanova JL, Blanche S, Emile JF, Jouanguy E, Lamhamedi S, Altare F, et al. Idiopathic disseminated bacillus Calmette-Guerin infection: a French national retrospective study. Pediatrics 1996;98(4 Pt 1):774–778.

25. Rodrigues LC, Diwan VK, Wheeler JG. Protective effect of BCG against tuberculous meningitis and military tuberculosis: a meta-analysis. Int J Epidemiol 1993;22(6):1154–1158.

26. Fomukong NG, Dale JW, Osborn TW, Grange JM. Use of gene probes based on the insertion sequence IS986 to differentiate between BCG vaccine strains. J Appl Bacteriol 1992;72(2):126–133.

27. Li H, Ulstrup JC, Jonassen TO, Melby K, Nagai S, Harboe M. Evidence for absence of the MPB64 gene in some substrains of Mycobacterium bovis BCG. Infect Immun 1993;61(5):1730–1734.

28. Yuan Y, Zhu Y, Crane DD, Barry CE, 3rd. The effect of oxygenated mycolic acid composition on cell wall function and macrophage growth in Mycobacterium tuberculosis. Mol Microbiol 1998;29(6):1449–1458.

29. Mahairas GG, Sabo PJ, Hickey MJ, Singh DC, Stover CK. Molecular analysis of genetic differences between Mycobacterium bovis BCG and virulent M. bovis. J Bacteriol 1996;178(5):1274–1282.

30. Brosch R, Gordon SV, Buchrieser C, Pym AS, Garnier T, Cole ST. Comparative genomics uncovers large tandem chromosomal duplications in Mycobacterium bovis BCG Pasteur. Yeast 2000;30;17(2):111–123.

31. Behr MA, Wilson MA, Gill WP, Salamon H, Schoolnik GK, Rane S, et al. Comparative genomics of BCG vaccines by whole-genome DNA microarray. Science 1999;284(5419):1520–1523.

32. Jungblut PR, Schaible UE, Mollenkopf HJ, Zimny-Arndt U, Raupach B, Mattow J, et al. Comparative proteome analysis of Mycobacterium tuberculosis and Mycobacterium bovis BCG strains: towards functional genomics of microbial pathogens. Mol Microbiol 1999;(6):1103–1117.

33. Horwitz MA, Harth G, Dillon BJ, Maslesa-Galic' S. Recombinant bacillus calmetteguerin (BCG) vaccines expressing the Mycobacterium tuberculosis 30-kDa major secretory protein induce greater protective immunity against tuberculosis than conventional BCG vaccines in a highly susceptible animal model. Proc Natl Acad Sci USA 2000;97(25):13,853–13,858.

7
Bacterial "Genes-to-Screens" in the Post-Genomic Era

Michael J. Pucci, John F. Barrett, and Thomas J. Dougherty

INTRODUCTION

In recent years, it has become increasingly apparent that the effectiveness of our antibiotic armamentarium is becoming severely eroded by microbial resistance *(1–3)*. The breadth of resistance mechanisms is astonishing and alarming. Genes for inactivating antibiotics on transmissible elements, antibiotic target modifications, and efflux pumps are only a few examples of a bewildering array of resistance strategies employed by microbes. At the same time, the search for novel antimicrobial agents has slowed dramatically as pharmaceutical companies turned their drug development efforts elsewhere. It is also apparent that whereas the early years of antibiotic discovery led to a number of antibiotics of differing chemical classes, these "classical" methods of antimicrobial identification yielded diminishing returns. Most of these antibiotics were derived from natural product sources, and the screens to identify their presence were relatively crude growth-inhibition assays. Although this offered advantages in terms of finding potent inhibitors that could reach their cellular targets, it ruled out moderately active compounds (that might be dramatically improved) or compounds present in lower concentrations. Indeed, it has been argued that the few soil organisms that are sources of antibiotics are overproducing mutants. Whatever the ultimate explanation may be, the fact remains that all clinically useful antibiotics are members of a very limited number of structural classes that were discovered over 30 years ago.

Resistance surveillance studies paint a somewhat grim picture of drug resistance, as it becomes clear that a number of pathogens continue to acquire multiple resistance, and the number of resistant isolates for many pathogens continues to climb. Even more disturbing are the recent findings on compensatory mutations in resistant bacteria *(4)*. Upon acquisition of resistance, the resistant bacteria are often at a growth disadvantage relative to the parental wild-type strain. However, recent studies demonstrate that fitness is rapidly restored by secondary compensatory mutations. These effectively act to "lock in" resistance, as either loss of the resistance mutation or the compensatory mutation results in a "less fit" organism. The hope that "antibiotic class cycling" may offer a respite from antibiotic resistance has been diminished by these studies. It is clear that the long-term strategy for control of

From: *Pathogen Genomics: Impact on Human Health*
Edited by: K. J. Shaw © Humana Press Inc., Totowa, NJ

infectious diseases demands that novel antibiotic classes be identified. If the obvious antibiotic classes have already been identified, we are then faced with the much more difficult task of identifying novel, validated antimicrobial targets for screening against large libraries of compounds to identify novel antibiotics. It is here that microbial genomics offers an unprecedented opportunity to search for fundamentally new targets and inhibitors.

With the publication of the genome of the first free-living organism in 1995, the bacterium *Haemophilus influenzae (5)*, a new era was initiated—the age of genomics *(6)*. The current availability of dozens of bacterial genomes has released a wealth of new information to the scientific community, and promises to greatly accelerate our knowledge of a wide variety of microbes. In addition to microorganisms, which offer the potential for immediate scientific benefits, informatic tools and experimental strategies developed in the microbial arena have the potential to assist in the study of the human genome. We now have a better opportunity to learn how living organisms function from information obtained in the simpler microbial context.

Along with a wealth of new genomic information, new methodologies and tools have either been improved or developed *de novo* in order to better make use of and analyze the new data. Biologists have suddenly found themselves utilizing very powerful computational resources previously used only by the high-energy physics community. For example, bioinformatics, the melding of biology and modern computer tools, has become a crucial part of the genomic process, both in assembling and interpreting vast amounts of sequence information. The shift from examining individual genes to examining the entire genetic complement of one or more organisms has been abrupt, and computer visualization methods are still under development. New approaches such as EcoCyc, MAGPIE, and other pathway tools *(7,8)* allow rationalization of the genomic information by arraying the data for further exploration of metabolic pathways. Web-based interfaces have also emerged to facilitate analyses. DNA microarray technology offers insights into gene expression *(9,10)* and the advance of proteomics allows the study of the "proteome," the products of gene expression *(11)*. Developments in structural biology and new screening techniques have also advanced alongside the progression of genomics *(12–14)*.

It is important to consider the evolution of microbiology over the past century. What began as "basic microbiology" eventually acquired key knowledge of microbial physiology and microbial genetics. The result was a number of important scientific discoveries such as the establishment of DNA as the key genetic material, elucidation of the genetic code, and the discovery of genetic exchange and recombination *(15–17)*. Beginning in the 1970s, the molecular era ushered in plasmid vectors, restriction enzymes, and cloning, which had implications well beyond simple microbes *(18,19)*. We are now several years into the next phase of this evolution—the genomics era. New microbial genomes are currently being completed and added to databases with increasing rapidity, and over the next few years, this revolutionary period will evolve into the post-genomics era. This could arguably be the most important period in our history, as we strive to decipher and interpret the vast array of information made available to the scientific community. This post-genomics period will probably last for many years to come, and is sure to usher in numerous significant scientific discoveries.

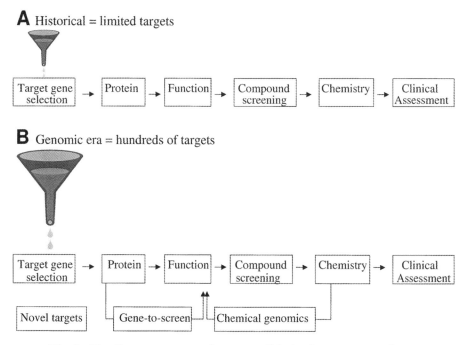

Fig. 1. The discovery process for new antibiotics from targets to drugs.

One of the greatest anticipated benefits of bacterial genomics is the promise of new antibacterial targets that will lead to the discovery of new antibiotics. The process of drug discovery is changing compared to past methods of finding new chemotypes (Fig. 1). Perhaps the biggest impact is in the identification of possibly hundreds of new and essential bacterial targets. The challenge will be in converting these genes into screens and finding inhibitors that can be developed into safe and efficacious drugs.

BACTERIAL GENOMIC INFORMATION: A SUMMARY

At the time of this writing, approximately 69 bacterial genomes, including 12 archaebacteria, have been completely sequenced by numerous groups with publicly available data. Other sequencing efforts continue in various stages, often with data available for viewing while the work is in progress. Several websites display this type of information including TIGR (The Institute for Genomic Research; www.tigr.org), and GOLD (Genomes On-Line Database, Integrated Genomics; http://igweb.integratedgenomics. com/GOLD). One can assume that within just a few years, more than 100 bacterial genomes will be completely sequenced with the predicted identification of more than 300,000 genes. Many of these genes will be novel and of unknown function. A summary of some key organisms whose DNA sequences are completed and published is shown in Table 1. It is apparent that the sizes of bacterial genomes are relatively small, ranging from 580 Kb to 6264 Kb. The smallest genome to date, that of *Mycoplasma genitalium,* appears to have 468 open reading frames (ORFs), and has been the subject of studies to determine the minimum genome required for a free-living organism *(20).*

What has been learned thus far from genome analysis of bacteria? Nearly all of the protein-coding regions of a bacterium can be identified with reasonable confidence

Table 1
Selected completed bacterial genomes

Organism	Strain	Size (kb)	ORFs	Source	Year
Haemophilus influenzae	KW20	1830	1850	TIGR	1995
Mycoplasma genitalium	G-37	580	468	TIGR	1996
Mycoplasma pneumoniae	M129	816	677	University of Heidelberg	1996
Escherichia coli	K12-MG1655	4639	4289	University of Wisconsin	1997
Helicobacter pylori	26695	1667	1590	TIGR	1997
Bacillus subtilis	168	4214	4099	European Consortium Japanese Consortium	1997
Borrelia burgdorferi	B31	1230	1256	Brookhaven Natl Lab TIGR	1997
Mycobacterium tuberculosis	H37Rv (lab strain)	4411	4402	Sanger Centre	1998
Treponema pallidum	Nichols	1138	1041	University of Texas TIGR	1998
Chlamydia trachomatis	serovar D	1042	896	Stanford University UC Berkeley	1998
Rickettsia prowazekii	Madrid E	1111	834	University of Uppsala	1998
Chlamydia pneumoniae	CWL029	1230	1052	Stanford University UC Berkeley	1999
Campylobacter jejuni	NCTC 11168	1641	1654	Sanger Centre LSHTM University of Leicester	2000
Neisseria meningitidis	MC58 (serogroup B)	2272	2158	TIGR	2000
Vibrio cholerae	Serotype O1, Biotype El Tor, strain N16961	4000	3885	TIGR	2000
Pseudomonas aeruginosa	PAO1	6264	5570	Pathogenesis University of Washington-Seattle	2000
Escherichia coli	O157:H7 EDL933	4100	5283	University of Wisconsin	2001
Mycobacterium leprae	TN	3268	1604	Sanger Centre Institut Pasteur	2001
Streptococcus pyogenes	SF370 (M1)	1852	1696	University of Oklahoma	2001
Lactococcus lactis	IL1403	2365	2266	Genoscope INRA	2001
Staphylococcus aureus	N315	2813	2595	NITE, ONRI, RIKEN Juntendo University University of Tsukuba University of Tokyo Kyushu University Kyoto University Kitasato University	2001

through several techniques such as similarity searches and Markov models *(21)* and, unlike eucaryotes, there is approximately one gene per kb with little intergenic space. Examination of the occurrence of horizontal or lateral gene transfer shows that the extent of exogenous DNA acquisition appears to be greater than originally believed *(22)*. Possibly the most intriguing and important finding is that, in general, 30–60% of hypothetical ORFs have no putative assigned functions *(22,23)*. In addition, some of the so-called identified genes may have problems with their annotations and may not be correctly identified *(24)*. Also, up to 25% of an organism's ORFs appear to be unique to that genus or species, indicating tremendous diversity among microorganisms. These unique genes are what make an *E. coli* an *E. coli* or a staphylococcus a staphylococcus.

To this point, bioinformatics has led the way in our analyses and interpretation of genomic data. Database comparisons have assigned putative functions to a large number of genes through various similarity searching tools such as BLAST (Basic Linear Alignment Search Tool; 25) and FASTA (FAST-ALL; 26). These assignments are based largely on vast genetic and physiological studies with two well-characterized bacteria, *E. coli* and *Bacillus subtilis,* along with specialized information from a number of other bacterial species. Nucleotide frequencies, repeats, regulatory regions, gene predictions, and pathway reconstructions are among the types of information that have been developed. One can also identify operons, which consist of clusters of genes transcribed from a common promoter *(27)*. Operons usually encode genes for serial steps in biochemical pathways. Valuable studies, such as comparisons between pathogenic and nonpathogenic strains within the same species, are now possible *(28)*. These offer insights into the pathogenic processes by which specific bacteria cause disease. Perhaps one of the biggest surprises has been the disparity between the genomes of *E. coli* K-12 and pathogenic strains of this organism which possess a megabase of additional genetic information *(29)*. However, despite the power of recent computational techniques, there are limitations as to how much we can learn from such data. Genes of unknown function or genes with incorrect annotations require more than what bioinformatics alone can presently offer. There is, and will continue to be, a need for experimental approaches,—so-called "wet biology"—to complement and extend the data gathered from *in silico* biology.

Even after the sequence of a key bacterium is completed, opportunities remain for additional sequencing projects. Comparative genomics projects and inter- and intraspecies comparisons promise to provide data that cannot be ascertained from the sequence information from just one strain of a given species. Such studies have already been initiated in such organisms as Helicobacter, Mycoplasma, and Mycobacteria *(30–32)*. As described for *E. coli* here, there may be significant variations in the gene content among strains. Allelic variations and polymorphisms require additional sequencing efforts. Finally, one can anticipate from early studies that organisms that readily undergo genetic exchange (e.g., transformation) may be particularly polymorphic, exchanging genes with closely related organisms.

GENOMICS AND MICROBIAL PHYSIOLOGY

As discussed here, genomic information coupled with bioinformatic analyses have resulted in a wealth of new information about bacteria. However, such analyses have also led to renewed attention to the field of microbial physiology. The advances of the molecular era beginning in the 1970s seemed to result in a concomitant decline of interest in classical microbial physiology. Genomics has illuminated both the importance of these studies and their unfinished nature. The ability to classify many genes with a function is largely the direct result of "classical" microbial physiology, biochemistry, and genetic studies stretching back over half a century. The annotation of microbial genomes is built on the framework of these studies. The one constant revelation in the genomes sequenced to date has been that a significant fraction of putative ORFs do not have functional assignments. A recently reported and detailed genomic analysis of *E. coli* categorized genes into classes such as enzymes, transporters, and structural *(33)*. Of the 4406 genes listed, 1408 remain unidentified, and an additional 954 require experimental verification. Another interesting finding was the presence of multiple enzymes. For 79 enzymatic reactions, there are from two to nine enzymes that catalyze identical or very closely related reactions. A sequence analysis applied to *Streptococcus pneumoniae (34)* was also able to identify a variety of bacterial metabolic functions, including genes encoding tRNA synthetases, ribosomal proteins, amino acids and cofactors, cell-wall enzymes, and DNA replication and repair. Studies such as these can reveal much important metabolic data. However, in order to verify questionable functional assignments, determine gene essentiality, or to establish biochemical assays, additional experiments in microbial physiology, genetics, and/or biochemistry are required. Genomics often enables such research to move more rapidly than previously possible, since less time is usually required for genetic experiments. More precise directed experiments can be made to focus in on a particular gene or genes. For example, with a map available of the bacterium under study and PCR techniques, genes can be rapidly cloned to the vector of choice, site-directed mutagenesis can be rapidly performed, transcriptional profiling under diverse growth conditions can be monitored, or targeted gene disruptions can be constructed and analyzed. Analysis of the protein sequence may suggest motifs and protein folds that may indicate potential functions.

In addition, with the seemingly large number of unidentified genes, functional genomics—the assignment of function to gene products—becomes a crucial area for research. Microbial physiology and biochemistry experimental approaches are clearly keys for success. In the past, mutants, often randomly generated, were identified by their phenotypes, followed by attempts at genetic characterization. It is now possible to use the reverse approach of first generating a specific mutant and then looking for a phenotype—i.e., one creates a specific mutation and then looks for the effects on the cell. The finding that there are essential function genes among the unknown function genes testifies to the inadequacy of past "mutant hunts" using restrictive conditions (e.g., auxotrophic or temperature-sensitive mutants). Systems for in vitro transposon saturation mutagenesis of overlapping cloned segments of a genome (GAMBIT) as well as other transposon-based methodologies are examples of new approaches to essential gene identification strategies *(35,36)*. The availability of genomic information can also assist the use of older standard genetic techniques such as phage transduction, transposon insertion linkage, and the use of various markers. Structural genomics, the application of sophisticated computational programs to gene analysis, can suggest among the following: possible functions based on motifs, a specific gene encodes an enzyme, and/or that a protein interacts with macromolecules *(37)*. In addition, it may identify binding ligands. NMR-based small-molecule binding studies and related technologies can also provide structural data that can be applied to model a protein's potential function. The requirement remains for microbial physiology experiments to verify such assignments. With genomic information, the physiology experiments can be designed to ask precise questions about the role of a protein in the cell.

Finally, genomic information will be of great assistance in the understanding of the integrated processes of the cell. We are on the verge of unraveling metabolic networks and identifying important cellular responses and controls *(38)*. Several recent reports describe *in silico* metabolic modeling in attempts to integrate genomic data at the whole-cell level *(39)*. These data will provide insights as to how a bacterium responds to the immediate environment and how it deals with various forms of stress. Bioinformatics, combined with microarray transcriptional analysis and proteomic analyses, will suggest numerous laboratory experiments for the microbial physiologist and biochemist to obtain corroborative data to identify function. Currently, one interesting observation is that there is only a modest correlation between microarray data and proteomic analysis of expression. It is unclear whether this signals a larger role for post-transcriptional control in microbes, or experimental artifact. It will be a challenging task to understand the bacterial cell at a global level, as sets of interacting metabolic networks will probably require many additional years of research. Such integration of multiple sources of information will be a roadmap to our understanding of the working of the far more complex eukaryotic cells and the total expression capacity of the human genome.

TARGET IDENTIFICATION

An important result of the microbial genomics era is that it will provide a number of essential, validated targets as possible candidates for new antimicrobials. These valid drug targets encode proteins either required for cell growth in vitro or for survival or virulence in the host. Properties of the ideal new antibacterial target may include the following. It would be present in multiple bacterial species, which might lead to discovery of broad-spectrum agents that would have wider potential usage and therefore could satisfy the marketing criteria for the expensive drug development process. The encoded function would be essential, with an inhibition leading to bacteriostatic or bactericidal growth arrest and/or killing of the pathogen. Presumably, screening against novel targets for inhibitors would result in the discovery of novel compounds active against current clinically antibiotic-resistant strains. The potential should exist for selectivity that would result in few or no side effects for a compound in the clinic, as genome comparisons can assist in eliminating eukaryotic proteins with significant similarity. However, as discussed here, use of homology data alone can sometimes be misleading.

The use of bioinformatics can lead to the putative identification of several classes of targets. Genes for potential targets can be sorted and classified based on several criteria. For example, genes can be grouped based on their distribution among a variety of Gram-negative and Gram-positive bacteria at a given level of similarity of their gene products. Inhibitors of these targets would possess the greatest opportunity for broad specificity. Alternatively, genes specific to either Gram-negative or Gram-positive bacteria can be identified. There are several successful, currently marketed antibacterial agents with such specificities *(40)*. Comparison with human and other eukaryotic databases can determine sequence identities and, therefore give an indication of possible selectivity of inhibitors. This may reduce the possibility of obtaining mechanism-based toxic compounds. Finally, this approach can also be used to find organism-specific targets. Organisms such as the Mycobacteria are rich in potential targets not present in other pathogens. These could still be of substantial commercial interest, with *Helicobacter pylori* or *Mycobacterium tuberculosis* drugs as examples.

An example of one such bioinformatic application was reported recently in a concordance analysis of microbial genomes *(41)*. This system performs a FASTA comparison of multiple genomes at the amino-acid level, and builds tables for access by a web-based interface. This particular concordance demonstration compared the *E. coli* genome against *B. subtilis, H. influenzae, H. pylori,* and *M. tuberculosis,* using a BLOSUM62 matrix and subtracted out sequences with similarity greater than a selected exclusion criterion with the yeast *Saccharomyces cerevisiae.* Almost 2000 sequences were found with a match to at least one of the five species under the selected criterion; however, only 265 matched all species. The final result was the selection of 89 sequences in common with all five bacterial species, with an additional 176 sequences eliminated because of similarity to yeast sequences. The value of such an approach was demonstrated by examination of the sequences selected. For example, the *gyrA* gene encoding DNA gyrase, the target of the quinolone class of antibiotics, was identified as well as *murA,* the target for fosfomycin. Several other previously reported essential genes were found, including *dnaA, ftsZ,* and *mraY.* Various organisms and more or less stringent criterion can be used for such analyses, depending on the desired end point. Also, organism-specific sequences can be revealed with this approach.

The study of smaller genomes such as *H. influenzae* and *M. genitalium* can also offer the potential of identifying targets with broad specificity. With their relatively small numbers of genes, chances are increased of identifying a core subset of genes common to pathogens that are also essential in function. It has been estimated that about 25% of a bacterium's gene complement are essential for normal growth in rich medium *(42,43)*. If genes with eukaryotic orthologs are subtracted (e.g., TCA enzymes), approximately 10% of the remaining genes encode potential selective antibacterial proteins. By this estimation, the number would be approximately 400 genes in *E. coli* and 200 in staphylococci. If only 5–10% of these targets actually lead to new antibacterials, the result could be 10–40 new classes of antibiotics. This type of informatics analysis provides one possible prioritization of targets by extracting potential conserved, selective gene products. Further experimental validation is required to confirm essentiality.

Target similarities should not be an absolute criterion for prioritization. Ribosomal inhibitors are highly selective despite strong similarities between prokaryotes and eukaryotes. Relatively slight differences in the structures of prokaryotic and eukaryotic ribosomes translate into different classes of protein synthesis inhibitors that largely do not crossreact. Other examples include human and *E. coli* dihydrofolate reductase, the target for trimethoprim (28% identical at the amino-acid level; ref. *14*) and human and *E. coli* topoisomerase II, the target for quinolones (20% identical).

From a different perspective, the penicillin-binding proteins (PBPs) show low overall identity at the amino-acid level to each other, but inhibitors often show broad specificity with strong affinities for PBPs across numerous bacterial species *(44)*. This is because of the high structural similarities at small conserved regions that make up both the active site and the site of inhibition by β-lactam antibacterial compounds. Therefore, it is possible to have selective targets despite similarities to eukaryotic orthologs or broad-spectrum targets, although the level of overall identity of proteins among various bacterial species appears low.

Despite the best of bioinformatic approaches, it is highly desirable to validate the essentiality of antibacterial targets by experimental means. Several methods have been previously described. One long-standing method is the conditional mutant, most of which are temperature-sensitive *(45)*. Such strains grow under permissive conditions, but are not viable under nonpermissive conditions such as elevated temperature. This type of data suggests an important function for the gene product in regard to cellular growth, and therefore, essentiality. Large collections of temperature-sensitive mutants have been generated, and many of the genes responsible for the phenotype have been identified. Indeed, at least one company has integrated the temperature sensitivity into a system to search for inhibitors. Another approach facilitated by the availability of genomic information is targeted gene disruption or "gene knockouts." One can attempt to specifically disrupt the desired gene in the chromosome using a selectable marker with success implying non-essentiality. It is possible to pursue a high-throughput approach to gene disruption. Caveats for this approach include that one is looking for a negative result, i.e., no colonies found with a disruption in the selected gene. Even with tight controls, technical issues cannot always be ruled out. Use of tightly regulated inducible promoters driving the gene of interest offers an alternative means of conducting these experiments *(46)*. An additional complication of targeted gene disruption is that many bacterial genes are found in operons, and disruption of a gene near the promoter could lead to a reduction in or lack of transcription of downstream genes, an effect known as polarity. It would be possible to be misled if one of the downstream nonexpressed genes is the essential one instead of the disrupted gene.

SCREENING FOR NEW INHIBITORS

The next step following the identification of validated essential targets is to discover inhibitors with the potential to be developed into new antibacterial drugs. A percentage of such targets will be amenable to some type of biochemical assay, based on functional annotation in the databases whereby inhibitory compounds can be readily sought by screening and subsequently characterized. Others will be found for which HTS assays will be developed after additional experimental work. However, the remaining targets, perhaps 40% or more, will either have an unknown function or will have no obvious assay method. This latter group of gene products offers great promise, as they comprise a pool of previously unexploited antibacterial targets.

The past history of screening for new antibacterials in the pharmaceutical industry focused primarily on testing large compound libraries—including natural products—against test bacterial strains, using cell death as a measure of success. Most of the current drugs on the market today were discovered this way. This type of random screening continues today, employing an expanded sampling of natural products and increased chemical diversity through combinatorial chemistry *(47)*. However, this approach suffers from the drawbacks of low sensitivity and no immediate knowledge of the target inhibited. Genomics provides several advantages in its potential to screen for new inhibitors. First, it allows the establishment of direct biochemical screens against certain selected targets. This increases the sensitivity of the assay and provides an early verification of proof-of-principle for the inhibitor. Also, genomic information can be used to aid in the determination of the previously unknown identity of a target for which an inhibitor has been discovered by other means, such as cell-based screening. This latter approach has been termed "chemical screening" *(48)* or, alternatively can be considered as "reverse functional genomics."

Another screening approach facilitated by genomic information is the use of surrogate markers in cell-based assays *(49)*. These surrogate markers are genes that are either positively or negatively regulated as a response to the inhibition of a particular essential target. When there are no known inhibitors of a desired target, conditional mutants or genes under the control of a tightly regulated promoter can simulate the effects that such an inhibitor would have on the bacterial cell *(50)*. This coupled with genomic technologies such as microarray-expression profiling and proteomic analysis can lead to the identification of such surrogate markers of inhibition. Such surrogate markers can be linked through gene fusions to produce proteins with measurable readouts such as β-galactosidase or green fluorescent protein (GFP). Several technologies have also been developed to indicate the presence of a potential ligand on a target protein. Displacement of surrogate ligands is one means of screening for inhibitors against targets of unknown function. Peptide ligands can be identified using phage display technology *(51)*, and can lead to peptide displacement assays. Displacement of the peptide by a small molecule can be detected, indicative of a potential inhibitor. These assays can include homogeneous time-resolved fluorescence (HTRF; ref. *52*) or fluorescence depolarization *(53)* to measure peptide displacement.

Other assay formats facilitated by genomic information include the use of hypersensitive strains. One reported approach employs strains with temperature-sensitive alleles of the target genes *(14)*. One drawback of this type of screen is that it appears that not all temperature-sensitive alleles exhibit hypersensitivity to an inhibitor of that target. Downregulation of the target gene can also lead to hypersensitivity, and such strains can be created through the use of gene fusions under the control of an inducible promoter *(54)*.

The use of virtual screening of compounds against selected targets is now becoming an important part of efforts to discover new inhibitors. Structural bioinformatics can identify the putative active site of a protein. Databases of small molecules then can be targeted to the surface of this active site in an attempt to determine which compounds may bind there based on shape or charge. Computational programs such as DOCK or CAVEAT can be used to "dock" hundreds of thousands of compounds in an attempt to identify a structure that can be used as a starting point for further chemistry programs *(55,56)*.

CHALLENGES AND SUMMARY

Knowledge of the complete genomes of bacterial pathogens should accelerate the development of new antibiotics, diagnostics, and vaccines. For each pathogen, we will know the number of genes, the chromosomal positions of these genes, and whether these genes are conserved within other pathogens or unique to the particular microorganism. We will learn more about the evolution of genes and whether they were recently acquired by sequence-based phylogenetic analyses. We will also know whether the gene has human homologs that could have possible implications ranging from selectivity of inhibitors to induction of autoimmunity in the host. However, the single most important contribution of bacterial genomics may be the identification of new targets that will lead to needed new drugs in the future. We have accelerated the shift away from empirical screening to a more targeted approach.

Along with this wealth of information come new challenges and issues that need to be addressed. With whole-cell empirical screening, the ability of the inhibitor to penetrate into the cell usually was not a major concern. However, with target-based approaches, potent in vitro inhibitors may not be able to reach their targets inside the bacterial cell. A better understanding of the physical properties that allow molecules to penetrate the bacterial membrane, which has a composition distinct from that of the eukaryotic membrane, is needed. Additional chemistry efforts may be required in attempts to discover analogs with improved cellular penetration. Some of those inhibitors that do manage to access the intracellular environment may be rapidly pumped back out of the cell by any of a number of efflux systems *(57)*. Recent analysis of genomic data has assisted in the identification of additional efflux pumps, indicating their prevalence in bacteria *(58)*. It may be necessary to either initiate chemistry efforts to identify inhibitor analogs with reduced susceptibility to efflux or to embark on programs to find inhibitors of the pumps themselves *(59)*.

Other areas in which genomics may eventually have major impacts include the development of targeted spectrum antibacterials through the identification of organism-specific targets. Thus, it may be possible to discover compounds specific for *H. pylori* or additional compounds for use against *M. tuberculosis.* Use of genomic information to develop rapid and specific diagnostics could even lead to selective therapeutic agents against a variety of troublesome, frequently encountered pathogens, reducing effects on normal flora and improving clinical outcomes. Also, genomic information on the organisms that produce the antibacterial secondary metabolites could lead to genetic modification of synthetic pathways and to the synthesis of numerous compound analogs.

As we continue in the genomics era and evolve into the post-genomics era, it is clear that our understanding of bacteria will be significantly enhanced. More will be known about the genetics and physiology of the bacterial cell than any time in history. However, the true impact of genomics in regard to the discovery of new classes of antibacterial agents remains to be determined. Since the discovery and development of such new drugs by the pharmaceutical industry typically takes 5–10 years before there is approval for human use, it may not be until 2010 or beyond before the first antibiotics of the genomic age begin to benefit mankind. However, it does raise hope that such agents will become available to combat the increasing rate of resistance reported in most of our key pathogens. Hopefully, the continued use of genomic information in the coming years will keep us ahead in this battle of man vs bacterial pathogens.

REFERENCES

1. Dougherty TJ, Pucci MJ, Bronson JJ, Bonner DP, Barrett JF. Antimicrobial resistance—why do we have it and what can we do about it? Exp Opin Invest Drugs 2000;9:1707–1709.

2. Breithaupt H. The new antibiotics. Nat Biotechnol 1999;17:1165–1169.
3. Moellering RC Jr. Antibiotic resistance: lessons for the future. Clin Inf Dis 1998;27(Suppl 1):S135–S140.
4. Bjorkland J, Anderson DI. The cost of antibiotic resistance from a bacterial perspective. Drug Res Updates 2000;3:237–245.
5. Fleischmann RD, Adams MD, White O, Clayton RA, Kirkness EF, Kerlavage AR, et al. Whole genome random sequencing and assembly of Haemophilus influenzae Rd. Science 1995;269:496–512.
6. McKusick VA. Genomics: structural and functional studies of genomes. Genomics 1997;45:244–249.
7. Karp PD. EcoCyc: encyclopedia of Escherichia coli genes and metabolism. Nucleic Acids Res 1999;27:55–58.
8. Gaasterland T, Sensen CW. Fully automated genome analysis that reflects user needs and preferences. A detailed introduction to the MAGPIE system architecture. Biochimie 1996;78:302–310.
9. Derisi JL, Iyer VR, Brown PO. Exploring the metabolic and genetic control of gene expression on a genomic scale. Science 1997;278:680–686.
10. Lashkari DA, Derisi JL, McCusker JH, Namath AF, Gentiles C, Hwang SY, et al. Yeast microarrays for genome wide parallel genetic and gene expression technology. Proc Natl Acad Sci USA 1997;94:13,057–13,062.
11. VanBogelen RA, Schiller EE, Thomas JD, Neidhardt FC. Diagnosis of cellular states of microbial organisms using proteomes. Electrophoresis 1999;20:2149–2159.
12. Shapiro L, Harris T. Finding function through structural genomics. Curr Opin Biotechnol 2000;11,31–38.
13. Eisenstein E, Gilliland GL, Herzberg O, Moult J, Orban J, Poljak RJ, et al. Biological function made crystal clear—annotation of hypothetical proteins via structural genomics. Curr Opin Biotechnol 2000;11:25–30.
14. Moir DT, Shaw KJ, Hare RS, Vovis GF. Genomics and antimicrobial drug discovery. Antimicrobiol Agents Chemother 1999;43:439–446.
15. Avery OT, MacLeod CM, McCarty M. Studies on the chemical nature of the substance inducing transformation of pneumococcal types. Induction of transformation by a deoxyribonucleic acid fraction from Pneumococcus Type III. J Exp Med 1944;79:137–158.
16. Nirenberg MW, Matthei JH. The dependence of cell-free protein synthesis in E. coli upon naturally occurring or synthetic polypeptides. Proc Natl Acad Sci USA 1961;47:1588–1602.
17. Lederberg J, Tatum EL. Gene recombination in E. coli. Nature 1946;158:558.
18. Chang AC, Cohen SN. Construction and characterization of amplifiable multicopy DNA cloning vehicles derived from the P15A cryptic miniplasmid. J Bacteriol 1978;134:1141–1156.
19. Boyer HW, Goodman HM, Helling RB. Analysis of endonuclease R-EcoRI fragments of DNA from lambdoid bacteriophages and other viruses by agarose-gel electrophoresis. J Virol 1974;14:1235–1244.
20. Fraser CM, Gocayne JD, White O, Adams MD, Clayton RA, Fleischmann RD, et al. The minimal gene complement of Mycoplasma genitalium. Science 1995;270:397–403.
21. Audic S, Claverie J-M. Self-identification of protein-coding regions in microbial genomes. Proc Natl Acad Sci USA 1998;95:10,006–10,031.
22. Fraser CM, Eisen JA, Salzberg SL. Microbial genome sequencing. Nature 2000;408:816–820.
23. Kotra LP, Vakulenko S, Mobashery S. From genes to sequences to antibiotics: prospects for future developments from microbial genomics. Microbes and Infection 2000;2:651–658.
24. Kyrpides NC, Ouzounis CA. Whole-genome sequence annotation: 'Going wrong with confidence'. Mol Microbiol 1999;32:886–887.

25. Altschul SF, Gish W, Miller W, Myers EW, Lipman DJ. Basic local alignment search tool. J Mol Biol 1990;215:403–410.

26. Pearson WR, Lipman DJ. Improved tools for biological sequence comparison. Proc Natl Acad Sci USA 1988;85:2444–2448.

27. Jacob F, Monod J. Genetic regulatory mechanisms in the synthesis of proteins. J Mol Biol 1961;3:318–356.

28. Behr MA, Wilson MA, Gill WP, Salamon H., Schoolnik GK, Rane S, et al. Comparative genomics of BCG vaccines by whole-genome DNA microarrays. Science 1999;284:1520–1523.

29. Hayashi T, Makino K, Ohnishi M, Kurokawa K, Ishii K, Yokoyama K, et al. Complete genome sequence of enterohemorrhagic Escerichia coli O157:H7 and genomic comparison with a laboratory strain K-12. DNA Res 2001;8:11–22.

30. Chalker AF, Minehart HW, Hughes NJ, Koretke KK, Lonetto MA, Brinkman KK, et al. Systematic identification of selective essential genes in Helicobacter pylori by genome prioritization and allelic replacement mutagenesis. J Bacteriol 2001;183:1259–1268.

31. Herrmann R, Reiner B. Mycoplasma pneumoniae and Mycoplasma genitalium: a comparison of two closely related bacterial species. Curr Opin Microbiol 1998;1:572–579.

32. Domenich P, Barry III CE, Cole ST. Mycobacterium tuberculosis in the post-genomic age. Curr Opin Microbiol 2001;4:28–34.

33. Riley M, Serres MH. Interim report on genomics of Escherichia coli. Annu Rev Microbiol 2000;54:341–411.

34. Baltz RH, Norris FH, Matsushima P, DeHoff BS, Rockey P, Porter G, et al. DNA sequence sampling of the Streptococcus pneumoniae genome to identify novel targets for antibiotic development. Microbiol Drug Res 1998;4:1–9.

35. Akerley BJ, Rubin EJ, Camilli A, Lampe DJ, Robertson HM, Mekalanos JJ. Systematic identification of essential genes by in vitro mariner mutagenesis. Proc Natl Acad Sci USA 1998;95:8927–8932.

36. Judson N, Mekalanos JJ. Transposon-based approaches to identify essential bacterial genes. Trends Microbiol 2000;8:521–526.

37. Shapiro L, Harris T. Finding function through structural genomics. Curr Opin Biotechnol 2000;11:31–35.

38. Edwards JS, Ibarra RU, Palsson BO. In silico predictions of Escherichia coli metabolic capabilities are consistent with experimental data. Nat Biotechnol 2001;19:125–130.

39. Couvert MW, Schilling CH, Famili I, Edwards JS, Goryanin II, Selkov E, et al. Metabolic modeling of microbial strains in silico. Trends Biochem Sci 2001;26:179–186.

40. Chu DTW, Plattner JJ, Katz L. New directions in antibacterial research. J Med Chem 1996;39:3853–3874.

41. Bruccoleri RE, Dougherty TJ, Davison DB. Concordance analysis of microbial genomes. Nucl Acids Res 1998;26:4482–4486.

42. Winzeler EA, Shoemaker DD, Astromoff A, Liang H, Anderson K, Andre B, et al. Functional characterization of the S. cerevisiae genome by gene deletion and parallel analysis. Science 1999;285:901–906.

43. Black T, Hare R. Will genomics revolutionize antimicrobial drug discovery? Curr Opin Microbiol 2000;3:522–527.

44. Goffin C, Ghuysen JM. Multimodular penicillin-binding proteins: an enigmatic family of orthologs and paralogs. Microbiol Mol Biol Rev 1998;62:1079–1093.

45. Schmid MB, Kapur N, Isaacson DR, Lindroos P, Sharpe C. Genetic analysis of temperature-sensitive lethal mutants of Salmonella typhimurium. Genetics 1999;123:625–639.

46. Khlebnikov A, Risa O, Skaug T, Carrier TA, Keasling JD. Regulatable arabinose-inducible gene expression system with consistent control in all cells of a culture. J Bacteriol 2000;182:7029–7034.

47. Silen JL, Lu AT, Solas DW, Gore MA, Maclean D, Shah NH, et al. Screening for novel antimicrobials from encoded combinatorial libraries using a two-dimensional agar format. Antimicrob Agents Chemother 1998;42:1447–1453.

48. King RW. Chemistry or biology: which comes first after the genome is sequenced? Chem Biol 1999;6:R327–R333.

49. Kirsch DR, Lai MH, McCullogh J, Gillum AM. The use of β-galactosidase gene fusions to screen for antibacterial antibiotics. J Antibiots 1991;44:210–217.

50. Arigoni F, Talabot F, Peitsch M, Edgerton MD, Meldrum E, Allet E, et al. A genome-based approach for the identification of essential bacterial genes. Nat Biotechnol 1998;16:851–856.

51. Hyde-DeRuyscher R, Paige LA, Christensen DJ, Hyde-DeRuyscher N, Lim A, Fredericks ZL. Detection of small-molecule enzyme inhibitors with peptides isolated from phage-displayed combinatorial peptide libraries. Chem Biol 2000;7:17–25.

52. Kolb JM, Yamanaka G, Manly S. Use of a novel homogeneous fluorescent technology in high throughput screening. J Biomol Screening 1996;1:203–210.

53. Rogers MV. Light on high throughput screening: fluorescence based assay technologies. Drug Discov Today 1997;2:156–160.

54. Khlebnikov A, Risa O, Skaug T, Carrier TA, Keasling JD. Regulatable arabinose-inducible gene expression system with consistent control in all cells of a culture. J Bacteriol 2000;182:7029–7034.

55. Connolly ML. Solvent-accessible surfaces of proteins and nucleic acids. Science 1983;221:709–713.

56. Lauri G, Bartlett PA. CAVEAT: a program to facilitate the design of organic molecules. J Comput-Aided Mol Des 1994;8:51–66.

57. Nikaido H. Multiple antibiotic resistance and efflux. Curr Opin Microbiol 1998;1:516–523.

58. Paulsen IT, Chen J, Nelson KE, Saier MH Jr. Comparative genomics of microbial drug efflux systems. J Mol Microbiol Biotechnol 2001;3:145–150.

59. Renau TE, Leger R, Flamme EM, Sangalang J, She MW, Yen R, et al. Inhibitors of efflux pumps in Pseudomonas aeruginosa potentiate the activity of the fluoroquinolone antibacterial levofloxacin. J Med Chem 1999;2;42:4928–4931.

DNA Microarray Expression Analysis in Antibacterial Drug Discovery

Brian J. Morrow and Karen Joy Shaw

INTRODUCTION

Bacteria have been the workhorses of biochemical, physiological, genetic, and molecular genetic investigations throughout the modern scientific era. In the era of whole-genome sequencing, attention is still focused on bacteria. Because of their relative ease of culture and vast wealth of supporting genetic data, commonly manipulated laboratory strains of bacteria were initially used as model organisms for developing and validating technologies for large-scale DNA sequencing projects, including the shotgun sequencing approach used to complete the human genome sequence. The relatively small genome size of bacteria allows for a rapid progression from initiating the sequencing project to completing annotation of the genome. For comparison, a bacterial species with a smaller genome such as *Helicobacter pylori* contains 1.66 million basepairs (bp) *(1)*, and a larger bacterial genome such as *Pseudomonas aeruginosa* contains 6.30 million bp *(2)*. The human genome measures 2.91 billion bp *(3)*. These smaller genomes, coupled with the importance of bacteria as causative agents of human, animal, and plant diseases, as well as their utility in industrial applications, have contributed to a large international effort yielding publicly available complete genome sequences for more than 40 prokaryotic species to date. The extent of this effort and the relative ease of sequencing bacterial genomes is exemplified in the United States Department of Energy's Joint Genome Institute's *(JGI)* "microbial marathon," in which 15 bacterial genomes were sequenced in a single month. On a single day—May 9, 2000—the JGI sequenced all 2.1 million bp of the genome of the multiple drug-resistant human pathogen *Enterococcus faecium*. The list of completed prokaryotic genomes includes species from diverse evolutionary backgrounds encompassing members of the Archae and Eubacteria. This ever-growing database of microbial genomes now includes the complete genomes for different strains within a species, including multiple strains of *Escherichia coli*, *H. pylori*, *Staphylococcus aureus*, *Neisseria meningitidis*, and *Mycobacterium tuberculosis*, to name only a few (http://www.jgi.doe.gov/tempweb.JGI_microbial/html).

The availability of whole-genome nucleotide sequence data has the potential to fulfill the promises of molecular genetics and biotechnology to meet the challenges presented by the emergence of bacterial pathogens that are resistant to many of the antibiotics

From: *Pathogen Genomics: Impact on Human Health*
Edited by: K. J. Shaw © Humana Press Inc., Totowa, NJ

developed to combat disease. Large-scale sequencing efforts and genomic technologies were developed at a time when antimicrobial drug discovery efforts were faced with increasing bacterial resistance to antibiotics that were developed almost exclusively from natural products identified decades ago to possess antimicrobial properties. Linezolid, an oxazolidinone, is the only novel class of antibacterials to be introduced in the last 30 years *(4),* leaving clinicians with a series of antibacterials that act against a small number of different bacterial targets. Whole-genome sequencing provides a list of all characterized genes and all predicted genes within the genome, allowing for the first time a global view of a prokaryotic genome without the limitations of individually cloning, sequencing, and characterizing genes identified through genetic screens. Genomic technologies continue to be developed to examine every gene within a genome, with the purpose of understanding the organism as a whole. DNA microarrays, in which the expression of every gene can be determined in a single hybridization experiment, constitute a primary technology in the functional characterization of a genome. Many of the genes present in a bacterial genome, and the proteins they encode, may serve as novel drug targets for the discovery and development of drugs to combat the emergence of multiple drug-resistant bacterial pathogens.

This chapter focuses on the development of DNA microarray technologies and how microarray expression analysis can be used to select novel targets for antimicrobial drug discovery, as well as to characterize the inhibitor mechanism of action. The use of DNA microarrays in the study of bacterial mechanisms of drug resistance is also examined.

BACTERIAL DNA MICROARRAY TECHNOLOGIES

DNA Microarray Design and Fabrication

DNA microarrays are an extension of the technology developed in the 1970s to detect specific nucleic-acid sequences, either DNA fragments in Southern blots *(5)* or RNA transcripts in Northern blots *(6).* Microarrays have resulted from a miniaturization of the process to examine thousands of different sequences in a single hybridization experiment. The complete nucleotide sequence and annotation of a bacterial genome provide the information needed to manufacture a DNA microarray containing every gene or predicted open reading frame (ORF) in the genome, as well as noncoding regions potentially transcribed as small or anti-sense RNAs. DNA microarray is used as a general term for arrays consisting of either single-stranded oligonucleotides or double-stranded DNA fragments, typically polymerase chain reaction (PCR) products or cDNAs, representing each gene or ORF. Unless specifically designated, the term "microarray" is used in this chapter to include oligonucleotide arrays as well as DNA microarrays and macroarrays. These technologies were recently reviewed by Schena et al. *(7)* and Freeman et al. *(8).*

Oligonucleotide arrays were developed through the adaptation of photolithography techniques used in the semiconductor industry. Standard solid-phase DNA synthesis chemistry is used to sequentially synthesize oligonucleotides of defined sequence directly onto the microarray substrate *(9).* Photomasks are used to direct light that activates modified phosphoramidite-containing deoxynucleotides, making them available for participation in synthesis reactions. Sequential changes in the photomask facilitates reactions in which each step results in the addition of a single base in a sequence-specific manner *(10)*. Multiple oligonucleotides of approximately 25 bp are synthesized to represent each ORF in the genome in such a way that groups of oligonucleotides, or probe sets, are complementary to a single transcript. Each ORF has an average of 15 probes designed to hybridize throughout the transcript length *(9)*. Mismatch probes, which contain a single base difference, are also synthesized for each probe set, to account for nonspecific hybridization.

Microarrays consisting of double-stranded DNAs are fabricated through use of ink-jet technology or mechanical microspotting, in which printheads containing microspotting pins are used to directly transfer solutions containing DNA to the microarray surface, typically a glass slide *(8)*. DNAs are printed in guanidine-containing buffer to denature the double-stranded DNA for subsequent hybridization. The nonporous glass substrate allows the DNA to be spotted in a discrete location without subsequent diffusion, and serves as the basis for miniaturization of the entire process, including hybridization. These same DNA solutions can also be printed onto nylon membranes to generate macroarrays. Oligonucleotide arrays and DNA microarrays are both hybridized to fluorescently labeled DNA probes, and the hybridization signals are read in a modified confocal scanning microscope *(8)*. Nylon macroarrays are hybridized to radiolabeled probes, and the hybridization signals are detected by a phosphoimager.

Challenges of Analyzing Bacterial RNA

The adaptability of bacteria and the nature of bacterial mRNA combine to present substantial challenges to the accurate analysis of the mRNA pool. Bacteria quickly adapt to changes in environmental conditions, and these responses frequently result in rapid alterations in the mRNA levels of specific genes, such as the induction of heat-shock genes in *E. coli (11)*. Levels of specific mRNAs can also change as a result of the half-lives of bacterial messages, which can be as short as 10 s *(12)*, but more typically vary between 40 s and 20 min *(13)*. Rapid alterations in mRNA levels necessitate the use of RNA extraction methods that quickly lyse the cells to preserve the RNA transcripts present in the cell population. RNA extraction methods that employ centrifugation steps of live bacteria or incubations of even a few minutes in enzymatic solutions to lyse the cells should be avoided. Tao et al. *(14)* purified *E. coli* RNA by directly pipetting growing cultures into boiling lysis buffer, a technique that effectively precludes adaptive transcriptional responses by the bacteria. Instantaneous lysis methods useful in Gram-negative bacteria may not be applicable to Gram-positive organisms, which are more difficult to lyse. High-quality RNA may be purified from these bacteria by use of a snap-freeze step in liquid nitrogen *(15)*, followed by disruption with glass beads *(16)* or use of an RNA stabilization reagent, such as RNALater (Ambion). Following purification, RNA preparations should be treated with a high-quality RNase-free DNase to ensure that the RNA is free from contaminating genomic DNA that could confound DNA microarray analysis.

Bacterial cDNA Probe Synthesis

DNA microarray probes are generated through the incorporation of radiolabeled or dye-conjugated nucleotides into cDNA by reverse transcriptase. Limited message polyadenylation in bacteria prevents the direct application of RNA and cDNA methodologies developed for use with eukaryotic RNA to the study of prokaryotic RNA. Only a small percentage of each specific bacterial mRNA is polyadenylated *(17),* and polyadenylated messages are targeted for destruction by mRNA-degrading complexes *(18).* This precludes the use of oligo(dT)-based methods to purify native bacterial mRNAs away from ribosomal and transfer RNAs. A method to selectively purify *E. coli* mRNA from total RNA has been developed, in which *E. coli* poly(A) polymerase is used to polyadenylate messages following RNA purification *(19).* The in vitro polyadenylated mRNA can then be purified by oligo(dT) chromatography. Purified *E. coli* mRNA was more sensitive than total RNA in DNA microarray hybridization, and both purified mRNA and total RNA exhibited similar *lacZYA* transcript levels subsequent to isopropyl-β-D-thiogalactopyranoside induction *(19).* Methods to prime bacterial cDNA synthesis include the use of random primers, a collection of primers specific to each ORF, or a minimal set of primers with sequences likely to be enriched in the 3′ end of each ORF. Random primers, typically hexamers, have been widely used to prime total RNA for cDNA synthesis, since they are universally applicable to all species. Random hexamers should prime all RNA species present in total RNA, including the 90–95% of total RNA that is comprised of rRNAs and tRNAs. DNA microarrays probed with randomly primed cDNAs would be expected to yield higher backgrounds than those probed with labeled cDNA primed with a complete set of oligonucleotides specific for the 3′ end of each ORF (a set of 25-bp gene-specific oligos is commercially available for the *E. coli,* K-12 genome from Sigma-Genosys). In a direct comparison of *E. coli* total RNA primed with either random hexamers or gene-specific primers, the randomly primed cDNA probes detected more specific mRNAs than did the gene-specific primer set *(20).* Additionally, the random primed cDNA probes generated hybridization signals that were more reproducible than the gene-specific primed cDNA probes *(20).* The inferior expression data generated by gene-specific primed cDNAs may be explained by different hybridization efficiencies of each primer in the collection, primer-primer interactions, ORF length, and ORF position in the operon as well as the potential loss of the primer binding sites caused by mRNA degradation. Each of these effects may be minimized by use of random primers that are capable of priming cDNA synthesis from any position in the polycistronic mRNA. An alternate method for priming total RNA for cDNA synthesis involves the use of genome-directed primers, which are comprised of a minimal number of primers predicted by an algorithm to specifically anneal to the 3′ ends of all genes within a given genome. A collection of 37 oligonucleotides that should prime all genes in the *M. tuberculosis* genome was directly compared with random primed cDNAs as microarray hybridization probes. Probes synthesized with the genome-directed primer set yielded higher hybridization signal intensities than the random primed cDNA probes, although the random primers generated a higher percentage of hybridization signals above the background threshold *(21).* Only a subset of the *M. tuberculosis* genome was tested in these arrays *(21),* and it remains to be demonstrated that the genome-directed primers can effectively prime cDNAs from all genes in the genome.

Microarray Hybridization and Detection

The small genome size of bacteria easily permits the deposition or synthesis of DNAs or oligonucleotides representing all ORFs in the genome onto a single array in duplicate, and expression data from every ORF can be generated in a single hybridization experiment. Direct comparisons of identical RNA samples that were either radio-labeled and hybridized to nylon macroarrrays or fluorescently labeled and hybridized to microarrays on glass slides have been made with *E. coli* total RNA *(22)*. Microarrays printed on glass slides generated hybridization data that were more reproducible than data generated by the hybridization of macroarrays on nylon filters. A comparison of data from oligonucleotide arrays and macroarrays that were each probed with the same RNA purified from THP-1 tissue-culture cells infected with *Listeria monocytogenes* demonstrated comparable results—both types of arrays detected the expression of common genes *(23)*.

The use of microarrays and macroarrays for global-expression analysis is dependent upon quantitative hybridization and the reproducibility of both the target DNA on the array and the cDNA probe synthesis. Since the amount of target DNA on the array should exceed the quantity of any specific cDNA sequence in the probe, the quantity of bound probe represents the message abundance within the total RNA sample. If target DNA is spotted onto the microarray in limiting quantities, the resulting hybridization signals will underestimate the mRNA levels present in the RNA and will lead to data compression *(24)*. Excess target DNA also allows for simultaneous hybridization of two differentially labeled cDNAs, facilitating comparative hybridization in a single step. It is important to accurately quantify input RNAs to ensure that probes are synthesized from equivalent masses of RNA, otherwise skewing of the data can result *(24)*. Typically, RNA from an untreated sample is labeled with one fluor, Cy5, and RNA from an experimentally manipulated sample is labeled with a different fluor, Cy3 (Amersham Pharmacia). The two fluors have different excitation and emission spectra, allowing independent detection of hybridization signals from each probe and direct comparisons of the abundance of a single mRNA species present in the two RNA samples. Direct comparisons of two RNAs on a single microarray have the advantage of eliminating variability in the amount of DNA spotted onto each microarray. However, the use of different fluors also introduces additional sources of variability. The two dyes have different quenching characteristics, complicating microarray scanning, and the differential incorporation of Cy3 or Cy5 by reverse transcriptase into specific genes can create gene-specific effects *(25,26)*. These gene-specific effects require double experiments, in which both the control and treated cDNAs are labeled with different fluors in the first experiment, and the fluors are reversed in the second experiment to ensure that the results are accurate. The direct comparison of RNAs in double-label experiments is only justified when the combined variability of the different dye properties and the differential dye incorporation into cDNA are less than the spot-to-spot variability introduced in printing each microarray. The necessity of labeling each probe with both dyes requires the same number of microarrays for each experiment as a single-label experiment in which all probes are labeled with the same dye.

Microarray hybridization sensitivity is determined by the amount of target DNA on the array and the quantity and quality of the RNA used to synthesize the labeled cDNA probe. Increasing the input RNA mass generates a corresponding increase in the labeled cDNA probe and microarray hybridization signal, although this signal can reach saturation *(24)*. Unless bacterial RNA is treated with poly(A) polymerase in vitro to facilitate mRNA purification *(19)*, limited message polyadenylation in bacteria dictates that total RNA must be used as a substrate for cDNA synthesis. The method of priming cDNA probe synthesis can affect the subsequent hybridization signal intensity. cDNA probes primed with a collection of gene-specific primers are highly sensitive, requiring only one to two µg of total RNA to achieve a strong hybridization signal *(14,20)*, whereas cDNA probes primed with random primers are much less sensitive, requiring as much as 20 µg of total RNA *(20,22)*. Under optimal conditions—for example, when both target DNA and probe RNA are not in limiting quantities—the dynamic range of hybridization signals is linear over three to four orders of magnitude *(20,27)*. In the case of oligonucleotide arrays containing an average of one 25 mer per every 30 bp over the entire *E. coli* genome, twofold changes in mRNA levels could be detected at 0.2 mRNA copies per cell *(9)*. The sensitivity of cDNA microarrays probed with complex mammalian probes is such that any specific mRNA could be detected at 2 pg with a signal to background ratio above 2.5 *(24)*. The sensitivity of oligonucleotide arrays raises some interesting questions. A reverse complement array detected anti-sense transcripts for at least 70% of all predicted *E. coli* ORFs *(9)*, suggesting that most of the chromosome is transcribed at a low level. The physiologic significance of these low-level transcripts has not yet been addressed.

Analysis of Microarray Data

The simultaneous determination of thousands of data points in microarray hybridization experiments necessitates the use of statistical analysis to differentiate true changes in hybridization signals that reflect biologically relevant changes in transcript levels from those variations that are inherent to the methodology. Experimental replication is essential to obtain statistically reliable data. A direct comparison of microarray hybridization data generated by different probes requires that the background is subtracted from the hybridization signals, and the signals are then normalized with respect to the specific activity of each probe. Normalization is typically performed through the expression of the hybridization intensity of a specific gene as a percentage of the total signal from all genes on the array *(14,20,22)*. The comparison of normalized signals from two arrays generates ratios that reflect the relative transcript levels. The magnitude of change in gene expression between two conditions is typically used to interpret comparisons of microarray data, with a twofold or greater difference in expression levels considered significant, although the statistical significance of a twofold change should be tested. Equating fold differences in expression with the accuracy of the measurement may not be valid, since the statistical significance of measurements can be higher for differential expression ratios of less than two than it is for ratios larger than two *(20)*. It is important to verify conclusions drawn concerning changes in gene expression from microarray data using an independent experimental method, such as quantitative reverse-transcriptase polymerase chain reaction (RT-PCR) or Northern blots *(16,28)*.

There are several caveats to consider when interpreting microarray hybridization data. Experimental variation arising from cross-hybridization or from the labile nature of RNA is always problematic in hybridization experiments, and microarray hybridization is not an exception. Microarrays are intrinsically limited because they only allow for an estimation of the steady-state level of transcripts present in the sampled population. Microarrays cannot provide data concerning rates of transcription initiation or changes in mRNA stability. Unless many RNA samples are purified over time, transient changes in mRNA levels, such as the induction of cold-shock genes in *E. coli(29),* may be missed. The need for total RNA masses between one and 20 μg for probe synthesis requires a population of bacteria containing at least 10^9 cells *(30).* The resulting microarray data represent an average of the transcriptional states of each bacterium in the sampled population. Gene-expression changes occurring in only a subset of the population, such as the spatial expression of alkaline phosphatase in *Klebsiella pnuemoniae* and *Pseudomonas aeruginosa* biofilms *(31),* would be averaged over all bacteria in the biofilm. Additionally, subtle changes in gene expression, such as changes less than twofold, may be discounted in microarray data as statistically insignificant, yet still have major physiologic consequences. Microarrays printed with double-stranded DNA are not capable of differentiating which DNA strand is transcribed, in the case of overlapping ORFs. Hydrogen peroxide treatment of *E. coli* induced transcript levels for numerous genes, including *ybjM,* but primer-extension analysis suggested that the *ybjM* signal actually corresponded to a gene on the opposite DNA strand *(32).* A major consideration in data analysis is that RNA levels do not always reflect changes in protein levels or in protein activity *(33).* In general, there is a positive correlation between changes in mRNA and protein abundance, but this correlation is incomplete *(20,33–37).* Studies directly comparing transcriptional and translational analyses of bacteria show that for the majority of genes, there is a positive correlation in qualitative, but not necessarily quantitative, changes between transcript levels and protein levels *(36,37).* In a few cases, clear discrepancies between the transcriptome and the proteome were observed, such as the accumulation of the protein CbpA in an *E. coli hns* mutant, for which no differences in transcript levels between mutant and wild-type strains could be detected *(37).*

BACTERIAL MICROARRAY EXPRESSION ANALYSIS AND DRUG TARGET SELECTION

Computational Approaches to Target Selection

The resource of complete microbial genome sequences presents the opportunity to use these data in the discovery of novel antimicrobial compounds. With these genomic sequences in hand, the antimicrobial drug discovery process is no longer limited to the bacterial targets that have been previously cloned and characterized, and an expansion of the number of bacterial drug targets should lead to increased diversity in the repertoire of antimicrobials available to clinicians. This, in turn, should assist in combating the microbial resistance that has developed in part because of the limited number of bacterial targets against which current drugs act. Genomic comparisons of the numerous bacterial species sequenced to date, in combination with DNA microarray global-expression analysis, can be used to prioritize the entire genome complement now available as potential antimicrobial targets. Computational approaches can be used to identify genes conserved across a defined set of microbial genomes *(38–40),* potentially yielding broad-spectrum targets or targets specific to a group of related pathogens, or perhaps even a single pathogen. Bacterial pathogens with unique physiologies that occupy exclusive niches, such as *H. pylori* and *M. tuberculosis,* may support efforts to develop selective narrow-spectrum drugs. The list of conserved genes is lengthy and contains many genes of unknown function, since approximately 30–45%

of sequenced microbial genomes are comprised of previously uncharacterized ORFs *(2,41,42)*. With the completion of the human genome sequence *(3)*, lists of genes conserved in a selected set of bacteria can be compared to eliminate those with human homologs, possibly increasing the selectivity of inhibitors developed against the bacterial targets. Evolutionary conservation of a gene implies that the gene product may be essential for viability, but it is not proof in and of itself. Of 26 *E. coli* genes of unknown function that are conserved in *Mycoplasma genitalium,* only six were shown to be essential *(43)*. Direct evidence for essentiality must be provided through the mutation or inactivation of the gene of interest, and the determination of essentiality is dependent upon the specific growth conditions under which it is tested. Genes essential for bacterial viability during the course of infection may not be essential for growth on rich medium in vitro. Evolutionarily conserved bacterial genes that are required for viability under all growth conditions are likely to represent optimal targets for antimicrobial drug discovery.

Validation of Microarray Expression Analysis

DNA microarrays effectively serve as high-throughput Northern blots, and the analysis of RNAs from numerous cultures that have been exposed to a wide variety of treatments or growth conditions can lead to the generation of a large database of global-expression profiles. When combined with a computational approach to identify evolutionarily conserved genes, the global-expression database can be used to prioritize potential drug targets through the analysis of transcriptional responses of individual genes as well as biochemical pathways and regulatory networks. These expression data can also be used for functional annotation of the large proportion of each genome that remains uncharacterized, a class of genes representing a pool of potential drug targets that have not yet been exploited.

Initial experiments validating whole-genome microbial microarrays analyzed the expression of the extensively studied bacterium *E. coli,* which is well-characterized genetically and biochemically and provides an excellent model for validating microarray-expression analysis. The first published reports compared transcript profiles of a laboratory strain of *E. coli* K-12 cultured in rich or minimal medium *(14,28)* or following treatment with either isopropyl-β-D-thiogalactopyranoside (IPTG) or heat shock *(22)*. The tremendous number of physiological experiments conducted on *E. coli* effectively corroborated the comparative transcriptional profiles observed for *E. coli* cultured in rich or minimal medium. As expected, when cultured in rich medium, *E. coli* contained elevated transcript levels of genes involved in macromolecule synthesis, particularly protein synthesis, and much lower transcript levels of genes encoding proteins that are needed for the biosynthesis of amino acids, vitamins, and various cofactors *(14)*. The transcriptional profile of *E. coli* was reversed in cells cultured in minimal medium *(14)*. The ability of DNA microarray-expression analysis to predict a cell's physiologic state was further validated through analysis of the treatment of *E. coli* with IPTG. The majority of gene expression was unchanged between IPTG-treated and untreated cultures, but the genes of the *lacZYA* operon were expressed at much higher levels following IPTG treatment *(22,28)*. Another example of the selective induction of a single operon, the tryptophan biosynthesis operon, was also detected by microarray analysis of RNA from an *E. coli* culture starved for tryptophan *(35)*. The analysis of more complex transcriptional changes, such as the pleiotropic effects resulting from heat-shock treatment of *E. coli (22),* anaerobic culture of *Bacillus subtilis (44),* or acid stress of *H. pylori (45)* has also been validated for DNA microarrays. In each of these studies, transcript levels for the majority of genes did not change as a result of treatment, as expected, but the transcript levels of genes known to respond to treatment were observed to change in a manner consistent with previous studies. These studies both confirm that the technology can reproducibly detect known transcriptional response, and provide novel observations concerning the transcriptional response of both characterized and uncharacterized genes to environmental perturbations. The organization of prokaryotic genomes into operons, in which groups of genes are regulated by a single promoter and transcribed into a single mRNA, provides a series of positive internal controls for expression analysis. The positive correlation of gene expression within an operon was observed in *E. coli* cultures starved for tryptophan in which elevated mRNA levels were observed for all five genes in the tryptophan biosynthetic operon, *trpEDCBA (35).* However, microarray analysis does not always detect coordinated changes in transcript levels from every gene in an operon *(20,35).* In general, there is a positive correlation between changes in the expression levels of all genes in an operon, although the magnitude of induction or repression of individual genes does not always correlate completely *(22,28,44).* The differences in magnitude between genes in an operon may be attributable to differences in DNA target concentration on the array, differences in the relative efficiencies of probe synthesis, differences in rates of mRNA degradation for each operon member, transcriptional attenuation, and transcription initiation from internal promoters.

Analysis of Co-Expressed Genes

A microarray-expression database can be efficiently screened to identify genes whose RNA levels are dramatically increased or decreased. Such analyses do not account for the more subtle changes in gene expression that may correlate with or provide the basis for phenotypic alterations. To address these more subtle complexities, computational analysis of expression data can be performed with a variety of algorithms to identify clusters of genes with similar expression patterns throughout the experimental data set *(46,47).* Cluster analysis provides an efficient means to comprehend the massive amounts of data generated in microarray experiments, since genes that are functionally related tend toward similar transcriptional regulation. The organization of genes into functional categories provides a global view of the transcriptional state of the bacteria and represents their physiological state, although the clustering of genes with similar transcriptional patterns does not necessarily imply direct regulation by a common element. The examination of the DNA sequences upstream of co-expressed genes can lead to the identification of common regulatory sites and confirmation of coregulation. This approach was used to identify putative integration host factor (IHF)-binding sites upstream of ORFs observed to be differentially expressed between isogenic *E. coli* IHF⁺ and IHF⁻ strains *(20).* Clusters of cell-cycle-dependent genes in *Caulobacter crescentus* identified in comparisons of wild-type and *ctrA* mutant strains were screened for CtrA-binding sites to identify those genes that are directly regulated, confirming the coregulation of those genes clustered by microarray-expression data *(48).*

Comparisons of the transcriptional profiles of wild-type strains and isogenic strains carrying mutations within a specific transcriptional regulator have resulted in an expansion of the number of genes classified within each regulon and a broadening of the physiologic role for each transcriptional regulator studied. DNA microarray analysis has augmented the list of *E. coli* genes known to be regulated, either directly or indirectly, by MarA *(49)*, IHF *(20)*, OxyR *(32)*, LexA *(50)*, and H-NS *(37)*. Despite the extensive characterization of each of these regulons prior to DNA microarray analysis, the global transcriptional profile of each mutant provided evidence for an expanded physiologic role for each of these proteins, enhancing our understanding of bacterial responses to growth conditions and environmental stresses. These studies also provide the opportunity to more completely understand the mechanism of action of antimicrobial agents.

The identification of co-expressed and coregulated genes serves an important role in the determination of regulatory networks governing cell functions *(51)*, as well as the functional annotation of unknown genes that comprise a large percentage of microbial genomes. In this role, DNA microarrays can augment the extensive genetic and biochemical data used to establish these networks *(33)*. Integration of microarray hybridization data with biochemical pathway databases, such as EcoCyc *(52)*, KEGG *(53)*, and WIT *(54)*, will advance the comprehensive understanding of *E. coli* biology, and also serve to prioritize potential drug targets. The countless genetic screens performed on model organisms such as *E. coli* and *B. subtilis* would suggest that all of the genes essential for growth under defined conditions and most of the important nonessential genes have been identified and characterized. Analysis of the genome sequences of these model organisms indicates that this assumption is not true. A study of unknown ORFs that are evolutionarily conserved identified five previously uncharacterized genes that are essential for growth of both *E. coli* and *B. subtilis (43)*. Characterization of unknown ORFs can proceed from nucleotide sequence analysis to expression analysis, promoter searches, and mutational analysis. The pleiotropic effects of heat shock *(22)*, acid stress *(45)*, growth in minimal medium *(14,28)*, and anaerobiasis *(44)* each resulted in changes in transcript abundance for genes previously known to be members of each respective stimulon, as well as changes in mRNA levels for a set of previously uncharacterized ORFs. These expression data provide the first functional information about an uncharacterized ORF that lacks meaningful sequence similarity to assign function on that basis. The clustering of unknown ORFs with genes of known function or with genes belonging to a common metabolic pathway is a first step in provisionally assigning function. The use of a diverse set of experimental conditions from which RNA is purified is valuable in assessing the degree of correlation of co-expression. Similar patterns of the transcriptional regulation of previously characterized genes and unknown ORFs induced by heat shock of *E. coli* cultures *(22)* or by anaerobic culture of *B. subtilis (44)* only provide a hypothesis that the known genes and unknown ORFs are functionally related. The identification of consensus binding sites for known transcriptional regulators upstream of the co-expressed ORFs *(20,48)* is the next logical step in functional annotation. A whole-genome in vivo approach to identifying protein-DNA interactions based upon methylase protection has also been used to identify DNA-binding sites upstream of uncharacterized ORFs *(51)*. Further validation of the function assigned to each ORF will require genetic studies, including mutational analysis. Microarray analysis of the transcriptional profiles of wild-type and isogenic strains carrying a mutation in an unknown ORF, in conjunction with phenotypic analysis, can provide valuable information concerning the role played by a gene in the cell *(20,44)*. The selection of unknown ORFs as targets for traditional screens to identify small-molecule inhibitors requires functional information beyond what can be provided through expression analysis. New technologies, such as high-throughput nuclear magnetic resonance screening *(55)* can identify protein binding without knowledge of functional inhibition. The use of these technologies may justify the selection of previously uncharacterized ORFs based upon genetic comparisons, essentiality, and DNA microarray expression data alone.

BACTERIAL TRANSCRIPTIONAL RESPONSES TO ANTIMICROBIALS

Expression Analysis: Target Validation and Inhibitor Mechanism of Action

Successful antimicrobial drugs frequently inhibit an enzyme or principal component of an essential pathway, resulting in metabolic disturbances brought about by an accumulation of reaction intermediates or alterations in the concentrations of other products in the pathway. Analysis of transcriptional profiles of bacteria treated with an inhibitor can provide valuable information for both pathway characterization and the mechanism of action of the inhibitor. Transcriptional analysis of inhibitor effects should focus on early responses and biologically relevant concentrations of the inhibitor, since later responses and responses to high inhibitor concentrations are likely to contain secondary effects of inhibition. Microarray analysis of *M. tuberculosis* cultures that were either untreated or treated with isoniazid, an inhibitor of mycolic acid biosynthesis, revealed a rapid and high level of induction of five genes involved in type II fatty acid synthesis and an enzyme involved in mycolate maturation *(16)*. A different mycolate biosynthesis inhibitor, ethionamide, induced these same five *M. tuberculosis* genes *(16)*. DNA microarray expression analysis also had the potential to distinguish the responses of *Haemophilus influenzae* to two different classes of DNA gyrase inhibitors, ciprofloxacin, or novobiocin. Ciprofloxacin, a quinolone, inhibits DNA gyrase in a manner that leads to double-stranded DNA breaks and the inhibition of DNA replication *(56)*, and novobiocin, a coumarin, inhibits DNA gyrase without causing DNA damage *(57)*. At the minimum inhibitory concentration (MIC), ciprofloxacin treatment of *H. influenzae* increased transcript levels for several genes involved in DNA repair and the SOS response including RecA recombinase, single-stranded DNA-binding protein, a DNA repair protein and the Holiday junction DNA helicase *(36)*. In contrast to ciprofloxacin, treatment with novobiocin at the MIC increased transcript levels for DNA gyrase subunit B and decreased transcript levels for topoisomerase I, ribosome releasing factor, and two ORFs of unknown function *(36)*. At higher inhibitor concentrations, many more genes showed altered transcript levels than at the MIC. These results raise the possibility of secondary or nonspecific effects of the gyrase inhibitors *(36)*. Transcriptional induction of the DNA repair systems distinguished the response of *H. influenzae* to ciprofloxacin from the response to novobiocin and may be viewed as a molecular marker of gyrase inhibitors that cause DNA damage. The creation of a large database of transcriptional responses to a variety of antimicrobials should allow for the identification of characteristic alterations or signatures in the transcriptional profile that are indicative of mechanism of action. These expression signatures should prove valuable in the characterization of novel compounds that lack a known mechanism of action. Additionally, the induction of essential genes or uncharacterized ORFs by an inhibitor may identify these ORFs as potential novel drug targets. A conditional mutation inactivating the gene encoding the target of an inhibitor should produce a transcriptional profile similar or identical to that observed following exposure of a wild-type strain to the drug, since the same step in the metabolic pathway is affected in both cases. Comparisons of transcript profiles of both wild-type and mutant strains treated with the same inhibitor should serve to validate the drug target, the mechanism of action, and to potentially indicate the presence of nonspecific effects *(16,58,59)*.

Expression Analysis: Mechanisms of Bacterial Resistance to Inhibitors

A logical extension of microarray expression analysis for the characterization of the mechanism of action of an inhibitor is the expression analysis of resistant strains to reveal an understanding of the development of resistance to a drug. The use of microarray expression analysis to characterize the mechanism of resistance was validated using a known case of resistance. The mycolate biosynthesis inhibitors isoniazid and ethionamide differ in that isoniazid requires oxidation by catalase to be active in *M. tuberculosis (16)*. An isoniazid-resistant, catalase-negative *M. tuberculosis* strain increased transcript levels for the fatty-acid biosynthesis genes in response to ethionamide treatment but not to isoniazid *(16)*. In *E. coli,* resistance to mitomycin C, an inhibitor that damages DNA *(60),* is conferred through overexpression of the positive transcriptional regulator *sdiA*. Microarray expression analysis of an *sdiA*-overexpressing strain revealed a pleiotropic effect, with elevated transcript levels for many genes involved in DNA replication, repair, and cell division *(28),* providing evidence for the mechanism of mitomycin C resistance. The overexpression of *sdiA* also increased transcript levels for the *acrAB* operon that encodes a drug efflux pump, and may explain the increased resistance of the overexpressing strain to antibiotics with such disparate mechanisms of action as tetracycline and nalidixic acid *(28)*.

CONCLUSIONS AND FUTURE DIRECTIONS

The growing database of complete genome sequences from a diverse collection of microorganisms provides the foundation for a rapid expansion in our understanding of prokaryotic biology. Genomics research has had a profound impact on all areas of microbiology, including molecular evolution, physiology, genetics, and bacterial pathogenesis. An understanding of the functions of every gene in a bacterium, as well as the pathways and regulatory networks through which they interact, is the goal of functional genomics. This understanding will be greatly advanced through the use of whole-genome DNA microarrays and genomic-scale protein technologies or proteomics. Protein-protein interaction maps, such as that initiated for *H. pylori (61),* will play an integral role along with genome sequences and DNA microarrays in the complete understanding of an organism.

For bacterial pathogens, DNA microarray-expression analysis can help to define the bacterial-host interactions that lead either to disease or resistance to disease. Microarray analysis of mRNAs purified from tissue-culture cells inoculated with bacterial pathogens have already been used to study the host response to infection *(23,62–65)*. Because of the technical difficulties associated with bacterial mRNA, the bacterial response to the interaction with mammalian cells has yet to be examined using DNA microarrays. A more complete understanding of the responses of bacterial pathogens and mammalian hosts to each other should identify new targets for therapeutic treatment of infections or new vaccine candidates to prevent infection.

The implementation and further development of DNA microarray technology will positively impact all aspects of human health. Expression analysis of pathogenic bacteria will assist the functional characterization of microbial genomes, the identification of novel drug targets for antimicrobial drug discovery, and the study of inhibitor mechanisms of action. DNA microarrays will also play a vital role in identifying the genes involved in the evolution of drug resistance and in efforts to combat drug-resistant pathogens. Clinical use of DNA microarrays will influence the diagnosis and treatment of infectious diseases. The identification of specific bacterial strains as the cause of an infection, combined with an improved understanding of bacterial-host interactions, will facilitate decisions regarding drug selection, both in terms of efficacy against the infecting strain and the physiology of the individual patient. The greatly expanded knowledge base of both bacterial and human genetics and physiology resulting from the application of DNA microarrays and other genomic technologies will significantly advance and accelerate efforts to develop novel therapeutics for the treatment of human infectious diseases.

REFERENCES

1. Tomb JF, White O, Kerlavage AR, et al. The complete genome sequence of the gastric pathogen Helicobacter pylori. Nature 1997; 388:539–547.
2. Stover CK, Pham XQ, Erwin AL, et al. Complete genome sequence of Pseudomonas aeruginosa PA01, an opportunistic pathogen. Nature 2000; 406:959–964.
3. Venter JC, Adams MD, Myers EW, et al. The sequence of the human genome. Science 2001; 291:1304–1351.
4. Bhavnani SM, Ballow CH. New agents for Gram-positive bacteria. Current Opinion in Microbiology 2000; 3:528–534.
5. Southern EM. Detection of specific sequences among DNA fragments separated by gel electrophoresis. Journal of Molecular Biology 1975; 98:503–517.
6. Alwine JC, Kemp DJ, Stark GR. Method for detection of specific RNAs in agarose gels by transfer to diazobenzyloxymethyl-paper and hybridization with DNA probes. Proc Natl Acad Sci USA 1977; 74:5350–5354.
7. Schena M, Shalon D, Davis RW, Brown PO. Quantitative monitoring of gene expression patterns with a complementary DNA microarray. Science 1995; 270:467–470.
8. Freeman WM, Robertson DJ, Vrana KE. Fundamentals of DNA hybridization arrays for gene expression analysis. Biotechniques 2000; 29:1042–1046, 1048–1055.
9. Selinger DW, Cheung KJ, Mei R, et al. RNA expression analysis using a 30 base pair resolution Escherichia coli genome array. Nat Biotechnol 2000; 18:1262–1268.
10. Fodor SP, Read JL, Pirrung MC, Stryer L, Lu AT, Solas D. Light-directed, spatially addressable parallel chemical synthesis. Science 1991; 251:767–773.
11. Yura T, Kanemori M, Morita MT. The heat shock response: regulation and function. In: Storz G, Hengge-Aronis R (eds). Bacterial Stress Responses. Washington, DC: ASM Press, 2000:3–18.

12. Goldenberg D, Azar I, Oppenheim AB. Differential mRNA stability of the cspA gene in the cold-shock response of Escherichia coli. Mol Microbiol 1996; 19:241–248.

13. Pedersen S, Reeh S. Functional mRNA half lives in E. coli. Molecular & General Genetics 1978; 166:329–336.

14. Tao H, Bausch C, Richmond C, Blattner FR, Conway T. Functional genomics: expression analysis of Escherichia coli growing on minimal and rich media. J Bacteriol 1999; 181:6425–6440.

15. de Saizieu A, Gardes C, Flint N, et al. Microarray-based identification of a novel Streptococcus pneumoniae regulon controlled by an autoinduced peptide. J Bacteriol 2000; 182:4696–4703.

16. Wilson M, DeRisis J, Kristensen H-H, Imboden P, Rane S, Brown PO. Exploring drug-induced alterations in gene expression. In: Mycobacterium tuberculosis by microarray hybridization. Proc Natl Acad Sci. USA 1999; 96:12,833–12,838.

17. Cao GJ, Sarkar N. Poly(A) RNA in Escherichia coli: nucleotide sequence at the junction of the lpp transcript and the polyadenylate moiety. Proc Natl Acad Sci USA 1992; 89:7546–7550.

18. O'Hara EB, Chekanova JA, Ingle CA, Kushner ZR, Peters E, Kushner SR. Polyadenylylation helps regulate mRNA decay in Escherichia coli. Proc Natl Acad Sci USA 1995; 92:1807–1811.

19. Wendisch VF, Zimmer DP, Khodursky A, Peter B, Cozzarelli N, Kustu S. Isolation of Escherichia coli mRNA and comparison of expression using mRNA and total RNA on DNA microarrays. Anal Biochem 2001; 290:205–213.

20. Arfin SM, Long AD, Ito ET, et al. Global gene expression profiling in Escherichia coli K12 the effects of integration host factor. J Biol Chem 2000; 275:29,672–29,864.

21. Talaat AM, Hunter P, Johnston SA. Genome-directed primers for selective labeling of bacterial transcripts for DNA microarray analysis. Natl Biotechnol 2000; 18:679–682.

22. Richmond CS, Glasner JD, Mau R, Jin H, Blattner FR. Genome-wide expression profiling in Escherichia coli K-12. Nucleic Acids Res 1999; 27:3821–3835.

23. Cohen P, Bouaboula M, Bellis M, et al. Monitoring cellular responses to Listeria monocytogenes with oligonucleotide arrays. J Biol Chem 2000; 275:11,181–11,190.

24. Yue H, Eastman PS, Wang BB, et al. An evaluation of the performance of cDNA microarrays for detecting changes in global mRNA expression. Nucleic Acids Res 2001; 29(8):41e.

25. Bartosiewicz M, Trounstine M, Barker D, Johnston R, Buckpitt A. Development of a toxicological gene array and quantitative assessment of this technology. Arch Biochem Biophys 2000; 376:66–73.

26. Taniguchi M, Miura K, Iwao H, Yamanaka S. Quantitative assessment of DNA microarrays—comparison with Northern blot analyses. Genomics 2001; 71:34–39.

27. Schena M, Heller RA, Theriault TP, Konrad K, Lachenmeier E, Davis RW. Microarrays: biotechnology's discovery platform for functional genomics. Trends in Biotechnology 1998; 16:301–306.

28. Wei Y, Lee J-M, Richmond C, Blattner FR, Rafalski JA, LaRossa RA. High-density microarray-mediated gene expression profiling of Escherichia coli. J Bacteriol 2001; 183:545–556.

29. Goldstein J, Pollitt NS, Inouye M. Major cold shock protein of Escherichia coli. Proc Natl Acad Sci USA 1990; 87:283–287.

30. Bremer H, Dennis PP. Modulation of chemical composition and other parameters of the cell by growth rate. In: Neidhardt FC (ed). Escherichia coli and Salmonella: cellular and molecular biology. Vol. 2. Washington, DC. ASM Press, 1996:1553–1569.

31. Huang CT, Xu KD, McFeters GA, Stewart PS. Spatial patterns of alkaline phosphatase expression within bacterial colonies and biofilms in response to phosphate starvation. Appl Environ Microbiol 1998; 64:1526–1531.

32. Zheng M, Wang X, Templeton LJ, Smulski DR, LaRossa RA, Storz G. DNA microarray-mediated transcriptional profiling of the Escherichia coli response to hydrogen peroxide. J Bacteriol 2001; 183:4562–4570.

33. VanBogelen RA, Greis KD, Blumenthal RM, Tani TH, Matthews RG. Mapping regulatory networks in microbial cells. Trends in Microbiology 1999; 7:320–328.

34. Vind J, Sorensen MA, Rasmussen MD, Pedersen S. Synthesis of proteins in Escherichia coli is limited by the concentration of free ribosomes. Expression from reporter genes does not always reflect functional mRNA levels. J Mol Biol 1993; 231:678–688.

35. Khodursky AB, Peter BJ, Cozzarelli NR, Botstein D, Brown PO, Yanofsky C. DNA microarray analysis of gene expression in response to physiological and genetic changes that affect tryptophan metabolism in Escherichia coli. PNAS 2000; 97:12,170–12,175.

36. Gmuender H, Kuratli K, Padova KD, Gray CP, Keck W, Evers S. Gene expression changes triggered by exposure of Haemophilus influenzae to novobiocin or ciprofloxacin: combined transcription and translation Analysis. Genome Res 2001; 11:28–42.

37. Hommais F, Krin E, Laurent-Winter C, et al. Large-scale monitoring of pleiotropic regulation of gene expression by the prokaryotic nucleoid-associated protein, H-NS. Mol Microbiol 2001; 40:20–36.

38. Mushegian AR, Koonin EV. A minimal gene set for cellular life derived by comparison of complete bacterial genomes. Proc Natl Acad Sci USA 1996; 93:10,268–10,273.

39. Koonin EV, Mushegian AR, Galperin MY, Walker DR. Comparison of archaeal and bacterial genomes: computer analysis of protein sequences predicts novel functions and suggests a chimeric origin for the archaea. Mol Microbiol 1997; 25:619–637.

40. Bruccoleri RE, Dougherty TJ, Davison DB. Concordance analysis of microbial genomes. Nucleic Acids Res 1998; 26:4482–4486.

41. Blattner FR, Plunkett G, 3rd, Bloch CA, et al. The complete genome sequence of Escherichia coli K-12. Science 1997; 277:1453–1474.

42. Ferretti JJ, McShan WM, Ajdic D, et al. Complete genome sequence of an M1 strain of Streptococcus pyogenes. Proc Natl Acad Sci USA 2001; 98:4658–4663.

43. Arigoni F, Talabot F, Peitsch M, et al. A genome-based approach for the identification of essential bacterial genes. Nat Biotechnol 1998; 16:851–856.

44. Ye RW, Tao W, Bedzyk L, Young T, Chen M, Li L. Global gene expression profiles of Bacillus subtilis grown under anaerobic conditions. J Bacteriol 2000; 182:4458–4465.

45. Ang S, Lee C-Z, Peck K, et al. Acid-induced gene expression in Helicobacter pylori: study in genomic scale by microarray. Infect Immun 2001; 69:1679–1686.

46. Ben-Dor A, Shamir R, Yakhini Z. Clustering gene expression patterns. Journal of Computational Biology 1999; 6:281–297.

47. Eisen MB, Spellman PT, Brown PO, Botstein D. Cluster analysis and display of genome-wide expression patterns. Proc Natl Acad Sci USA 1998; 95:14,863–14,868.

48. Laub MT, McAdams HH, Feldblyum T, Fraser CM, Shapiro L. Global analysis of the genetic network controlling a bacterial cell cycle. Science 2000; 290:2144–2148.

49. Barbosa TM, Levy SB. Differential expression of over 60 chromosomal genes in Escherichia coli by constitutive expression of MarA. J Bacteriol 2000; 182:3467–3474.

50. Courcelle J, Khodursky A, Peter B, Brown PO, Hanawalt PC. Comparative gene expression profiles following UV exposure in wild-type and SOS-deficient Escherichia coli. Genetics 2001; 158:41–64.

51. Tavazoie S, Hughes JD, Campbell MJ, Cho RJ, Church GM. Systematic determination of genetic network architecture. Nat Genet 1999; 22:281–285.

52. Karp PD, Riley M, Paley SM, Pellegrini-Toole A, Krummenacker M. Eco Cyc: encyclopedia of Escherichia coli genes and metabolism. Nucleic Acids Res 1999; 27:55–58.

53. Ogata H, Goto S, Sato K, Fujibuchi W, Bono H, Kanehisa M. KEGG: Kyoto encyclopedia of genes and genomes. Nucleic Acids Res 1999; 27:29–34.

54. Selkov E, Galimova M, Goryanin I, et al. The metabolic pathway collection: an update. Nucleic Acids Res 1997; 25:37–38.

55. Hajduk PJ, Gerfin T, Boehlen JM, Haberli M, Marek D, Fesik SW. High-throughput nuclear magnetic resonance-based screening. J Med Chem 1999; 42:2315–2317.

56. Hooper DC. Quinolone mode of action—new aspects. Drugs 1993; 45:8–14.

57. Kampranis SC, Gormley NA, Tranter R, Orphanides G, Maxwell A. Probing the binding of coumarins and cyclothialidines to DNA gyrase. Biochemistry 1999; 38:1967–1976.

58. Marton MJ, DeRisi JL, Bennett HA, et al. Drug target validation and identification of secondary drug target effects using DNA microarrays. Nat Med 1998; 4:1293–1301.

59. Bammert GF, Fostel JM. Genome-wide expression patterns in Saccharomyces cerevisiae: comparison of drug treatments and genetic alterations affecting biosynthesis of ergosterol. Antimicrob Agents Chemother 2000; 44:125–1265.

60. Tomasz M, Palom Y. The mitomycin bioreductive antitumor agents: cross-linking and alkylation of DNA as the molecular basis of their activity. Pharmacol Ther 1997; 76:73–87.

61. Rain JC, Selig L, De Reuse H, et al. The protein-protein interaction map of Helicobacter pylori. Nature 2001; 409:211–215.

62. Eckmann L, Smith JR, Housley MP, Dwinell MB, Kagnoff MF. Analysis by high density cDNA arrays of altered gene expression in human intestinal epithelial cells in response to infection with the invasive enteric bacteria Salmonella. J Biol Chem 2000; 275:14,084–14,094.

63. Rosenberger CM, Scott MG, Gold MR, Hancock RE, Finlay BB. Salmonella typhimurium infection and lipopolysaccharide stimulation induce similar changes in macrophage gene expression. J Immunol 2000; 164:5894–5904.

64. Ichikawa JK, Norris A, Bangera MG, et al. Interaction of Pseudomonas aeruginosa with epithelial cells: identification of differentially regulated genes by expression microarray analysis of human cDNAs. Proc Natl Acad Sci USA 2000; 97:9659–9664.

65. Belcher CE, Drenkow J, Kehoe B, et al. The transcriptional responses of respiratory epithelial cells to Bordetella pertussis reveal host defensive and pathogen counter-defensive strategies. PNAS 2000; 97:13,847–13,852.

9

The Influence of Genomics on the Molecular Epidemiology of Nosocomial Pathogens

Richard V. Goering

INTRODUCTION

Historically, epidemiology has been fundamentally linked to the discovery of infectious disease. As it became clear that specific etiological agents could be transferred between hosts, it was equally apparent that logical inquiry could be used to better understand—and hopefully prevent—the transmission process. As with all scientific investigation, the nature of this inquiry has changed over time, depending on the investigative tools available. Recent years have seen advances leading to genome sequencing that is either completed or in progress for an increasing number of bacterial pathogens (Table 1). This genomic database represents a powerful resource with enormous potential application for the understanding and treatment of infectious disease. This chapter explores the potential impact of genomics on issues related to epidemiological analysis, focusing particularly on problem bacterial pathogens in the nosocomial setting.

DEFINING EPIDEMIOLOGICAL INTERRELATIONSHIPS

It is important to emphasize that epidemiological investigation is essentially a context-driven process. Potential interactions between host, etiological agent, and environment *(1)* are assessed to determine causal interrelationships and define the nature of the outbreak—common source or continuing *(2)*. However, episodes of nosocomial infection are not characterized by advance warning. The index patient and associated bacterial isolates in a particular outbreak may be difficult or impossible to identify. Thus, the analysis must be conducted within the context of data from the available epidemiological window, *(3)* which may or may not include the outbreak source. Working backward in time, the result is conclusions that are often necessarily based on probabilities rather than absolutes. These constraints are important to remember when assessing the epidemiological interrelationships of bacterial isolates. In this context, it is important to look beyond attempts at rigid definitions of bacterial strain or type to highlight the true issue at hand: whether or not a series of clinical isolates represents the result of patient-to-patient transfer. In addressing this question, microbial characterization is only one piece of the epidemiological puzzle that must

From: *Pathogen Genomics: Impact on Human Health*
Edited by: K. J. Shaw © Humana Press Inc., Totowa, NJ

Table 1
Genomes of representative bacterial pathogens currently sequenced or in progress

Organism	Reference or Internet Link
Acinetobacter baumannii	http://www.genomecorp.com/programs/organisms.shtml
Bacillus anthracis	http://www.tigr.org
Bacteroides fragilis	http://www.sanger.ac.uk/Projects
	http://www.genomecorp.com/programs/organisms.shtml
Bordetella bronchiseptica	http://www.sanger.ac.uk/Projects
Bordetella parpertussis	http://www.sanger.ac.uk/Projects
Bordetella pertussis	http://www.sanger.ac.uk/Projects
Borrelia bergdorferi	(48)
	http://www.genomecorp.com/programs/organisms.shtml
Brucella abortus	http://www.cbc.umn.edu/ResearchProjects/Pm/index.html
Burkholderia cepacia	http://www.sanger.ac.uk/Projects
Burkholderia mallei	http://www.tigr.org
Burkholderia pseudomallei	http://www.sanger.ac.uk/Projects
Campylobacter jejuni	(49)
	http://www.genomecorp.com/programs/organisms.shtml
Chlamydia pneumoniae	(50–52)
	http://www.genomecorp.com/programs/organisms.shtml
Chlamydia psittaci	http://www.tigr.org
Chlamydia trachomatis	(50,51,53)
	http://www.genomecorp.com/programs/organisms.shtml
Clostridium botulinum	http://www.sanger.ac.uk/Projects
Clostridium difficile	http://www.sanger.ac.uk/Projects
Corynebacterium diphtheriae	http://www.sanger.ac.uk/Projects
Coxiella burnetii	http://www.tigr.org
Enterobacter cloacae	http://www.genomecorp.com/programs/organisms.shtml
Enterococcus faecalis	http://www.tigr.org
	http://www.genomecorp.com/programs/organisms.shtml
Enterococcus faecium	http://www.genomecorp.com/programs/organisms.shtml
Escherichia coli	(54–56)
	http://www.genomecorp.com/programs/organisms.shtml
Francisella tularensis	(57)
Haemophilus influenzae	(47)
	http://www.genomecorp.com/programs/organisms.shtml
Helicobacter pylori	(33,58)
	http://www.genomecorp.com/programs/organisms.shtml
Klebsiella pneumoniae	http://genome.wustl.edu/gsc/Projects/bacteria.shtml
	http://www.genomecorp.com/programs/organisms.shtml
Legionella pneumophila	http://genome3.cpmc.columbia.edu/~legion
Listeria monocytogenes	http://www.tigr.org
	http://www.pasteur.fr/recherche/unites/gmp
Moraxella catarrhalis	http://www.genomecorp.com/programs/organisms.shtml
Mycobacterium avium	http://www.tigr.org
Mycobacterium bovis	http://www.sanger.ac.uk/Projects
Mycobacterium leprae	(59)

(continued)

Table 1
(Continued)

Organism	Reference or Internet Link
Mycobacterium tuberculosis	*(60)*
	http://www.tigr.org
	http://www.genomecorp.com/programs/organisms.shtml
Mycoplasma genitalium	*(61)*
	http://www.genomecorp.com/programs/organisms.shtml
Mycoplasma pneumoniae	*(62)*
	http://www.genomecorp.com/programs/organisms.shtml
Neisseria gonorrhoeae	http://www.genome.ou.edu
Neisseria meningitidis	*(63)*;http://www.tigr.org
	http://www.genomecorp.com/programs/organisms.shtml
Pasteurella multocida	*(64)*
	http://www.cbc.umn.edu/ResearchProjects/Pm/index.html
Proteus mirabilis	http://www.genomecorp.com/programs/organisms.shtml
Pseudomonas aeruginosa	*(65)*
	http://www.genomecorp.com/programs/organisms.shtml
Rickettsia prowazekii	*(66)*
	http://www.genomecorp.com/programs/organisms.shtml
Salmonella dublin	http://salmonella.utmem.edu/
Salmonella enteritidis	http://salmonella.utmem.edu/
Salmonella paratyphi	http://genome.wustl.edu/gsc/Projects/bacteria.shtml
Salmonella typhi	http://www.sanger.ac.uk/Projects
Salmonella typhimurium	http://genome.wustl.edu/gsc/Projects/bacteria.shtml
Staphylococcus aureus	*(67)*;http://www.tigr.org;
	http://www.sanger.ac.uk/Projects
	http://www.genome.ou.edu
Staphylococcus epidermidis	http://www.tigr.org
	http://www.genomecorp.com/programs/organisms.shtml
Streptococcus agalactiae	http://www.pasteur.fr/recherche/unites/gmp
Streptococcus pneumoniae	*(68)*;http://www.tigr.org
	http://www.genomecorp.com/programs/organisms.shtml
Streptococcus pyogenes	*(69)*;http://www.sanger.ac.uk/Projects
Treponema pallidum	*(70)*
	http://www.genomecorp.com/programs/organisms.shtml
Ureaplasma urealyticum	*(71)*
Vibrio cholerae	*(72)*
Yersinia enterocolitica	http://www.sanger.ac.uk/Projects
Yersinia pestis	http://www.sanger.ac.uk/Projects

be put together with all the other available clinical data for accurate analysis. Thus, no matter how sophisticated (e.g., molecular) the approach, the utility of a method employed to characterize and assign isolate interrelationships must always ultimately be validated within the context of the total epidemiological picture. It must make (clinical) epidemiological sense.

EPIDEMIOLOGICAL ANALYSIS: MOVING
FROM PHENOTYPE TO GENOTYPE

Tests aimed at identifying epidemiologically related isolates have always reflected then-current technology, moving from phenotypic characterization to genotypic methods adapted from the molecular biology laboratory. In turn, the molecular approaches have evolved through several iterations *(3)*. As first-generation molecular epidemiology, plasmid fingerprinting had widespread use in isolate analysis. However, an emerging view of the bacterial chromosome as the fundamental molecule of cellular identity led to methods designed to more directly assess the genomic relatedness of isolates. Second-generation molecular epidemiology utilized restriction enzymes and probes for genomic comparisons, usually by characterizing the location and/or distribution of specific chromosomal sequences, such as insertion sequences or restriction-fragment-length polymorphisms (RFLP). This was followed by (third-generation) methods based on polymerase chain reaction (PCR) and pulsed-field gel electrophoresis (PFGE), currently the most common molecular approaches to epidemiological analysis.

PCR-based Genome Characterization

Random Chromosomal Analysis

PCR found initial epidemiological application utilizing primers and PCR conditions generally designed for low-stringency (and thus random) amplification of chromosomal sequences (i.e., randomly amplified polymorphic DNA (RAPD), arbitrarily primed PCR (APPCR) *(4,5)*. In theory, clinical isolates resulting from patient-to-patient transfer would be expected to exhibit a similar degree of randomness. Thus, this approach was expected to provide discrimination by producing a uniform set of random amplicons from the genomes of epidemiologically related vs unrelated isolates. However, the procedure has proven to be extremely susceptible to experimental variables such as template and primer concentrations, choice of thermocycler, and PCR reagents *(6)*. Difficulties with reproducibility and interpretation of amplicon-banding patterns on agarose gels have thus discouraged routine epidemiological use of this method. Binary typing is a process that begins with RAPD analysis, using bacterial isolates of the same species that are known to be epidemiologically unrelated. Unique amplicons, capable of strain differentiation, are cloned to produce a set of probe sequences. In subsequent isolate analysis, hybridization with each of the unique probes has a yes or no (plus or minus; binary) outcome that constitutes the binary type. This approach, which has thus far been validated only with *Staphylococcus aureus (7)*, appears suitable for data storage, portability, and analysis, but at the cost of significant up-front effort in probe construction and validation for various organisms to be analyzed.

Repetitive Sequence Distribution Analysis

Repeated sequences have been found in the genomes of numerous clinically important bacteria. For example, enterobacteria are known to contain several hundred copies of repetitive extragenic palindromic (REP) elements and enterobacterial repetitive intergenic consensus (ERIC) sequences *(8)*. BOX element sequences are repeated in the chromosome of *Streptococcus pneumoniae (9)*. Multiple IS256 copies are found in staphylococcal genomes *(10)*. These and other repeat elements represent genomic landmarks of known sequence to which PCR primers may be specifically anchored in an outwardly oriented fashion. The result is amplicon production, in which inter-repeat distances do not exceed the capability of the thermostable polymerase. Performed under relatively stringent conditions, these methods approach the epidemiological typing of isolates by comparing the chromosomal distribution of repeated elements as reflected by amplicon-banding patterns on agarose gels.

Epidemiological typing by Amplified Fragment Length Polymorphism (AFLP) analysis *(11)* is based on the genomic distribution of restriction enzyme sites combined with PCR. Originally developed for use with eukaryotic organisms, this method has been applied to the epidemiological analysis of several bacterial pathogens *(12–14)*. In this approach, chromosomal DNA is digested with two different restriction endonucleases, usually chosen so that one cuts more frequently than the other. Although a large group of restriction fragments is created, only specific subsets are utilized for isolate comparison. This is accomplished by linking adapter sequences to the ends of the restriction fragments, which extend the length of the known terminal sequences. PCR primers are designed to specifically hybridize with the adapter-restriction site sequence. However, the primer design incorporates one or two additional nucleotides (chosen at random) extending beyond the known sequence into the restriction fragment. Each primer nucleotide beyond the known adapter-restriction site reduces the potential size of the fragment subset that will be amplified. The specificity of the process is further controlled through labeled primers, ultimately leading to an electrophoretic pattern of amplified products that is used to analyze isolate interrelationships. The recent automation of the AFLP process (Autograph Microbial Characterization Systems; PE Biosystems, Foster City, California) has increased the appeal of this otherwise potentially demanding approach to epidemiological typing.

The molecular typing of *Mycobacterium tuberculosis* illustrates the effective use of another combined approach to epidemiological analysis. In most instances, isolate interrelationships in this organism are assessed by the strain-specific genomic distribution of the insertion sequence IS*6110*. This is accomplished by second-generation RFLP analysis, using chromosomal restriction-enzyme digests hybridized with an IS*6110* probe *(15)*. However, in instances of low IS*6110* copy number, isolates may be compared by splogiotyping *(16)*. This method is based on a polymorphism located within a unique Direct Repeat (DR) genomic region of *M. tuberculosis* complex bacteria. Within this locus, the directly repeated sequences are interspersed by DNA spacers, which generally are not repeated (e.g., >40 different spacer sequences). PCR amplicons of the DR region probed against a grid of various spacer sequences results in a pattern of hybridization (the splogiotype), which can be used to assess epidemiological interrelationships.

PFGE-Based Genome Characterization

Restriction enzymes with rare recognition sites in bacterial chromosomes have been described since the late 1970s. However, it was not until the 1980s that the large restriction fragments they produce were routinely resolved by an electrophoretic current pulsed in alternating directions for different lengths of time, (i.e., PFGE) *(17)*. As with second-generation chromosomal restriction-enzyme analysis (REA), restriction-fragment patterns from PFGE result from the specific spatial distribution of repeated restriction sequences around the bacterial chromosome. However, in contrast to REA, the ability of PFGE to resolve the large fragments produced by rare-cutting restriction enzymes yields patterns representing >90% of the bacterial chromosome *(18)*. Genomic differences between isolates that affect distances between rare restriction sites are visualized by PFGE as changes in restriction-fragment patterns which provide a sense of global chromosomal comparison (see ref. 4 for a detailed review of the influence of various genetic events on PFGE patterns). Present concerns regarding PFGE as an epidemiological tool relate to the time and expertise involved in DNA preparation and the interpretation of data *(3,4,19)*. Nevertheless, since chromosomal similarity is expected to correlate with epidemiological relatedness, the ability of PFGE to provide a general sense of genomic comparison has made it a powerful epidemiological tool, currently considered the method of choice (the gold standard) for the analysis of most bacterial pathogens *(3)*.

BEYOND PFGE AND PCR: *SEQUENCE-BASED MOLECULAR EPIDEMIOLOGY*

As stated previously, the bacterial chromosome represents the most fundamental molecule of identity in the cell. Thus, one would expect some form of chromosomal sequence analysis to be the most fundamental means of assessing potential interrelationships in nosocomial isolates. In theory, a comparison of total chromosomal sequence could be envisioned as the ultimate iteration of this approach. However, in practice this objective cannot presently be achieved in an epidemiologically relevant time frame. In addition, such a goal is probably not desirable because the data would include potentially confusing genomic noise (wobble), which would accumulate in even a single isolate over time. Nevertheless, rapid cycle sequencing and the random shotgun approach to total genome sequencing have clearly ushered in at least the beginning phase of fourth-generation molecular epidemiology, based on the search for nucleotide sequences with epidemiological relevance *(3)*. In comparison to previous typing methods, a sequence-based approach is attractive for several reasons.

Issues of Simplicity and Reproducibility

At present, molecular methods for epidemiological analysis involve a myriad of experimental variables including types of equipment, reagents, and differences in experimental protocols, all of which affect inter- and intra-laboratory reproducibility. With enough time and effort, any epidemiological method can be standardized as evidenced by classical bacteriophage typing of staphylococci *(20)* or the success of the nationwide PFGE Pulse-Net System for the investigation of food-borne outbreaks designed by the United States Centers for Disease Control and Prevention *(21)*. However, nucleotide-sequence analysis is a more straightforward process that can be performed in a more controlled, uniform, and reproducible manner with specific chromosomal loci.

Data Sharing and Storage

In most instances, data from third-generation epidemiological methods is generated as banding patterns of DNA fragments electrophoretically separated in agarose or acrylamide gels. Electronic storage and sharing of such data is possible through the use of bitmapped (e.g., .tiff, .jpeg) computer images. But the larger the number of isolates being surveyed, the more unwieldy the process can become. In addition, some form of nomenclature must be used to identify and interrelate isolate banding patterns, because it may be difficult to retrieve specific raw data in a large group of images (i.e., the banding pattern for an individual isolate). With large data sets, the use of appropriate computer software such as the GelCompar and BioNumerics programs (Applied Maths BVBA, Sint-Martens-Latem, Belgium) is essential to effectively manage this process. However, the framework within which the data is shared, stored, and retrieved is necessarily in the form of visual images and the limits that format imposes. Conversely, nucleotide sequences represent simple, highly portable, quaternary data that can be shared, stored, and retrieved with ease.

Detecting Significant Difference

The most crucial parameter of any typing method is its ability to detect significant (epidemiologically relevant) differences. Thus, with genotypic tests, one is attempting to utilize chromosomal similarity as a discriminator of isolate relatedness. Most genotypic methods, including PCR and PFGE, allow only indirect chromosomal comparisons, for which differences are related to changes in electrophoretic banding patterns. Despite computer programs (mentioned previously), which can assist in this process, there is always an element of end-user judgment that can affect the final evaluation. This situation is illustrated in Fig. 1, lane 1, with a PFGE gel, where one must decide whether the intensity of a specific (highlighted) band may represent a co-migrating doublet. In addition, with electrophoretic data, judgments must also commonly be made as to whether specific bands exhibit equivalent migration distances (highlighted in Fig. 1, lanes 4–5). In contrast, nucleotide sequence data represents a direct and unambiguous chromosomal comparison of the genomic region being analyzed.

Data Interpretation

Although related to the detection of significant difference, the interpretation of typing data poses an additional set of challenges common to all genotypic typing methods. As noted previously, nosocomial outbreaks are usually discovered in progress without a clearly defined original index isolate. The foundation for epidemiological assessment, the bacterial chromosome, is a dynamic molecule that can change over time through such processes as mutation or horizontal gene transfer. Thus, epidemiological typing is a study in interrelationships that becomes potentially more complicated the longer the organism persists in (and moves between) patients in a given clinical setting. Over time, the goal is no longer trying to interrelate parents and offspring, but isolates potentially much further down the family tree. The differences between these are the sum of the changes each exhibits from the parental type. With PFGE, for example, a single chromosomal change can alter the position of up to four restriction-fragments in a particular banding pattern *(4)*. Two such isolates, each independently derived from a common ancestor by different genetic events, would thus exhibit a discrepancy of eight band positions when compared by PFGE. Sequence-based molecular typing must deal with the same molecular dynamics, but simpler chromosomal events are monitored (e.g., single-base sequence changes). As shown theoretically in Fig. 2, the result is that single-mutation subtypes, differing from the original index isolate by one characteristic

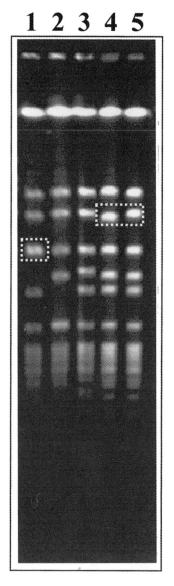

Fig. 1. Chromosomal macro-restriction fragments analyzed by PFGE. The boxed areas represent issues of interpretation (discussed in the text) related to (lane 1) single vs co-migrating fragments and (lanes 4–5) relative band-migration distances.

(nucleotide base), would vary from each other by only two base changes. In this example, even second-step subtypes would differ by only four nucleotides, thus making the reconstruction of interrelationships potentially less confusing, assuming that the chromosomal region being monitored exhibits an epidemiologically relevant rate of change (i.e., clock speed). Thus, for sequence-based characterization, the challenge is one of identifying a chromosomal region (or regions) that exhibits the proper balance of conserved vs variable sequence.

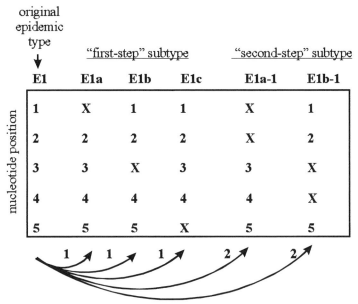

Fig. 2. Diagrammatic representation of nucleotide-sequence interrelationships in bacterial isolates, which differ from a common epidemic type by either one or two sequential mutations, indicated by an X at specific nucleotide positions. Bottom numbers and arrows indicate total nucleotide differences between individual subtypes and the original parent.

CURRENT APPROACHES TO SEQUENCE-BASED EPIDEMIOLOGICAL ANALYSIS

In recent years, the rapidly expanding database of sequence data on microbial genomes has served as the foundation for a variety of typing approaches. These efforts have focused on both single and multiple chromosomal loci.

Single-Locus Sequence Typing (SLST)

A comparison of sequence data for specific loci from different strains of the same organism has revealed several instances of variability, such as single-nucleotide polymorphisms (SNPs) or repeated regions, with potential epidemiological application. This has led to SLST protocols for microorganisms (Table 2) utilizing loci related to a variety of microbial characteristics including virulence, pathogenicity, and drug resistance. However, a number of these methods either await or show discrepancies in comparative evaluation with other molecular typing techniques such as PFGE *(22),* and require validation with isolates of known epidemiological interrelationships. Others such as *spa* typing in *S. aureus (23),* appear quite robust, with benefits in throughput and ease of use that tend to balance a level of epidemiological discrimination that may be somewhat less than that of established genotypic methods such as PFGE *(24).* At present, no specific SLST protocol has emerged as an unequivocal stand-alone approach to epidemiological typing. Nevertheless, SLST is attractive in its singular

Table 2
Examples of sequence-based epidemiological analysis

Chromosomal region	Organism	Reference
single-locus sequence typing		
flaA	*Camphylobacter jejuni*	*(25)*
omp1	*Chlamydia trachomatis*	*(73)*
gyrA, parC	*Klebsiella oxytoca*	*(74)*
gyrA, parC	*Klebsiella pneumoniae,*	*(74)*
gyrA	*Legionella pneumophila*	*(75)*
pvpA	*Mycoplasma gallisepticum*	*(76)*
porA, porB	*Neisseria meningitidis*	*(77,78)*
coa	*Staphylococcus aureus*	*(79,80)*
mec	*Staphylococcus aureus*	*(81)*
spaA	*Staphylococcus aureus*	*(23,24,82)*
emm	*Streptococcus pyogenes*	*(83,84)*
toxRS	*Vibrio parahaemolyticus*	*(85)*
multi-locus sequence typing		
aspA, glnA, gltA, glyA pgm, tkt, uncA	*Campylobacter jejuni*	*(86)*
adk, fuc, mdh, pgi, rec	*Haemophilus influenzae*	
http://www.mlst.net		
atpD, glnA, scoB, recA	*Helicobacter pylori*	*(87)*
abcZ, adk, aroE, funC, gdh, pdhC, pgm	*Neisseria meningitidis*	*(26)*
aroE, gdh, gki, recP, spi, xpt, ddl	*Streptococcus pneumoniae*	*(88)*
gki, gtr, murl, mutS, recP, xpt, yqiL	*Streptococcus pyogenes*	*(28)*
arcC, aroE, glpF, gmk, pta, pti, yqil	*Staphylococcus aureus*	*(27)*
16S–23S intergenic rDNA	various	*(89)*

focus and, at a minimum, currently represents an important potential means of preliminary characterization that can serve as an adjunct to more definitive genotyping
methods *(25)*.

Multi-Locus Sequence Typing (MLST)

Derived in principle from multi-locus enzyme electrophoresis (MLEE), MLST uti-
lizes a larger, and potentially more representative, portion of the genome than SLST.
MLST was originally described for *Neisseria meningitidis (26)*. However, the approach
has now been applied to a variety of other pathogens (Table 2), surveying a series of
housekeeping genes (usually seven) which, by their essential nature, are present with a
degree of stability in all isolates of a particular species. In evaluating MLST as a typing
method, it is important to remember that, like MLEE, the method was originally
designed to assess genetic interrelationships in bacterial populations with sufficient
opportunity over time for the sequence of housekeeping genes to diversify. As discussed previously, the epidemiological window of investigation often represents a relatively short time period. For this reason, one could expect MLST to be somewhat less
discriminating than typing methods in which surveillance is based on a more rapid
genomic clock. In the analysis of *S. aureus (27)* and *Streptococcus pyogenes (28)*, for

example, MLST has proven to be less sensitive than PFGE and *emm*-typing, respectively. Nevertheless, studies to date have shown that this method is capable of identifying general epidemiological interrelationships in bacterial populations. MLST thus demonstrates the potential of sequenced-based typing to generate consistent and reproducible isolate profiles that are highly amenable to standardization and database cataloging. However, as noted by others *(29)*, it is difficult to envision the present form of MLST in a real-time clinical setting because of the expense (i.e., equipment and sequencing costs), labor, and time involved in surveying greater than 2,500 bp of sequence for each isolate.

Although it is not commonly referred to as MLST, variable 16S-23S intergenic (ISR) spacer regions in the multiple rRNA operons of numerous bacterial species, have also served as a basis for epidemiological typing *(30)*. As with other MLST approaches, ISR typing surveys a region within an essential gene that is present in multiple locations around the genome. However, the method tends to suffer from the disadvantages of multiple-loci sequencing cited here, including cost, labor, and time. In addition, this approach has not been rigorously evaluated in comparison to currently used genotyping approaches such as PFGE and PCR.

THE FUTURE OF SEQUENCE-BASED TYPING IN THE AGE OF GENOMICS

In a sense, current SLST and MLST methods represent a first iteration of sequence-based typing developed, for the most part, without benefit of the currently available and rapidly expanding database of completed genomes. However, advances in genomics such as sequencing technology and bioinformatics in the years ahead will undoubtedly have a profound effect on epidemiological typing. At a minimum, one can envision this influence in two key areas: the discovery of epidemiologically relevant sequences and data throughput and analysis.

Sequence Discovery

The future will undoubtedly see genomes of numerous additional pathogens added to the current database (Table 1). This will obviously serve to broaden the scope of sequence-based typing. However, in addition to new organisms, there will be great value in analyzing additional strains of currently sequenced bacteria. Such data provides the investigator with a head start in the search for epidemiologically relevant loci, which should show disparity in unrelated, but not related, isolates. Complete and fully annotated genomes are the gold standard for analysis, because they allow comparison not only of individual loci, but overall gene organization and distribution, which could also have potential epidemiological significance. This is illustrated in Fig. 3, where the MUMmer *(31)* approach to whole-genome alignment (accessible at http://www.tigr.org) has been utilized to compare *Escherichia coli* 0157:H7 strains VT2-Sakai and EDL933. By varying the window size for minimum alignment length, one can move from a general genomic overview to higher-resolution comparison. Regions of interest can then be specifically examined for epidemiological utility by sequence analysis in additional bacterial strains. The years ahead will obviously see great advances in the throughput and computer-assisted analysis of complete genomes. However, it is important to note that high-quality draft sequences can also be

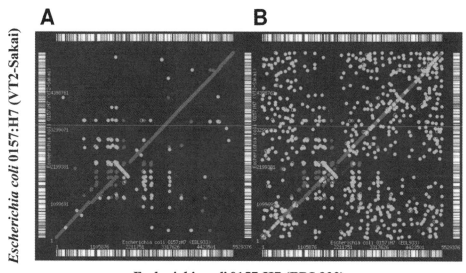

Escherichia coli 0157:H7 (EDL933)

Fig. 3. Graphic output of the MUMer computer algorithm for total genome alignment *(31)* comparing *Escherichia coli* 0157:H7 strain VT2-Sakai (vertical axis) and EDL933 (horizontal axis) using a minimum alignment length of either 100 or 20 bp (A and B, respectively). Alignments with the same orientation are shown in dark gray, and those with opposite orientations are shown in light gray. The output was originally generated on-line at *http://www.tigr.org*.

extremely useful in providing a multi-strain database of specific loci for comparison. Facilities such as the United States Department of Energy Joint Genome Institute (JGI) have demonstrated the present-day power of a dedicated effort in this area, producing 15 high-quality draft sequences from different microorganisms in a 1-mo period (http://www.jgi.doe.gov/News/news_11_2_00.htm). However, whether from draft or complete genomes, the ability to rapidly compare multiple copies of loci for potential epidemiological utility *(32,33)* is a process essential to the further development of sequence-based typing. For example, we have recently reported the potential usefulness of the DNA polymerase III gene in the epidemiological analysis of *S. aureus (34)*. As shown in Fig. 4, a comparison of this 4.3–kb region from complete (N315, Mu50) and draft (COL, 8325, GenBank D86727) sources demonstrates an interesting diversity moving toward the 3' direction. The potential epidemiological relevance of this observation is currently being validated in additional *S. aureus* isolates.

Data Throughput and Analysis

Although the assessment of isolate interrelationships in a specific outbreak may involve a relatively small number of samples, the desire to database information and survey larger populations (e.g., in a public health setting) is establishing a clear movement toward large data sets. This trend will drive sequence-based typing toward a minimum number of steps with the potential for automation (especially important in the clinical laboratory setting) while maintaining a high degree of accuracy. Once sequences are validated as epidemiologically relevant, the potential bottleneck clearly relates to data generation and analysis. This situation will probably be resolved by data

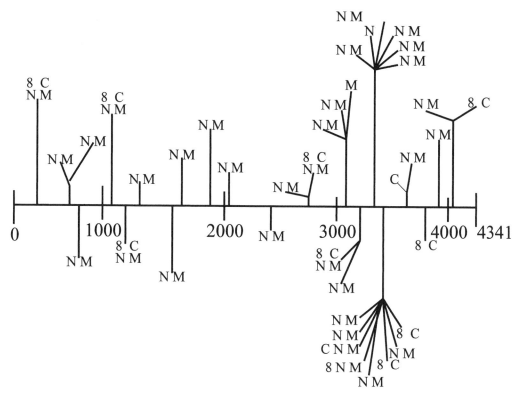

Fig. 4. Diagrammatic representation of nucleotide-sequence differences within the 4.3-kb DNA polymerase III gene in isolates of *Staphylococcus aureus.* Numbers on the horizontal line represent the sequence of GenBank accession number D86727. Letters indicate the relative position of nucleotide differences between D86727 and strains 8325 *(8),* COL **(C),** N315 **(N),** and Mu50 **(M)** (data obtained from *www.genome.ou.edu, www.tigr.org,* and ref. *(67),* respectively).

output in a form that reflects the sequence content with accuracy equivalent to or greater than direct sequencing, but with faster throughput. Advances in genomics will certainly drive the need for innovative approaches to sequence analysis, which may then find application in epidemiological typing. For example, new approaches for the detection of SNPs have been described, based on a variety of methods including allele-specific hybridization, allele-specific primer extension, allele-specific oligonucleotide ligation, allele-specific cleavage of a flap probe, molecular beacons, rolling-circle amplification, denaturing high-performance liquid chromatography (HPLC), and oligonucleotide microarrays, *(35–38).* Of these newer methods, microarrays appear especially promising for epidemiological application. Sequence-based typing will always involve the detection of more than one SNP or other genetic event in a group of isolates. Thus, the array format provides an important advantage in the simultaneous, rather than sequential, analysis of multiple genetic events. One can envision arrays designed in a reproducible organism-specific manner, in which the spatial distribution of the multicolored fluorescent output is not only an intuitive fingerprint to the naked eye, but is clearly amenable to computer analysis and databasing. In addition, the microchip may serve as a platform where previously separate elements of the typing process can be combined through methods such as on-chip amplification *(39,40)*, thus improving throughput and the potential for automation. Recent studies have reported the use of microarrays in viral epidemiology *(41,42)* and preliminary microbial typing based on the genomic distribution of insertion sequences *(43)*. Other non-epidemiological studies have reported whole-genome comparisons of bacteria using microarray analysis *(44–46)*, thus demonstrating the power of this technique to explore sequence-based microbial interrelationships. The refinement of this and other methods will undoubtedly have a major role in streamlining the process of sequence-based epidemiological typing in the future.

CONCLUSION: *MOLECULAR EPIDEMIOLOGY AND GENOMICS*

The first complete sequence of a microbial genome (i.e., *Haemophilus influenzae*), published by The Institute for Genomic Research in 1995 *(47)*, provided the incentive that has firmly ushered in sequence-based typing as the ultimate approach to epidemiological analysis. However, as stated previously, it is important to emphasize the point that, no matter how sophisticated the analytical method, epidemiology will always be a study in interrelationships without the intellectual satisfaction of an absolute yes-no answer. For this reason, it is essential that approaches to sequence-based typing are initially validated with epidemiologically characterized bacterial populations. Over the years, numerous collections of problem pathogens have been assembled where, by a combination of clinical, microbiological, and typing efforts, epidemiological interrelationships are known. To be of any value, at the outset, a typing method must affirm these interrelationships before being applied to the analysis of uncharacterized isolates. Sequence-based typing thus represents a quest for the most epidemiologically relevant loci, which current evidence suggests will vary between different bacterial species. Genomics has opened the door not only to the discovery of these sequences, but most certainly also to their optimized throughput and analysis. It is not an exaggeration to state that the result of this effort will have a major positive impact on the treatment of infectious disease worldwide.

REFERENCES

1. Jackson MM, Tweeten SM. General principles of epidemiology. APIC text of infection control and epidemiology. Washington, DC: Association for Professionals in Infection and Control and Epidemiology, Inc., 2000: 1–17.
2. Checko PJ. Outbreak investigation. APIC text of infection control and epidemiology. Washington, DC: Association for Professionals in Infection and Control and Epidemiology, Inc., 2000: 1–9.
3. Goering RV. The molecular epidemiology of nosocomial infection: past, present, and future. Rev Med Microbiol 2000; 11:145–152.
4. Goering RV. The molecular epidemiology of nosocomial infection: an overview of principles, application, and interpretation. In: Specter S, Bendinelli M, Friedman H, (eds). Rapid Detection of Infectious Agents. New York: Plenum Press, 1998, pp. 131–157.
5. Tenover FC, Arbeit RD, Goering RV. How to select and interpret molecular strain typing methods for epidemiological studies of bacterial infections: a review for healthcare epidemiologists. Infect Control Hosp Epidemiol 1997; 18:426–439.

6. Tyler KD, Wang G, Tyler SD, Johnson WM. Factors affecting reliability and reproducibility of amplification-based DNA fingerprinting of representative bacterial pathogens. J Clin Microbiol 1997; 35:339–346.

7. Van Leeuwen W, Verbrugh H, van der Velden J, van Leeuwen N, Heck M, Van Belkum A. Validation of binary typing for Staphylococcus aureus strains. J Clin Microbiol 1999; 37:664–674.

8. Versalovic J, Koeuth T, Lupski JR. Distribution of repetitive DNA sequences in eubacteria and application to fingerprinting of bacterial genomes. Nucleic Acids Res 1991; 19:6823–6831.

9. Van Belkum A, Sluijter M, De Groot R, Verbrugh H, Hermans PWM. Novel BOX repeat PCR assay for high-resolution typing of Streptococcus pneumoniae strains. J Clin Microbiol 1996; 34:1176–1179.

10. Deplano A, Vaneechoutte M, Verschraegen G, Struelens MJ. Typing of Staphylococcus aureus and Staphylococcus epidermidis strains by PCR analysis of Inter-IS256 spacer length polymorphisms. J Clin Microbiol 1997; 35:2580–2587.

11. Vos P, Hogers R, Bleeker M, Reijans M, Van de Lee T, Hornes M, et al. AFLP: A new technique for DNA fingerprinting. Nucleic Acids Res 1995; 23:4407–4414.

12. Van Eldere J, Janssen P, Hoefnagels-Schuermans A, Van Lierde S, Peetermans WE. Amplified-fragment length polymorphism analysis versus macro-restriction fragment analysis for molecular typing of Streptococcus pneumoniae isolates. J Clin Microbiol 1999; 37:2053–2057.

13. Nair S, Schreiber E, Thong KL, Pang T, Altwegg M. Genotypic characterization of Salmonella typhi by amplified fragment length polymorphism fingerprinting provides increased discrimination as compared to pulsed-field gel electrophoresis and ribotyping. J Microbiol Methods 2000; 41:35–43.

14. Rademaker JL, Hoste B, Louws FJ, Kersters K, Swings J, Vauterin L, et al. Comparison of AFLP and rep-PCR genomic fingerprinting with DNA-DNA homology studies: Xanthomonas as a model system. Int J Syst Evol Microbiol 2000; 50 Pt 2:665–677.

15. Van Embden JDA, Cave MD, Crawford JT, Dale JW, Eisenach KD, Gicquel B, et al. Strain identification of Mycobacterium tuberculosis by DNA fingerprinting: recommendations for a standardized methodology. J Clin Microbiol 1993; 31:406–409.

16. Goyal M, Saunders NA, van Embden JD, Young DB, Shaw RJ. Differentiation of Mycobacterium tuberculosis isolates by spoligotyping and IS6110 restriction fragment length polymorphism. J Clin Microbiol 1997; 35:647–651.

17. Schwartz DC, Saffran W, Welsh J, Haas R, Goldenberg M, Cantor CR. New techniques for purifying large DNA's and studying their properties and packaging. Cold Spring Harbor Symp Quant Biol 1983; 47:189–195.

18. Goering RV. Molecular strain typing for the clinical laboratory: current application and future direction. Clin Microbiol News 2000; 22:169–173.

19. Van Belkum A, Van Leeuwen W, Kaufmann ME, Cookson B, Forey F, Etienne J, et al. Assessment of resolution and intercenter reproducibility of results of genotyping Staphylococcus aureus by pulsed-field gel electrophoresis of SmaI macrorestriction fragments: a multicenter study. J Clin Microbiol 1998; 36:1653–1659.

20. Bannerman TL, Hancock GA, Tenover FC, Miller JM. Pulsed-field gel electrophoresis as a replacement for bacteriophage typing of Staphylococcus aureus. J Clin Microbiol 1995; 33:551–555.

21. Swaminathan B, Barrett TJ, Hunter SB, Tauxe RV. PulseNet: the molecular subtyping network for foodborne bacterial disease surveillance, United States. Emerg Infect Dis 2001; 7:382–389.

22. Winstanley C, Shina A, Dawson S, Gaskell RM, Hart CA. Variation in Bordetella bronchiseptica flaA does not correlate with typing by macro-restriction analysis by pulsed-field gel electrophoresis. J Med Microbiol 2001; 50:255–260.

23. Shopsin B, Gomez M, Montgomery SO, Smith DH, Waddington M, Dodge DE, et al. Evaluation of protein A gene polymorphic region DNA sequencing for typing of Staphylococcus aureus strains. J Clin Microbiol 1999; 37:3556–3563.

24. Oliveira DC, Crisostomo I, Santos-Sanches I, Major P, Alves CR, Aires-de-Sousa M, et al. Comparison of DNA sequencing of the protein A gene polymorphic region with other molecular typing techniques for typing two epidemiologically diverse collections of methicillin-resistant Staphylococcus aureus. J Clin Microbiol 2001; 39:574–580.

25. Fitzgerald C, Helsel LO, Nicholson MA, Olsen SJ, Swerdlow DL, Flahart R, et al. Evaluation of methods for subtyping Campylobacter jejuni during an outbreak involving a food handler. J Clin Microbiol 2001; 39:2386–2390.

26. Maiden MCJ, Bygraves JA, Feil E, Morelli G, Russell JE, Urwin R, et al. Multilocus sequence typing: a portable approach to the identification of clones within populations of pathogenic microorganisms. Proc Natl Acad Sci USA 1998; 95:3140–5145.

27. Enright MC, Day NP, Davies CE, Peacock SJ, Spratt BG. Multilocus sequence typing for characterization of methicillin-resistant and methicillin-susceptible clones of Staphylococcus aureus. J Clin Microbiol 2000; 38:1008–1015.

28. Enright MC, Spratt BG, Kalia A, Cross JH, Bessen DE. Multilocus sequence typing of Streptococcus pyogenes and the relationships between emm type and clone. Infect Immun 2001; 69:2416–2427.

29. Shopsin B, Kreiswirth BN. Molecular epidemiology of methicillin-resistant Staphylococcus aureus. Emerg Infect Dis 2001; 7:323–326.

30. Gurtler V, Stanisich VA. New approaches to typing and identification of bacteria using the 16S-23S rDNA spacer region. Microbiology 1996; 142:3–16.

31. Delcher AL, Kasif S, Fleischmann RD, Peterson J, White O, Salzberg SL. Alignment of whole genomes. Nucleic Acids Res 1999; 27:2369–2376.

32. Oggioni MR, Pozzi G. Comparative genomics for identification of clone-specific sequence blocks in Streptococcus pneumoniae. FEMS Microbiol Lett 2001; 200:137–143.

33. Alm RA, Ling LS, Moir DT, King BL, Brown ED, Doig PC, et al. Genomic-sequence comparison of two unrelated isolates of the human gastric pathogen Helicobacter pylori. Nature 1999; 397:176–180.

34. Cooper KLF, Goering RV, Robinson MJ, Schmitt TJ. A novel approach to the molecular strain typing of methicillin-resistant Staphylococcus aureus (MRSA) based on a comparative analysis of DNA polymerase III and DNA gyrase gene variability. Abstr Annu Meeting Amer Soc Microbiol 2001; C74 p. 164–165.

35. Shi MM. Enabling large-scale pharmacogenetic studies by high-throughput mutation detection and genotyping technologies. Clin Chem 2001; 47:164–172.

36. Kwok PY. High-throughput genotyping assay approaches. Pharmacogenomics 2000; 1:95–100.

37. Hecker KH, Asea A, Kobayashi K, Green S, Tang D, Calderwood SK. Mutation detection in the human HSP7OB′ gene by denaturing high-performance liquid chromatography. Cell Stress Chaperones 2000; 5:415–424.

38. Gilles PN, Wu DJ, Foster CB, Dillon PJ, Chanock SJ. Single nucleotide polymorphic discrimination by an electronic dot blot assay on semiconductor microchips. Nat Biotechnol 1999; 17:365–370.

39. Westin L, Miller C, Vollmer D, Canter D, Radtkey R, Nerenberg M, et al. Antimicrobial resistance and bacterial identification utilizing a microelectronic chip array. J Clin Microbiol 2001; 39:1097–1104.

40. Tillib SV, Strizhkov BN, Mirzabekov AD. Integration of multiple PCR amplifications and DNA mutation analyses by using oligonucleotide microchip. Anal Biochem 2001; 292:155–160.

41. Li J, Chen S, Evans DH. Typing and subtyping influenza virus using DNA microarrays and multiplex reverse transcriptase PCR. J Clin Microbiol 2001; 39:696–704.

42. Vinje J, Koopmans MP. Simultaneous detection and genotyping of "Norwalk-like viruses" by oligonucleotide array in a reverse line blot hybridization format. J Clin Microbiol 2000; 38:2595–2601.

43. Raychaudhuri S, Stuart JM, Liu X, Small PM, Altman RB. Pattern recognition of genomic features with microarrays: site typing of Mycobacterium tuberculosis strains. Proc Int Conf Intell Syst Mol Biol 2000; 8:286–295.

44. Fitzgerald JR, Sturdevant DE, Mackie SM, Gill SR, Musser JM. Evolutionary genomics of Staphylococcus aureus: insights into the origin of methicillin-resistant strains and the toxic shock syndrome epidemic. Proc Natl Acad Sci USA 2001; 98:8821–8826.

45. Behr MA, Wilson MA, Gill WP, Salamon H, Schoolnik GK, Rane S, et al. Comparative genomics of BCG vaccines by whole-genome DNA microarray. Science 1999; 284:1520–1523.

46. Salama N, Guillemin K, McDaniel TK, Sherlock G, Tompkins L, Falkow S. A whole-genome microarray reveals genetic diversity among Helicobacter pylori strains. Proc Natl Acad Sci USA 2000; 97:14,668–14,673.

47. Fleischmann RD, Adams MD, White O, Clayton RA, Kirkness EF, Kerlavage AR, et al. Whole-genome random sequencing and assembly of Haemophilus influenzae Rd. Science 1995; 269:496–512.

48. Fraser CM, Casjens S, Huang WM, Sutton GG, Clayton R, Lathigra R, et al. Genomic sequence of a Lyme disease spirochaete, Borrelia burgdorferi. Nature 1997; 390:580–586.

49. Parkhill J, Wren BW, Mungall K, Ketley JM, Churcher C, Basham D, et al. The genome sequence of the food-borne pathogen Campylobacter jejuni reveals hypervariable sequences. Nature 2000; 403:665–668.

50. Read TD, Brunham RC, Shen C, Gill SR, Heidelberg JF, White O, et al. Genome sequences of Chlamydia trachomatis MoPn and Chlamydia pneumoniae AR39. Nucleic Acids Res 2000; 28:1397–1406.

51. Kalman S, Mitchell W, Marathe R, Lammel C, Fan J, Hyman RW, et al. Comparative genomes of Chlamydia pneumoniae and C. trachomatis. Nat Genet 1999; 21:385–389.

52. Shirai M, Hirakawa H, Kimoto M, Tabuchi M, Kishi F, Ouchi K, et al. Comparison of whole genome sequences of Chlamydia pneumoniae J138 from Japan and CWL029 from USA. Nucleic Acids Res 2000; 28:2311–2314.

53. Stephens RS, Kalman S, Lammel C, Fan J, Marathe R, Aravind L, et al. Genome sequence of an obligate intracellular pathogen of humans: Chlamydia trachomatis. Science 1998; 282:754–759.

54. Blattner FR, Plunkett G, III, Bloch CA, Perna NT, Burland V, Riley M, et al. The complete genome sequence of Escherichia coli K-12. Science 1997; 277:1453–1474.

55. Perna NT, Plunkett G, III, Burland V, Mau B, Glasner JD, Rose DJ, et al. Genome sequence of enterohaemorrhagic Escherichia coli O157:H7. Nature 2001; 409:529–533.

56. Hayashi T, Makino K, Ohnishi M, Kurokawa K, Ishii K, Yokoyama K, et al. Complete genome sequence of enterohemorrhagic Escherichia coli O157:H7 and genomic comparison with a laboratory strain K-12 (supplement). DNA Res 2001; 8:47–52.

57. Karlsson J, Prior RG, Williams K, Lindler L, Brown KA, Chatwell N, et al. Sequencing of the Francisella tularensis strain Schu 4 genome reveals the shikimate and purine metabolic pathways, targets for the construction of a rationally attenuated auxotrophic vaccine. Microb Comp Genomics 2000; 5:25–39.

58. Tomb JF, White O, Kerlavage AR, Clayton RA, Sutton GG, Fleischmann RD, et al. The complete genome sequence of the gastric pathogen Helicobacter pylori. Nature 1997; 388:539–547.

59. Cole ST, Eiglmeier K, Parkhill J, James KD, Thomson NR, Wheeler PR, et al. Massive gene decay in the leprosy bacillus. Nature 2001; 409:1007–1011.

60. Cole ST, Brosch R, Parkhill J, Garnier T, Churcher C, Harris D, et al. Deciphering the biology of Mycobacterium tuberculosis from the complete genome sequence. Nature 1998; 393:537–544.

61. Fraser CM, Gocayne JD, White O, Adams MD, Clayton RA, Fleischmann RD, et al. The minimal gene complement of Mycoplasma genitalium. Science 1995; 270:397–403.

62. Himmelreich R, Hilbert H, Plagens H, Pirkl E, Li BC, Herrmann R. Complete sequence analysis of the genome of the bacterium Mycoplasma pneumoniae. Nucleic Acids Res 1996; 24:4420–4449.

63. Parkhill J, Achtman M, James KD, Bentley SD, Churcher C, Klee SR, et al. Complete DNA sequence of a serogroup A strain of Neisseria meningitidis Z2491. Nature 2000; 404:502–506.

64. May BJ, Zhang Q, Li LL, Paustian ML, Whittam TS, Kapur V. Complete genomic sequence of Pasteurella multocida, Pm70. Proc Natl Acad Sci USA 2001; 98:3460–3465.

65. Stover CK, Pham XQ, Erwin AL, Mizoguchi SD, Warrener P, Hickey MJ, et al. Complete genome sequence of Pseudomonas aeruginosa PA01, an opportunistic pathogen. Nature 2000; 406:959–964.

66. Andersson SG, Zomorodipour A, Andersson JO, Sicheritz-Ponten T, Alsmark UC, Podowski RM, et al. The genome sequence of Rickettsia prowazekii and the origin of mitochondria. Nature 1998; 396:133–140.

67. Kuroda M, Ohta T, Uchiyama I, Baba T, Yuzawa H, Kobayashi L, et al. Whole genome sequencing of methicillin-resistant Staphylococcus aureus. Lancet 2001; 357:1225–1240.

68. Dopazo J, Mendoza A, Herrero J, Caldara F, Humbert Y, Friedli L, et al. Annotated draft genomic sequence from a Streptococcus pneumoniae type 19F clinical isolate. Microb Drug Resist 2001; 7:99–125.

69. Ferretti JJ, McShan WM, Ajdic D, Savic DJ, Savic G, Lyon K, et al. Complete genome sequence of an M1 strain of Streptococcus pyogenes. Proc Natl Acad Sci USA 2001; 98:4658–4663.

70. Fraser CM, Norris SJ, Weinstock GM, White O, Sutton GG, Dodson R, et al. Complete genome sequence of Treponema pallidum, the syphilis spirochete. Science 1998; 281:375–388.

71. Glass JI, Lefkowitz EJ, Glass JS, Heiner CR, Chen EY, Cassell GH. The complete sequence of the mucosal pathogen Ureaplasma urealyticum. Nature 2000; 407:757–762.

72. Heidelberg JF, Eisen JA, Nelson WC, Clayton RA, Gwinn ML, Dodson RJ, et al. DNA sequence of both chromosomes of the cholera pathogen Vibrio cholerae. Nature 2000; 406:477–483.

73. Takourt B, de Barbeyrac B, Khyatti M, Radouani F, Bebear C, Dessus-Babus S, et al. Direct genotyping and nucleotide sequence analysis of VS1 and VS2 of the Omp1 gene of Chlamydia trachomatis from Moroccan trachomatous specimens. Microbes Infect 2001; 3:459–466.

74. Brisse S, Verhoef J. Phylogenetic diversity of Klebsiella pneumoniae and Klebsiella oxytoca clinical isolates revealed by randomly amplified polymorphic DNA, gyrA and parC genes sequencing and automated ribotyping. Int J Syst Evol Microbiol 2001; 51:915–924.

75. Feddersen A, Meyer HG, Matthes P, Bhakdi S, Husmann M. GyrA sequence-based typing of Legionella. Med Microbiol Immunol (Berl) 2000; 189:7–11.

76. Liu T, Garcia M, Levisohn S, Yogev D, Kleven SH. Molecular variability of the adhesin-encoding gene pvpA among Mycoplasma gallisepticum strains and its application in diagnosis. J Clin Microbiol 2001; 39:1882–1888.

77. Jelfs J, Munro R, Wedege E, Caugant DA. Sequence variation in the porA gene of a clone of Neisseria meningitidis during epidemic spread. Clin Diagn Lab Immunol 2000; 7:390–395.

78. Bash MC, Lynn F, Concepcion NF, Tappero JW, Carlone GM, Frasch CE. Genetic and immunologic characterization of a novel serotype 4, 15 strain of Neisseria meningitidis. FEMS Immunol Med Microbiol 2000; 29:169–176.

79. Shopsin B, Gomez M, Waddington M, Riehman M, Kreiswirth BN. Use of coagulase gene (coa) repeat region nucleotide sequences for typing of methicillin-resistant Staphylococcus aureus strains. J Clin Microbiol 2000; 38:3453–3456.

80. Kanemitsu K, Yamamoto H, Takemura H, Kaku M, Shimada J. Characterization of MRSA transmission in an emergency medical center by sequence analysis of the 3′-end region of the coagulase gene. J Infect Chemother 2001; 7:22–27.

81. Nahvi MD, Fitzgibbon JE, John JF, Dubin DT. Sequence analysis of dru regions from methicillin-resistant Staphylococcus aureus and coagulase-negative staphylococcal isolates. Microb Drug Resist 2001; 7:1–12.

82. Tang YW, Waddington MG, Smith DH, Manahan JM, Kohner PC, Highsmith LM, et al. Comparison of protein A gene sequencing with pulsed-field gel electrophoresis and epidemiologic data for molecular typing of methicillin-resistant Staphylococcus aureus. J Clin Microbiol 2000; 38:1347–1351.

83. Beall B, Gherardi G, Lovgren M, Facklam RR, Forwick BA, Tyrrell GJ Temm and sof gene sequence variation in relation to serological typing of opacity-factor-positive group A streptococci. Microbiology 2000; 146 (Pt 5):1195–1209.

84. Dicuonzo G, Gherardi G, Lorino G, Angeletti S, De Cesaris M, Fiscarelli E, et al. Group a streptococcal genotypes from pediatric throat isolates in Rome, Italy. J Clin Microbiol 2001; 39:1687–1690.

85. Matsumoto C, Okuda J, Ishibashi M, Iwanaga M, Garg P, Rammamurthy T, et al. Pandemic spread of an O3:K6 clone of Vibrio parahaemolyticus and emergence of related strains evidenced by arbitrarily primed PCR and toxRS sequence analyses. J Clin Microbiol 2000; 38:578–585.

86. Dingle KE, Colles FM, Wareing DR, Ure R, Fox AJ, Bolton FE, et al. Multilocus sequence typing system for Campylobacter jejuni. J Clin Microbiol 2001; 39:14–23.

87. Maggi SN, Bernasconi MV, Valsangiacomo C, Van Doorn LJ, Piffaretti JC. Population genetics of Helicobacter pylori in the southern part of Switzerland analysed by sequencing of four housekeeping genes (atpD, glnA, scoB and recA), and by vacA, cagA, iceA and IS605 genotyping. Microbiology 2001; 147:1693–1707.

88. Feil EJ, Smith JM, Enright MC, Spratt BG. Estimating recombinational parameters in Streptococcus pneumoniae from multilocus sequence typing data. Genetics 2000; 154:1439–1450.

89. Gurtler V. The role of recombination and mutation in 16S-23S rDNA spacer rearrangements. Gene 1999; 238:241–252.

Borrelia Genomics as a Tool for Studying Pathogenesis and Vaccine Development

Alireza Shamaei-Tousi and Sven Bergström

INTRODUCTION

The classical approach to vaccine development requires cultivation of the pathogenic microorganism and concomitant biochemical, serological, and microbiological methods to identify the components important for immunity. This scheme has been successful in many cases, although it is both time-consuming and time-intensive in terms of labor. Whole-genome sequencing has revolutionized the search for vaccine candidates, as it will be possible to predict all of the antigens, independent of their abundance and immunogenicity. This strategy will reduce the need for growth of the pathogen in vitro and for time-consuming biochemical, serological, and microbiological work. The resulting increase in our knowledge of the pathogenicity and virulence of pathogenic microorganisms will facilitate the ease and probability of success in vaccine development. Since this process of vaccine discovery uses sequence information rather than the biological characteristics of the pathogen, it has been named reverse vaccinology *(1–3)*. This approach to vaccine development could also be a tool to develop new vaccine candidates for infections caused by relapsing fever (RF) *Borrelia* spirochetes and for the development of second-generation vaccine candidates of Lyme disease (LD) *Borrelia*. This chapter examines how the genome sequence of *B. burgdorferi* has increased our understanding of the biology of *Borrelia* spirochetes, and how this knowledge can be used in vaccine development.

BRIEF HISTORY OF *BORRELIA*

RF is an arthropod-borne disease caused by spirochetes that belong to the genus *Borrelia*. Although described in ancient Greece *(4)*, it was not until 1868 that Otto Obermeier, a German scientist in Berlin, identified spirochetes as the cause of RF. These were named *Spirocheta obermeieri* after him, but were later renamed as *Borrelia recurrentis*.

During the second half of the nineteenth and first half the twentieth century, scientists in different parts of the world studied RF extensively. The disease was also used by earlier immunologists as a model for the study of the immune response, which attracted some of the pioneers in the fields such as Metchnikoff, Gabritchewsky, and Ehrlich.

From: *Pathogen Genomics: Impact on Human Health*
Edited by: K. J. Shaw © Humana Press Inc., Totowa, NJ

One reason for the interest in RF during the Second World War and thereafter is the seriousness of the disease and its resulting high mortality. Another reason for the attraction to this field was European colonization. During that time, Europeans experienced different epidemics of louse-borne disease in Asia and Africa. Interest in this field declined rapidly after the Second World War, until the beginning of the 1980s, when a new *Borrelia* infection—Lyme disease—was discovered.

The agent of LD, *B. burgdorferi,* was initially isolated in New York *(5),* yet there is evidence indicating that Lyme borreliosis was common in more ancient civilizations. For example, after macroscopic, radiographic, and histologic examination, Lewis could show that treponemal infection was present in the 16ST1 Tchefuncte Indian burial population, dated 500 BC–300 AD. Additionally, *B. burgdorferi* was the infectious agent responsible for the prevalence of adult rheumatoid arthritis in this population, and *B. burgdorferi* antibody provided partial immunity to the related spirochete *Treponema pallidum (6).*

GENERAL CLINICAL SIGNS

The first manifestation of LD is often a skin rash that grows radially from the site of the tick bite, the so-called erythema migrans (EM). EM is also associated with flu-like symptoms such as fever, muscle pain, and headache. Without treatment, the infection may disseminate and cause various neurological symptoms including meningitis and arthritis. In severe cases, the infection can become chronic and then become associated with neurological disorder, atrophy of the skin, or arthritis. A small percentage of patients with severe subacute Lyme arthritis will subsequently develop chronic arthritis, which is characterized by persistence in a single joint for greater than 12 mo and is unresponsive to antibiotic therapy.

The clinical hallmark of RF is a period of high fever followed by relative well-being. The incubation period is 5–8 d in louse-borne RF, whereas it varies extensively with the infecting species in tick-borne RF. During the febrile period, numerous spirochetes circulate in the blood (spirochetemia). Between fever peaks, no spirochetemia is detected. The fever pattern and recurrent spirochetemia are the consequence of antigenic variation of the bacteria's major outer surface proteins called Vmp (variable major protein). Patients often complain of headache, backache, muscle pain, arthralgia, and abdominal pain in addition of fever. Sometimes clinical examination can reveal jaundice, tenderness of the liver, and spleen with or without hepatosplenomegaly. Progressive weakness and weight loss can occur if successive relapses occur without sufficient treatment.

CHARACTERISTICS OF THE GENUS *BORRELIA*

General Characteristics

Borreliae are helical-shaped like all other spirochetes, with an outer membrane that surrounds the protoplasmic cylinder complex *(7).* Structural and genomic features clearly separate this phylum from other eubacteria. All *Borrelia* species are transmitted to vertebrates by hematophagous arthropods, and have a genomic DNA guanosine-cytosine content between 27% and 32%.

The classification of *Borrelia* has mostly been based on the specificity of the parasite-vector relationship. For example, *B. crocidurae* and *B. anserina* cannot be

Table 1
Human pathogenic relapsing fever *Borreliae* and Lyme disease *Borreliae*
with their respective vectors and geographical distribution

Borrelia species	Vector	Geographical district
B. burgdorferi	*Ixodes ricinus complex*	Europe and North America
B. garinii	*I. ricinus complex*	Europe and parts of Asia
B. afzelii	*I. ricinus complex*	Europe and parts of Asia
B. recurrentis	*Pediculus humanus*	Virtually worldwide
B. hispanica	*Ornithodoros erraticus*	Spain, Portugal, Greece, Cyprus, North Africa
B. crocidurae	*O. sonrai*	From West Africa to Northeast Africa, Middle East to Iran
B. persica	*O. tholozani*	Middle East
B. duttoni	*O. moubata*	East and Central Africa
B. hermsii	*O. hermsii*	Western US, British Columbia
B. turicatae	*O. turicata*	Mexico, Kansas, Texas
B. parkeri	*O. parkeri*	Western US
B. uzbekistania	*O. papillipes*	Tadjikstan, Uzbekistan
B. venezuelensis	*O. rudis*	Central America and northern South America
B. anserina	*Argas persicus*	Worldwide
B. coriaceae	*O. coriaceus*	US
B. lonestari[1]	Amblyomma americanum	Southern US
B. miyamotoi[1]	Ixodes persulcatus	Japan
Spanish isolate[2]	Unknown	Spain

[1] Not well-characterized and unknown pathogenicity

[2] Unknown pathogenicity

effectively transmitted by each other's natural vectors, *Ornitbodoros sonrai* and *Argas persicus,* respectively.

Phylogeny of Borrelia

Spirochetes within the genus *Borrelia* are divided into three pathogenic groups (Table 1): LD *Borrelia,* RF *Borrelia,* and the animal spirochetosis agent's *B. anserina* and *B. coriaceae (8,9).*

The members of the LD *Borrelia* complex consist of ten different species: *B. burgdorferi, B. afzelii, B. garinii, B. japonica, B. andersonii, B. valaisiana, B. turdii, B. tanukii, B. lusitaniae,* and *B. bissettii.* Among those, *B. burgdorferi, B. afzelii,* and *B. garinii* are known as human pathogens. *B. garinii* is the most heterogeneous species and has the largest geographical coverage, possibly resulting from being the most ancient species *(10).*

Using pulsed-field gel electrophoresis, *(PFGE),* PCR *(11),* and *osp*C gene-sequence analysis *(10)* of several *Borrelia* strains isolated in Europe and in the United States, it was shown that the North American strains were more heterogeneous than Europeans strains. These data suggest that the *B. burgdorferi* sensu stricto might have evolved in North America. Migrating birds may have served as a vehicle for the evolutionary divergence of these spirochetes. Once introduced into a new region, the spirochetes may have further evolved to adapt to new host reservoirs, ticks, and other ecological niches *(12)*.

To show the diversity of *Borrelia* species, Fukunaga et al. used the flagellin gene to construct a neighbor-joining phylogenetic analysis that showed that the genus *Borrelia* was divided into three clusters *(9)*. The LD borreliae, *B. burgdorferi, B. afzelii,* and *B. garinii* were tightly linked in one cluster. The second cluster contained the Old World tick-borne RF borreliae, *B. crocidurae, B. duttoni, B. hispanica,* and the *Borrelia* species from Spain *(9)*. In this group *B. crocidurae* and *B. duttoni* were 99.6% identical. The last group consisted of the New World tick-borne RF borreliae (*B. hermsii, B. turicatae,* and *B. parkeri*) and the animal spirochetosis agents, as well as *B. miyamotoi* and *B. lonestari*. The finding of the latter two borreliae within this group argue against the assumption that the hard-shelled ticks are the vectors for LD *Borrelia,* since the LD agents do not cluster with any other borreliae that are transmitted by hard-shelled ticks or lice. Thus, the RF borreliae may have evolved from a common ancestor, whereas *B. miyamotoi* and *B. lonestari* have adapted to ixodid ticks.

Genome Sequence and Organization

The etiological agent of LD, *B. burgdorferi,* has attracted great attention during the 1980s and 1990s. The nearly completed sequence of the eubacterial phylum spirochete was first reported by Fraser et al., 1997, and the completed sequence of *B. burgdorferi* containing additional circular and linear plasmids was published in 2000 *(13,14)*.

The genome size of *B. burgdorferi* is rather small compared to many known pathogens such as *Escherichia coli* and *Mycobacterium tuberculosis*. It has a low guanine and cytosine content of 28–30.5 mole % *(13,15,16)*, separating the *Borrelia* from the genera of *Treponema* and *Leptospira* *(17)*.

The sequencing of the *B. burgdorferi* B31 genome revealed a total genome size of 1.52 Mbp; 910,725 bp on a linear chromosome, and 610 kbp divided on 12 linear and 9 circular plasmids. This genetic organization is unusual among prokaryotes *(13,18–26)*. A linear chromosome has only been described in two other eubacteria, *Streptomyces lividans (27)* and *Agrobacterium tumefaciens (28),* yet linear plasmids have been observed in *Streptomyces* spp. *Rhodococcus fascians,* and *Thiobacillus versutus (29–31)*. The vast majority of bacterial species have a circular chromosome and circular plasmids. The ends of the *Borrelia* chromosome and linear plasmids are covalently closed loops similar to eukaryotic telomeres *(25,32)*.

Only 1283 putative genes were identified in *B. burgdorferi (13),* as compared with the 4405 genes present in *E. coli (33,34)*. The small number of genes in *B. burgdorferi* is similar to the number of genes in the related spirochete *T. pallidum (35)* and the obligate intracellular bacterium *Mycoplasma genitalium (36)*. As in *T. pallidum* and *M. genitalium,* a number of genes encoding cellular biosynthetic enzymes are missing in *B. burgdorferi* B31. Because *Mycoplasma* and spirochetes are only distantly related, the limited metabolic capacity probably reflects convergent evolution by the loss of genes, allowed by the parasitic lifestyle of these bacteria.

The linear chromosome of *B. burgdorferi* contains 853 genes, encoding proteins involved in fundamental processes such as replication, transcription, translation, energy metabolism, and transport across the membranes. The average size of the open reading frames (ORFs) was 992 bp, and 93% of the genome was found within coding sequences. The G-C content of only 28.6% of the *Borrelia* chromosome was confirmed, and all 61 possible codon triplets were used, with a marked bias toward the AU-rich triplets. *(13,15,17,37)*. The genome-sequence analysis revealed two surprising findings: first, a lack of ortholog of invasion genes, global regulatory systems, toxins, and two-component signal transduction seen in other bacteria, and second, the presence of a mystifying array of duplicated lipoproteins that are unique to *Borrelia,* and have no known function.

Each linear plasmid of *Borrelia* has a copy number of approximately one per chromosome *(22,38),* and many plasmids appear to contain homologous regions of DNA *(26,39–42).*

In vitro cultivation (10–17 passages) often results in the loss of some plasmids. Thus, it is likely that the many plasmid-encoded genes are nonessential for growth in vitro. However, plasmid loss mediates changes in protein expression and a loss of the ability to infect laboratory animals *(43–45).* Low-passage strains are therefore often more virulent than are high-passage strains; thus, these plasmids may encode key virulence determinants and/or proteins involved in infection and immune evasion. This hypothesis is supported by the observation that *B. burgdorferi* contains plasmid-encoded genes, which are selectively expressed during infection of mammalian hosts *(46–48).* The plasmids mainly contain unique *Borrelia* genes with unknown function. In fact, 14.5% of the plasmid-borne genes encode the putative lipoproteins that may be involved in host-parasite interactions. Some plasmids have a high fraction of pseudogenes, possibly reflecting an ongoing rapid evolution *(14).*

Genetic Tools

Despite the significance as human pathogens, the spirochete genetics is still in its infancy, and many future advances in *Borrelia* pathogenesis research will come from experimental observations in the laboratory. However, this will not be achieved until effective, reliable methods to mutagenize specific genes have been developed. Until recently, genetic studies in *Borrelia* have been hindered by the lack of an exogenous selectable marker, low transformation frequency, and difficulties in growing *Borrelia* on solid medium. The first selectable marker used for *B. burgdoferi* was *gyrB*[r], a mutated form of the chromosomal *gyrB* gene that encodes the B subunit of DNA gyrase and confers resistance to the antibiotic coumermycin A$_1$ *(49,50).* The use of coumermycin as selectable marker is limited by a high frequency of recombination with the endogenous *gyrB* gene. A major improvement by Bono and colleagues *(51)* was the development of an efficient marker for mutant selection in *B. burgdorferi.* By linking the *B. burgdorferi flaB* or *flgB* promoter with the *kan* gene from Tn*903,* transformants could be selected that were resistant to high levels of kanamycin. To date, gene inactivation has not been achieved in an infectious strain, and therefore analysis of phenotypes important in critical to infection has not been possible.

Shuttle vectors have also been developed for *B. burgdorferi,* and a broad-host-range plasmid that can function as a *B. burgdorferi-E. coli* shuttle vector was reported by Sartakova et al. *(52).* Stewart et al. successfully transformed infectious *B. burgdorferi* using a shuttle vector, including a 3.3-kb region of the *B. burgdorferi* circular plasmid 9, and this vector could be stably maintained in *B. burgdorferi.* However, infectious *B.*

burgdorferi isolates transformed with frequencies 100-fold lower than those found for high-passage, non-infectious strains *(53)*.

HOST-PARASITE INTERACTIONS

Lessons from the **Borrelia** Genomic Project

The genome sequence of *B. burgdorferi* and *T. pallidum* will not only add to our knowledge of the biology of these two spirochetes, but will also be important for the study of other spirochetes. For example, studies of the biosynthetic and transport limitations of *B. burgdorferi* and *T. pallidum* may suggest methods for cultivation of the *Borrelia* spp, thus far uncultivable.

The sequence information will also be important for future virulence studies, such as suggesting hypotheses about how the spirochete migrates from the midgut of the tick to the salivary gland, or from the skin (the site of tick bite) to a distant organ such as the brain. It is of particular importance and interest to determine which surface antigens are involved and how these genes are regulated, and to understand why different surface exposed proteins are expressed differently in the mammalian host and the tick.

It is also important in *Borrelia* to determine the association between genes and gene products on individual plasmids and infectivity. Two linear plasmids (lp25 and lp 28-1) were shown to affect the infectivity of *B. burgdorferi* B31 in C3H/HeN mice. Lp25 contains 31 predicted ORFs, each is either smaller than 200 bp, or closely related to paralogous sequences in other plasmids. Lp28-1 contains the *vls* locus, a *vmp*-like sequence *(54–56)* described for RF *B. hermsii (57)*. The relevance of this mechanism is not clear in *B. burgdorferi,* since *vls* appears to be a minor component of the bacterial surface. However, the decreased infectivity observed in the absence of this plasmid may be related to the loss of the *vls* system. It is likely that, analogous to RF *Borrelia,* the antigenic variation by the variable major protein-like sequence *(vls)* gene locus of *B. burgdorferi* is important for persistence in mammals and evasion of the host immune response. In a series of experiments, Anguita and colleagues demonstrated by differential immunoscreening and RT-PCR, that IFN-γ-mediated signals facilitate spirochete recombination at the *vls* sequence locus *(58)*. These results suggest that the immune response can promote the in vivo adaptation of *B. burgdorferi*.

Like other pathogens such as *Salmonella enterica* serovar *typhimurium, Yersinia,* and *Shigella flexneri (59),* it is known that infectivity of *B. burgdorferi* is plasmid-dependent, and loss of the virulence-associated plasmid leads to an attenuation or complete loss of pathogenicity *(40,43,45)*. Taking advantage of *B. burgdorferi* B31 genome-sequence information, Labandeira-Rey and Skare constructed PCR primers to 13 plasmids (11 linear and 2 circular) *(60)*. The authors established that a B31 strain lacking lp28-4 was modestly attenuated in all analyzed tissue, whereas a strain lacking lp25 was completely attenuated in all investigated tissues. Isolates without lp28-1 were able to infect the joint but not other tissues.

Inside the unfed Ixodes ticks, outer-surface protein (Osp) A is the main surface structure expressed by *B. burgdorferi*. As the tick sucks blood from the mammalian host, the expression of OspA decreases rapidly and the spirochete begins synthesis of OspC, another Osp. This change is at least partly regulated by temperature, since OspC is induced at 32–37°C, but not at 24°C *(61)*. This upregulation has been shown to occur at the transcriptional and translational levels *(62,63)*. The immune system of the infected host encounters large amounts of OspC expressed within the invading spirochetes, resulting in the production of anti-OspC antibodies. If the host has been immunized with an OspA-vaccine prior infection, the anti-OspA antibodies taken up by the ticks with the blood meal results in the killing of *Borrelia* spirochetes that produce OspA.

More recently, an analogous alternation in expression of surface proteins between ticks and mammals was observed in the North American RF *B. hermsii.* Similarly, upon the infection of the tick, the serotype-specific Vmps on the surface of *B. hermsii* became undetectable and was replaced by Vmp33 *(64)*. The process is inverted after tick-bite transmission back to the animal, when the *B. hermsii* spirochetes start to express the same Vmp present in the previous blood meal.

Using a proteomics approach with techniques such as mass spectrometric peptide fingerprinting (MALDI-TOF) mass spectrometry and immunoblotting/Southern blotting, 11 genes that were regulated by pH and encoded by linear plasmids of *B. burgdorferi* were identified *(65)*. An understanding of the mechanism of gene regulation by pH will help to elucidate how these spirochetes adapt to different environments, i.e. in the tick vector and in the mammalian host.

The Initial Host-Parasite Interaction

Bacterial adherence to the host cell or surface is the essential first step in the disease process, since the pathogenic microorganisms become localized to an appropriate target tissue *(66,67)*.

Borrelia spirochetes can adhere to and invade different cell types, including the apical side of human umbilical vein endothelial cell (HUVEC). This attachment is partly inhibited by monoclonal antibodies (MABs) directed against an outer membrane lipoprotein, OspB *(68)*. *Borrelia* spirochetes are also able to penetrate through the eukaryotic-cell monolayers by passing through the intercellular tight junctions *(69)*.

B. burgdorferi has been demonstrated to adhere to primary rodent-brain cultures and C6 glioma cells, and to have an affinity for the extracellular matrix produced by the primary brain cultures and by glioma cells *(70)*. This adherence has been shown to be harmful to oligodendrocytes in a neonatal rat-brain culture *(71)*. The *B. burgdorferi* spirochete is also known to bind to human platelets and endothelial cells through the platelet-specific integrin $\beta_{IIb}\beta_3$ and integrins $\beta_v\beta_3$ and/or $\beta_5\beta_1$, respectively *(72–75)*. In addition, it has been shown that LD *Borrelia* bind to GAG (glycosaminoglycan), and glycosphingolipids *(76–79)*. Binding of *B. burgdorferi* to GAG and to glycosphingolipids may represent very similar adhesion pathways, since both types of molecules may be present on a variety of cell types. Different GAGs (heparin, heparin sulfate, and dermatan sulfate) are responsible for the attachment of *Borrelia* sp. to various host-cell types; heparin sulfate mediates attachment to endothelial cells and heparin sulfate and dermatan sulfate are involved in attachment to glial cells *(77)*.

As *B. burgdorferi* disseminates to different organs, the spirochetes can also be seen in association with collagen fibers in the extracellular spaces of the tissues. *B. burgdorferi* expresses on its surface decorin-binding protein A and B (DbpA and DbpB), which bind to decorin, a collagen-associated extracellular matrix proteoglycan *(80–82)*. Blocking this binding may affect the host-parasite interaction during

Lyme borreliosis. Thus, Dbp is one of several intriguing candidates for the development of a second-generation vaccine.

Spread of Borrelia Throughout the Body

In order to enhance the possibility of transmission by an arthropod from one host to another, it is beneficial for *Borrelia* to persist in the host's vascular system as long as possible. The blood is also the most effective vehicle for the spread of microbes throughout the body. After entering the blood system, they can be transported within a few minutes to a vascular bed in any part of the body. In small vessels such as capillaries and sinusoids where blood flow is slow, the microorganism's movement is more likely to be arrested, facilitating the establishment of infection in neighboring tissues. The persistence of RF borreliae in the blood is in part accomplished by antigenic variation, and has been extensively studied in the North American species *B. hermsii (55,83,84)*. In conjunction with antigenic variation, the RF *B. crocidurae* can bind and become completely covered with erythrocytes *(85)*. This may facilitate immune evasion, as erythrocyte-covered spirochetes may avoid contact with the phagocytic cells and B cells of immune system, thereby delaying the onset of a specific immune response.

To establish a systemic infection, *Borrelia* spirochetes must transmigrate the endothelial layer of blood vessels. This migration is markedly enhanced if the spirochetes bind plasminogen and use the host's plasminogen activator, uPA, to form active plasmin on the spirochete's cell surface *(86–89)*. Plasmin is a serine protease, able to digest extracellular matrix *(90)*. *Streptococcus pyogenes, Staphylococcus aureus,* and *Yersinia pestis* can also activate plasminogen to plasmin, using their endogenous plasminogen activator. These data suggest that plasmin localized on the surface of pathogenic bacteria enables the microorganisms to disseminate from their cutaneous site of entry to the blood and other organs. Several *Borrelia* spp. including *B. burgdorferi, B. coriaceae, B. garinii, B. parkeri, B. anserine, B. turicatae,* and *B. crocidurae* also have the ability to bind uPA, plasminogen, or both on their surfaces *(91,92)*. In a series of experiments, Coleman et al. investigated the capacity of pathogenic *B. burgdorferi* coated with plasmin to degrade extracellular matrix (ECM) components and an interstitial ECM. They showed that plasmin-coated *B. burgdorferi* degraded fibronectin, laminin, and vitronectin, but not collagen *(88)*.

Innate Response

Humoral immunity seems to be the host's most effective defense against *B. burgdorferi,* as shown in several animal models. It has been demonstrated that passive or active immunizations using antibodies against whole-cell *B. burgdorferi* or an outer-surface antigen, especially OspA, can protect against infection *(93,94)*.

B. burgdorferi has a potent effect on the host immune defense because a few spirochetes are enough to induce tissue damage *(95)*. Neutrophils and macrophages appear to be relatively ineffective in limiting *B. burgdorferi* infection, but may be important in early inflammation *(96,97)*. In vitro, *B. burgdorferi* induces expression of E-selectin, intercellular adhesion molecule 1 (ICAM-1), and vascular-cell adhesion molecule 1 (VCAM-1) *(98,99)* on the endothelial-cell surface. This results in secretion of the chemokine IL-8 by the activated endothelium *(100)*, and subsequently promotes transendothelial migration of neutrophils *(99,100)*. These in vitro results were confirmed by the in vivo findings of Schaible et al., which showed an elevated expression of E-selectin, P-selectin, VCAM-1, and ICAM-1 on blood vessels of affected heart and joint tissue from mice infected with *B. burgdorferi (101)*.

Similarly to *B. burgdorferi,* the African RF *B. crocidurae* activated HUVEC, inducing E-selectin and ICAM-1 to become upregulated in a dose- and time-dependent fashion *(102)*. Furthermore, conditioned medium from HUVEC stimulated with *B. crocidurae* contained interleukin-8 (IL-8), and neutrophils added to *B. crocidurae*-stimulated HUVEC cultured on amniotic tissue migrated across the endothelial monolayer *(102)*.

Interestingly, Vidal et al., showed that a Vmp-like lipoprotien of *B. recurrentis,* the causative agent of louse-borne RF, is the principal factor that induces secretion of the pro-inflammatory cytokine tumor necrosis factor (TNF) α by human monocytes *(103)*. In Lyme borreliosis, increasing evidence indicates that primary stimulation of the lipoprotein OspA may induce production of pro- or anti-inflammatory cytokines by these cells, and thereby influence the severity of the symptoms of arthritis that develop *(104,105)*. The role of lipoprotein-stimulated monocytes for the development of symptoms in tick-borne RF has not yet been investigated.

ANIMAL MODELS OF *BORRELIA* INFECTION

Over the years, different animals have been essential as models for studying the pathogenesis and host-parasite interactions for different *Borrelia* species, although mice are most commonly used. Mice are the main source of many of the pathogenic borreliae, and their immune system is well understood—a factor important to studies of RF and LD. In addition, the existence of inbred strains, immunocompetent/ immunodeficient mice, and knockout strains provide good tools for studying RF or LD in detail.

Tissue Tropism

As discussed previously, some of the *Borrelia* species that cause RF (as well as LD *B. burgdorferi*) are neurotropic in humans *(106)*. Generally, the risk of neurological involvement is greater with tick-borne RF than louse-borne RF caused by *B. recurrentis (107,108)*.

During the 1990s Barbour and Colleagues *(107,109,110)* established different mouse models for investigation of brain invasion and histopathological effects by the North American species *B. hermsii* and *B. turicatae*. They found that *B. hermsii* invaded the brain and cerebrospinal fluid of immunodeficient Balb/c mice *(109)*. Severe combined immunodeficiency (SCID) mice were infected with *B. turicatae* serotype A or serotype B in order to investigate the histopathology of the disease *(110)*. No difference was observed in the spirochetemic burden in mice infected with serotype A or serotype B during the 31 days of study. However, serotype A invaded the central nervous system *(CNS),* whereas serotype B caused arthritis in mice. The authors suggested that the observed differences in tissue tropism are associated with the expression of different surface proteins, VmpA and VmpB, which are members of the Vsp-OspC family *(111,112)*. According to the previous suggested classification, the serotype-specific protein of RF *Borrelia* species can be divided in two groups based on their size. Namely the variable small proteins (Vsp) which are 20–23 kDa, and the variable large proteins (Vlp) ranging from 36 to 40 kDa in size *(111,113)*. By grouping the Vmps of RF and Osps of LD, an extensive catalog of the *vsp-vlp* genes can be made. However, the functions of Vsp and Vlp are still not well understood.

The agents of African RF, *B. crocidurae,* have the ability to establish infection in immunocompetent mice *(114)*. In these mice, spirochetes were observed extravascularly as early as d 2 after infection. Interestingly, these spirochetes were found in the parenchyma, leptominges, and plexus choroideus *(114)*. More surprisingly, in a rat model of *B. crocidurae* infection, it was shown that these spirochetes could penetrate the seminiferous tubules of the testes, and remain there for an extended period *(115)*. The testis is an immune-privileged site, where immune reactions are continuously suppressed in order to avoid immune reaction against germ cells that are potent antigens. The testes may therefore function as a possible reservoir for RF *Borrelia (115)*. During the course of infection in the testes, erythrocyte rosettes blocked pre- and postcapillary blood vessels and reduced the blood flow by 60%, resulting in an increase in apoptotic germ cells.

Clinical manifestations of LD vary between different geographical locations, yet both arthritis and neurological disorders are common. Several animal models of LD have been established in various laboratory mouse strains infected with *B. burgdorferi.* In these models, which include immunocompetent as well as immunocompromised animals, involvement of the joints and heart but little or no neurologic disorder were observed. Usually the brain infection was inconsistent and short-lived. However, the animal models for *B. turicatae* and *B. crocidurae* not only allowed the study of the pathogenic process during infection with this organism, but also allowed studies of the pathogenesis of the brain invasion in Lyme borreliosis and of other persistent spirochetal diseases. In addition, the rat model of *B. crocidurae* could be a promising system for the study of *Plasmodium falciparum,* the agent of human malaria. Malaria-infected erythrocytes display features similar to those induced by the presence of *B. crocidurae* in the blood system, although the rosetting properties are presented on the surface of infected erythrocytes instead of the parasite itself *(116–118)*. Thus, the use of in vivo microscopy and laser Doppler flowmetry may facilitate investigation of efficient antirosetting therapies.

Plasminogen-Knockout Mice as an Animal Model

The role of the host plasminogen activation system in transmission, development of spirochetemia, and tissue invasion of *Borrelia* has been studied by several investigators *(87,90–92)*. As outlined previously, *Borrelia* spirochetes can incorporate plasminogen on their surface, and in conjunction with host's plasminogen activator system (PAS), the attached plasminogen is transformed to active plasmin, which enables the microorganisms to transmigrate an endothelial monolayer more readily than "non-clothed" spirochetes *(86)*. Plasminogen could not be detected on spirochetes from unfed ticks, but after a blood meal, binding of spirochetes and plasminogen were observed *(86)*. A requirement for plasminogen was observed for the efficient dissemination of *B. burgdorferi* within the tick and for the enhancement of spirochetemia, whereas plasminogen was not necessary for systemic infection.

To examine the role of the PAS in the pathogenicity of RF *Borrelia,* Gebbia et al. used a RF *Borrelia* species from Spain *(119)* to infect *plg +/+* or *plg –/–* mice *(120)*. Plasminogen binding was shown to be important for organ invasion but not essential for spirochetemia, which was the opposite result obtained when LD *Borrelia* were used *(86)*. Moreover, the PAS had an effect on the invasion of the brain by the RF *Borrelia* and on invasion of the heart, but without a significant difference in the inflammatory response in heart tissue. The heart invasion results resembled those described earlier for *B. turicatae (110)* and *B. burgdorferi (121)*.

In a recent study by Nordstrand and colleagues, the role of the PAS system for the pathogenic capacity of *B. crocidurae* was investigated by infection of *plg –/–* and *plg +/+* mice *(92)*. The study was the first to analyze the importance of plasminogen for organ invasion at the early stage of *Borrelia* infection. No differences in spirochetal titers and peak patterns were observed in blood between the *plg –/–* and *plg +/+* mouse groups. Despite this fact, signs indicative of brain invasion, such as neurological symptoms and histopathological changes, were more common in *plg +/+* mice. The results from that study showed that invasion of the brain and kidney occurred as early as two days after infection, and that plasminogen was not required for establishment of spirochetemia by the organism, whereas it is involved in the invasion of the organs *(92)*.

In summary, these studies describe the involvement of the PAS in LD *Borrelia* and RF *Borrelia* infections, which is manifested in different ways. Although the reason for these differences remains to be elucidated, two factors could play important roles. First, the nature of tick—feeding, soft-bodied *Ornithodoros* ticks transmitting RF species require short feeding, whereas the hard-bodied *Ixodes* ticks of Lyme borreliosis spend a longer time period on the mammalian host for a blood meal. Secondly, there may be differences in the mechanisms used by the spirochetes to spread and to cross the endothelium of the blood vessel.

VACCINE DEVELOPMENT AGAINST *BORRELIA* SPIROCHETES

Two monovalent vaccines that utilize the borrelial outer surface protein A (OspA) as an antigen have been developed in the USA, and one of these vaccines was released for general use in 1999 *(122,123)*. A European polyvalent vaccine using the antigen OspC is currently undergoing clinical trials in Finland, yet results from this trial have not yet been published. Recently, another antigen, the decorin-binding proteins (Dbp), have been considered for prophylactic purposes.

The Current Vaccine and its Limitations

Recombinant OspA has been shown to be an efficient vaccine against LD *(122,123)*. This vaccine has been evaluated and approved in persons older than 15 years of age. Antibodies against OspA taken in with a blood meal kill spirochetes in the tick midgut before dispersal to the salivary glands. Thus transmission to the vertebrate host is blocked *(93,124)*. However, the apparent variability of OspA proteins limits the usefulness of the current monovalent vaccine in Europe *(125)*, since the borrelial flora in Europe is much more heterogeneous compared to the flora in the United States.

A second problem is that antibodies raised against OspA have crossreactivity with a particular major histocompatibility complex class II alleles (DRB1*0401). This crossreactivity may be associated with treatment-resistant Lyme arthritis, generation of synovial fluid T-cell responses to an immunodominant epitope of OspA, and a highly homologous region of the human-lymphocyte-function-associated antigen-1alphaL chain. This association was also revealed by a database homology search showing that the human leukocyte function-associated antigen-1 (hLFA-1) peptide was homologous to an epitope of OspA in *B. burgdorferi* s.s *(104,126).*

Second-Generation Vaccines Against Lyme Borreliosis

It is very likely that for optimum protection against LD morbidity at least one other antigen will be needed, either alone or in combination with the current vaccine, since the OspA vaccine, by itself functions solely to prevent infection. Once infection is initiated, OspA production is downregulated and may not resume until late in the disease. Consequently, antibodies to OspA may not be effective in stopping the infection once it begins in the host. Several different surface antigens of *B. burgdorferi* have been suggested as second-generation vaccine candidates.

The second reason for proposing that another antigen in the vaccine preparation would be desirable is the observation that antibodies to OspA may bind to the cell but are subsequently shed away from the cell on extracellular vesicles known as blebs, without killing the spirochete. Thus, in some vaccinees even high titers of anti-OspA antibodies may not be sufficient to provide protection. Antibodies to a second antigen may have greater access to the cell surface when their epitopes are newly exposed. The characteristics of a few novel second-generation vaccine candidates are discussed in the following sections.

OspC

The vaccine developed against OspC is recombinant polyvalent OspC produced in the yeast *Pichia pastoris.* To date, it has been shown to be nontoxic but immunogenic. This vaccine is believed to act when the spirochetes has entered the mammalian host,—i. e., when the spirochetes have an upregulated OspC expression *(127).*

OspC is very heterogeneous, and a large degree of molecular polymorphism of the *ospC* gene has been shown when comparing the different *Borrelia* genospecies *(128,129).* To date, 19 major OspC groups have been identified *(130).* The use of OspC as vaccines may therefore be limited by the apparent variability of the protein *(125).*

Decorin-Binding Protein

Adhesion and colonization are important events in the bacterial infection processes, and most pathogenic bacteria express one or several adhesins on their surface. These adhesins participate in the attachment to host cells, resulting in tissue colonization. Blocking the adhesion process would be an important mechanism in preventing the development of disease and a target for prophylactics. *Borrelia* spirochetes that are injected in the skin by a tick are usually found associated with collagen fibers in the ECM/LD *Borrelia* do not attach directly to collagen but to decorin, a small leucine-rich proteoglycan (SLRP) that is associated with collagen fibers *(80,81).* Decorin-binding protein (Dbp) A and DbpB are two adhesins on *B. burgdorferi* that can bind to decorin *(80,82).* Both DbpA and DbpB are outer-membrane associated and have been shown to elicit an antibody response in mice infected with *B. burgdorferi (131,132).* To further investigate the role of Dbp in Lyme borreliosis pathogenesis, a decorin-deficient (*dcn* –/–) mouse was developed and used in experimental Lyme borreliosis *(133)*. It was demonstrated that *dcn* –/– mice were more resistant to Lyme borreliosis, suggesting that decorin may be a limiting substrate for the adherence of *B. burgdorferi*. Induction of antibodies directed against DbpA and DbpB may therefore be an important vaccine strategy directed against both early and late LD.

Both DbpA and DbpB have been shown by several laboratories to be a protective antigen in murine models of *B. burgdorferi* infection *(133–135)*. Additionally, nonsecreted recombinant forms of DbpA exhibited better activity and antigenic potency effect than secreted lipoprotein DbpA. These data suggest that elicitation of a bactericidal and protective immune response to DbpA requires a specific conformation for the production of functional antibodies *(136)*.

The Integral Membrane Proteins P66 and P13

B. burgdorferi binds to glycosphingolipids *(79)*, fibronectin *(137,138)*, decorin *(80)*, glycosaminoglycans *(77,139)*, and integrin *(72,73)*. Thus, other binding proteins such as fibronectin-binding protein, are additional possible vaccine candidates against Lyme borreliosis. In a clinical study, the sera from 79 patients with early or late manifestations of LD were shown to have an IgM and/or IgG response to P66, a candidate integrin ligand β_3-chain integrins) *(140)*. Among the patients with late manifestation of the disease, antibody response against the C-terminal region of this protein was more prominent. Among the same group of the patients, those with late neuroborreliosis had a more prominent response, indicating that p66 may be expressed differently in the nervous system.

Correct localization of membrane proteins in most bacteria often results from the presence of transmembrane-spanning domains. However, proteins containing transmembrane-spanning domains appear to be rare in *Borrelia (141)*. Furthermore, freeze-fracture electron microscopy showed that these putative transmembrane proteins were relatively rare *(142,143)*. Thus, *B. burgdorferi* contains two classes of integral membrane proteins: abundant lipoproteins and rare transmembrane-spanning proteins.

Three characterized membrane proteins have been predicted to contain transmembrane-spanning domains, the previously mentioned P66 (Oms66), Oms28 (Oms refers to outer-membrane spanning), and P13, *(144–147)*. P66 and Oms28 both exhibit porin activities *(144,145)*. In Gram-negative bacteria, porins are known to form large water-filled channels, allowing the diffusion of hydrophilic molecules into the periplasmic space *(148)*, and thereby facilitating transport of molecules across the bacterial membrane. The third protein, P13, contains transmembrane-spanning domains and was shown to be surface exposed by immunofluorescence assay, immunoelectron microscopy, and protease sensitivity assays *(147,149)*. Mass spectrometry, in vitro translation, and N- and C-terminal amino-acid sequencing analyses indicated that P13 was post-translationally processed at both ends and modified by an unknown mechanism *(147)*. Therefore, in the development of a second-generation vaccine against Lyme borreliosis, it may be reasonable to include a minor outer-surface-exposed proteins, such as P13 and P66, in combination with one or two of the major Osp proteins, i.e., OspA and OspC.

FUTURE VACCINE STRATEGIES

Research in microbial pathogenicity and host response has fundamentally changed in the last few years, from the characterization of individual determinants to a comprehensive analysis of host-pathogen interactions. This has been fueled by the completion of over 100 genome sequences, mainly microbial, with hundreds more in progress. Thus, various post-genomic approaches have resulted in new methods for the identification and characterization of novel virulence genes in human pathogens. Through microarray analysis, it is now becoming possible to obtain a global picture of gene content and expression in the microbe as well as in the infected host during the disease process. The detailed understanding of possible virulence traits in different microorganisms can be used to identify important relationships in other microbial-host interactions in order to obtain a fuller understanding of eukaryotic- and prokaryotic-cell functions during disease. These technologies should increase our understanding of the pathogenesis and accelerate the development of more efficient prophylactic regimens against various microbial diseases.

The new genomics and proteomics era will be instrumental for future borreliosis vaccine development and virulence studies of *Borrelia* spirochetes. Several studies *(150)* using DNA microarrays have focused on the hosts' exposure to bacterial pathogens, and have identified a number of genes that have not previously been implicated in a host response to infection. Although each microarray study is independently valuable, the combination of data from different microorganisms has the potential of further increasing our knowledge of the pathogenesis of different microorganisms, including *Borrelia* spirochetes. In addition, the similarity of genome-wide host gene-expression responses induced by different pathogens under various circumstances can also be addressed. Thus, the approach will be important in the identification of central regulators of common host responses and the manner in which microbes attempt to defeat this process. Knowledge of the genes involved in this process will provide valuable tools for designing novel prophylactic methods.

ACKNOWLEDGMENT

This study was supported by the Swedish Medical Research Council (Projects 07922), the Swedish Council for Forestry and Agricultural Research grant No. 23.0161 and the J. C. Kempes Foundation (grant to A. S.-T.). We thank Rachel Cahill for critically reading the manuscript. We are also grateful to Annika Nordstrand, Pierre Martin, and Christer Larsson for fruitful discussions that have improved the manuscript.

REFERENCES

1. Rappuoli R. Reverse vaccinology. Curr Opin Microbiol 2000; 3:445–450.
2. Rappuoli R. Reverse vaccinology, a genome-based approach to vaccine development. Vaccine 2001; 19:2688–2691.
3. Rappuoli R. Conjugates and reverse vaccinology to eliminate bacterial meningitis. Vaccine 2001; 19:2319–2322.
4. Felsenfeld O. Borrelia, human relapsing fever, and parasite-vector-host relationships. Bacteriol Rev 1965; 342:1213–1215.
5. Burgdorfer W, Barbour AG, Hayes SF, Benach JL, Grunwaldt E, Davis JP. Lyme disease-a tick-borne spirochetosis? Science 1982; 216:1317–1319.

6. Lewis B. Treponematosis and Lyme borreliosis connections: explanation for Tchefuncte disease syndromes? Am J Phys Anthropol 1994; 93:455–475.

7. Johnson RC. The spirochetes. Annu Rev Microbiol 1977; 31:89–106.

8. Ras NM, Lascola B, Postic D, Cutler SJ, Rodhain F, Baranton G, et al. Phylogenesis of relapsing fever Borrelia spp. Int J Syst Bacteriol 1996; 46:859–865.

9. Fukunaga M, Okada K, Nakao M, Konishi T, Sato Y. Phylogenetic analysis of Borrelia species based on flagellin gene sequences and its application for molecular typing of Lyme disease borreliae. Int J Syst Bacteriol 1996; 46:898–905.

10. Marti Ras N, Postic D, Foretz M, Baranton G. Borrelia burgdorferi sensu stricto, a bacterial species "made in the U.S.A."? Int J Syst Bacteriol 1997; 47:1112–1117.

11. Foretz M, Postic D, Baranton G. Phylogenetic analysis of Borrelia burgdorferi sensu stricto by arbitrarily primed PCR and pulsed-field gel electrophoresis. Int J Syst Bacteriol 1997; 47:11–18.

12. Gylfe Å, Bergström S, Lundström J, Olsén B. Reactivation of Borrelia infection in birds. Nature 2000; 403:724–725.

13. Fraser CM, Casjens S, Huang WM, Sutton GG, Clayton R, Lathigra R, et al. Genomic sequence of a Lyme disease spirochaete, Borrelia burgdorferi. Nature 1997; 390:580–586.

14. Casjens S, Palmer N, Van Vugt R, Mun Huang W, Stevenson B, Rosa P, et al. A bacterial genome in flux: the twelve linear and nine circular extrachromosomal DNAs in an infectious isolate of the lyme disease spirochete Borrelia burgdorferi. Mol Microbiol 2000; 35:490–516.

15. Schmid GP, Steigerwalt AG, Johnson SE, Barbour AG, Steere AC, Robinson JM, et al. DNA characterization of the spirochete that causes Lyme disease. J Clin Microbiol 1984; 20:155–158.

16. Bergström S, Bundoc VG, Barbour AG. Molecular analysis of linear plasmid-encoded major surface proteins, OspA and OspB, of the Lyme disease spirochaete Borrelia burgdorferi. Mol Microbiol 1989; 3:479–486.

17. Hyde FW, Johnson RC. Genetic relationship of lyme disease spirochetes to Borrelia, Treponema, and Leptospira spp. J Clin Microbiol 1984; 20:151–154.

18. Baril C, Richaud C, Baranton G, Saint Girons IS. Linear chromosome of Borrelia burgdorferi. Res Microbiol 1989; 140:507–516.

19. Ferdows MS, Barbour AG. Megabase-sized linear DNA in the bacterium Borrelia burgdorferi, the Lyme disease agent. Proc Natl Acad Sci USA 1989; 86:5969–5973.

20. Bergström S, Olsen B, Burman N, Gothefors L, Jaenson TG, Jonsson M, et al. Molecular characterization of Borrelia burgdorferi isolated from Ixodes ricinus in northern Sweden. Scand J Infect Dis 1992; 24:181–188.

21. Davidson BE, MacDougall J, Saint Girons I. Physical map of the linear chromosome of the bacterium Borrelia burgdorferi 212, a causative agent of Lyme disease, and localization of rRNA genes. J Bacteriol 1992; 174:3766–3774.

22. Casjens S, Huang WM. Linear chromosomal physical and genetic map of Borrelia burgdorferi, the Lyme disease agent. Mol Microbiol 1993; 8:967–980.

23. Barbour AG, Garon CF. Linear plasmids of the bacterium Borrelia burgdorferi have covalently closed ends. Science 1987; 237:409–411.

24. Barbour AG. Plasmid analysis of Borrelia burgdorferi, the Lyme disease agent. J Clin Microbiol 1988; 26:475–478.

25. Casjens S, Murphy M, DeLange M, Sampson L, van Vugt R, Huang WM. Telomeres of the linear chromosomes of Lyme disease spirochaetes: nucleotide sequence and possible exchange with linear plasmid telomeres. Mol Microbiol 1997; 26:581–596.

26. Casjens S, van Vugt R, Tilly K, Rosa PA, Stevenson B. Homology throughout the multiple 32-kilobase circular plasmids present in Lyme disease spirochetes. J Bacteriol 1997; 179:217–227.

27. Lin YS, Kieser HM, Hopwood DA, Chen CW. The chromosomal DNA of Streptomyces lividans 66 is linear. Mol Microbiol 1993; 10:923–933.

28. Allardet-Servent A, Michaux-Charachon S, Jumas-Bilak E, Karayan L, Ramuz M. Presence of one linear and one circular chromosome in the Agrobacterium tumefaciens C58 genome. J Bacteriol 1993; 175:7869–7874.

29. Kinashi H, Shimaji M, Sakai A. Giant linear plasmids in Streptomyces which code for antibiotic biosynthesis genes. Nature 1987; 328:454–456.

30. Pisabarro A, Correia A, Martin JF. Pulsed-field gel electrophoresis analysis of the genome of Rhodococcus fascians: genome size and linear and circular replicon composition in virulent and avirulent strains. Curr Microbiol 1998; 36:302–308.

31. Crespi M, Messens E, Caplan AB, van Montagu M, Desomer J. Fasciation induction by the phytopathogen Rhodococcus fascians depends upon a linear plasmid encoding a cytokinin synthase gene. Embo J 1992; 11:795–804.

32. Hinnebusch J, Bergström S, Barbour AG. Cloning and sequence analysis of linear plasmid telomeres of the bacterium Borrelia burgdorferi. Mol Microbiol 1990; 4:811–820.

33. Blattner FR, Plunkett G, 3rd Bloch CA, Perna NT, Burland V, Riley M, et al. The complete genome sequence of Escherichia coli K-12. Science 1997; 277:1453–1474.

34. Blattner FR, Burland V, Plunkett G, 3rd, Sofia H, Daniels DL. Analysis of the Escherichia coli genome. IV. DNA sequence of the region from 89.2 to 92.8 minutes. Nucleic Acids Res 1993; 21:5408–5417.

35. Fraser CM, Norris SJ, Weinstock GM, White O, Sutton GG, Dodson R, et al. Complete genome sequence of Treponema pallidum, the syphilis spirochete. Science 1998; 281:375–388.

36. Fraser CM, Gocayne JD, White O, Adams MD, Clayton RA, Fleischmann RD, et al. The minimal gene complement of Mycoplasma genitalium. Science 1995; 270:397–403.

37. Johnson RC, Marek N, Kodner C. Infection of Syrian hamsters with Lyme disease spirochetes. J Clin Microbiol 1984; 20:1099–1101.

38. Hinnebusch J, Barbour AG. Linear- and circular-plasmid copy numbers in Borrelia burgdorferi. J Bacteriol 1992; 174:5251–5257.

39. Simpson WJ, Garon CF, Schwan TG. Borrelia burgdorferi contains repeated DNA sequences that are species specific and plasmid associated. Infect Immun 1990; 58:847–853.

40. Simpson WJ, Garon CF, Schwan TG. Analysis of supercoiled circular plasmids in infectious and non-infectious Borrelia burgdorferi. Microb Pathog 1990; 8:109–118.

41. Barbour AG, Carter CJ, Bundoc V, Hinnebusch J. The nucleotide sequence of a linear plasmid of Borrelia burgdorferi reveals similarities to those of circular plasmids of other prokaryotes. J Bacteriol 1996; 178:6635–6639.

42. Zuckert WR, Meyer J. Circular and linear plasmids of Lyme disease spirochetes have extensive homology: characterization of a repeated DNA element. J Bacteriol 1996; 178:2287–2298.

43. Schwan TG, Burgdorfer W, Garon CF. Changes in infectivity and plasmid profile of the Lyme disease spirochete, Borrelia burgdorferi, as a result of in vitro cultivation. Infect Immun 1998; 56:1831–1836.

44. Norris SJ, Howell JK, Garza SA, Ferdows MS, Barbour AG. High- and low-infectivity phenotypes of clonal populations of in vitro- cultured Borrelia burgdorferi. Infect Immun 1995; 63:2206–2212.

45. Xu Y, Kodner C, Coleman L, Johnson RC. Correlation of plasmids with infectivity of Borrelia burgdorferi sensu stricto type strain B31. Infect Immun 1996; 64:3870–3876.

46. Akins DR, Porcella SF, Popova TG, Shevchenko D, Baker SI, Li M, et al. Evidence for in vivo but not in vitro expression of a Borrelia burgdorferi outer surface protein F (OspF) homologue. Mol Microbiol 1995; 18:507–520.

47. Champion CI, Blanco DR, Skare JT, Haake DA, Giladi M, Foley D, et al. A 9.0-kilobase-pair circular plasmid of Borrelia burgdorferi encodes an exported protein: evidence for expression only during infection. Infect Immun 1994; 62:2653–2661.

48. Suk K, Das S, Sun W, Jwang B, Barthold SW, Flavell RA, et al. Borrelia burgdorferi genes selectively expressed in the infected host. Proc Natl Acad Sci USA 1995; 92:4269–4273.

49. Samuels DS, Marconi RT, Huang WM, Garon CF. gyrB mutations in coumermycin A1-resistant Borrelia burgdorferi. J Bacteriol 1994; 176:3072–3075.

50. Samuels DS, Mach KE, Garon CF. Genetic transformation of the Lyme disease agent Borrelia burgdorferi with coumarin-resistant gyrB. J Bacteriol 1994; 176:6045–6049.

51. Bono JL, Elias AF, Kupko JJ, 3rd Stevenson B, Tilly K, Rosa P. Efficient targeted mutagenesis in Borrelia burgdorferi. J Bacteriol 2000; 182:2445–2452.

52. Sartakova M, Dobrikova E, Cabello FC. Development of an extrachromosomal cloning vector system for use in Borrelia burgdorferi. Proc Natl Acad Sci USA 2000; 97:4850–4855.

53. Stewart PE, Thalken R, Bono, JL, Rosa P. Isolation of a circular plasmid region sufficient for autonomous replication and transformation of infectious Borrelia burgdorferi. Mol Microbiol 2001; 39:714–721.

54. Barbour AG. Immunobiology of relapsing fever. Contrib Microbiol Immunol 1987; 8:125–137.

55. Barbour AG. Antigenic variation of a relapsing fever Borrelia species. Annu Rev Microbiol 1990; 44:155–171.

56. Barbour AG. Linear DNA of Borrelia species and antigenic variation. Trends Microbiol 1993; 1:236–239.

57. Zhang JR, Hardham JM, Barbour AG, Norris SJ. Antigenic variation in Lyme disease borreliae by promiscuous recombination of VMP-like sequence cassettes. Cell 1997; 89:275–285.

58. Anguita J, Thomas V, Samanta S, Persinski R, Hernanz C, Barthold SW, et al. Borrelia burgdorferi-induced inflammation facilitates spirochete adaptation and variable major protein-like sequence locus recombination. J Immunol 2001; 167:3383–3390.

59. Portnoy DA, Martinez RJ. Role of a plasmid in the pathogenicity of Yersinia species. Curr Top Microbiol Immunol 1985; 118:29–51.

60. Labandeira-Rey M, Skare JT. Decreased infectivity in Borrelia burgdorferi strain B31 is associated with loss of linear plasmid 25 or 28-1. Infect Immun 2001; 69:446–455.

61. Schwan TG, Piesman J, Golde WT, Dolan MC, Rosa PA. Induction of an outer surface protein on Borrelia burgdorferi during tick feeding. Proc Natl Acad Sci USA 1995; 92:2909–2913.

62. Tilly K, Casjens S, Stevenson B, Bono JL, Samuels DS, Hogan D, et al. The Borrelia burgdorferi circular plasmid cp26: conservation of plasmid structure and targeted inactivation of the ospC gene. Mol Microbiol 1997; 25:361–373.

63. Ramamoorthy R, Philipp MT. Differential expression of Borrelia burgdorferi proteins during growth in vitro. Infect Immun 1998; 66:5119–5124.

64. Schwan TG, Hinnebusch BJ. Bloodstream- versus tick-associated variants of a relapsing fever bacterium. Science 1998; 280:1938–1940.

65. Carroll JA, Cordova RM, Garon CF. Identification of 11 pH-regulated genes in Borrelia burgdorferi localizing to linear plasmids. Infect Immun 2000; 68:6677–6684.

66. Isberg RR. Discrimination between intracellular uptake and surface adhesion of bacterial pathogens. Science 1991; 252:934–938.

67. Patti JM, Allen BL, McGavin MJ, Hook M. MSCRAMM-mediated adherence of microorganisms to host tissues. Annu Rev Microbiol 1994; 48:585–617.

68. Thomas DD, Comstock LE. Interaction of Lyme disease spirochetes with cultured eucaryotic cells. Infect Immun 1989; 57:1324–1326.

69. Szczepanski A, Furie MB, Benach JL, Lane BP, Fleit HB. Interaction between Borrelia burgdorferi and endothelium in vitro. J Clin Investia 1990; 85:1637–1647.

70. Garcia-Monco JC, Fernandez-Villar B, Benach JL. Adherence of the Lyme disease spirochete to glial cells and cells of glial origin. J Infect Dis 1989; 160:497–506.

71. Garcia-Monco JC, Fernandez Villar B, Szczepanski A, and Benach JL. Cytotoxicity of Borrelia burgdorferi for cultured rat glial cells. J Infect Dis 1991; 163:1362–1366.

72. Coburn J, Leong JM, Erban JK. Integrin alpha IIβ beta 3 mediates binding of the Lyme disease agent Borrelia burgdorferi to human platelets. Proc Natl Acad Sci USA 1993; 90:7059–7063.

73. Coburn J, Barthold SW, Leong JM. Diverse Lyme disease spirochetes bind integrin alpha IIβ beta 3 on human platelets. Infect Immun 1994; 62:5559–5567.

74. Coburn J, Chege W, Magoun L, Bodary SC, Leong JM. Characterization of a candidate Borrelia burgdorferi beta3-chain integrin ligand identified using a phage display library. Mol Microbiol 1999; 34:926–940.

75. Coburn J, Magoun L, Bodary SC, Leong JM. Integrins alpha(v)beta3 and alpha5beta1 mediate attachment of lyme disease spirochetes to human cells. Infect Immun 1998; 66:1946–1952.

76. Parveen N, Robbins D, Leong JM. Strain variation in glycosaminoglycan recognition influences cell-type- specific binding by lyme disease spirochetes. Infect Immun 1999; 67:1743–1749.

77. Leong JM, Wang H, Magoun L, Field JA, Morrissey PE, Robbins D, et al. Different classes of proteoglycans contribute to the attachment of Borrelia burgdorferi to cultured endothelial and brain cells. Infect Immun 1998; 66:994–999.

78. Garcia Monco JC, Fernandez Villar B, Rogers RC, Szczepanski A, Wheeler CM, Benach JL. Borrelia burgdorferi and other related spirochetes bind to galactocerebroside. Neurology 1992; 42:1341–1348.

79. Backenson PB, Coleman JL, Benach JL. Borrelia burgdorferi shows specificity of binding to glycosphingolipids. Infect Immun 1995; 63:2811–2817.

80. Guo BP, Norris SJ, Rosenberg LC, Hook M. Adherence of Borrelia burgdorferi to the proteoglycan decorin. Infect Immun 1995; 63:3467–3472.

81. Guo BP, Brown EL, Dorward DW, Rosenberg LC, Hook M. Decorin-binding adhesins from Borrelia burgdorferi. Mol Microbiol 1998; 30:711–723.

82. Hanson MS, Cassatt DR, Guo BP, Patel NK, McCarthy MP, Dorward DW, et al. Active and passive immunity against Borrelia burgdorferi decorin binding protein A (DbpA) protects against infection. Infect Immun 1998; 66:2143–2153.

83. Donelson JE. Mechanisms of antigenic variation in Borrelia hermsii and African trypanosomes. J Biol Chem 1995; 270:7783–7786.

84. Barbour AG, Restrepo BI. Antigenic variation in vector-borne pathogens. Emerg Infect Dis 2000; 6:449–457.

85. Burman N, Shamaei-Tousi A, Bergström S. The spirochete Borrelia crocidurae causes erythrocyte rosetting during relapsing fever. Infect Immun 1998; 66:815–819.

86. Colemanl JL, Sellati TJ, Testa JE, Kew RR, Furie MB, Benach JL. Borrelia burgdorferi binds plasminogen, resulting in enhanced penetration of endothelial monolayers. Infect Immun 1995; 63:2478–2484.

87. Coleman JL, Benach JL. Use of the plasminogen activation system by microorganisms. J Lab Clin Med 1999; 134:567–576.

88. Coleman JL, Roemer EJ, and Benach JL. Plasmin-coated Borrelia burgdorferi degrades soluble and insoluble components of the mammalian extracellular matrix. Infect Immun 1999; 67:3929–3936.

89. Boyle MD, Lottenberg R. Plasminogen activation by invasive human pathogens. Thromb Haemost 1997; 77:1–10.

90. Fuchs H, Wallich R, Simon MM, Kramer MD. The outer surface protein A of the spirochete Borrelia burgdorferi is a plasmin(ogen) receptor. Proc Natl Acad Sci USA 1994; 91:12,594–12,598.

91. Klempner MS, Noring R, Epstein MP, McCloud B, Rogers RA. Binding of human urokinase type plasminogen activator and plasminogen to Borrelia species. J Infect Dis 1996; 174:97–104.

92. Nordstrand A, Shamaei-Tousi A, Ny A, Bergström S. Delayed invasion of the kidney and brain by Borrelia crocidurae in plasminogen-deficient mice. Infect Immun 2001; 69:5832–5839.

93. de Silva AM, Telford SR, 3rd, Brunet LR, Barthold SW, Fikrig E. Borrelia burgdorferi OspA is an arthropod-specific transmission- blocking Lyme disease vaccine. J Exp Med 1996; 183:271–275.

94. Fikrig E, Barthold SW, Kantor FS, Flavell RA. Protection of mice against the Lyme disease agent by immunizing with recombinant OspA. Science 1990; 250:553–556.

95. Steere AC. Lyme disease. N Engl J Med 1989; 321:586–596.

96. Georgilis K, Steere AC, Klempner MS. Infectivity of Borrelia burgdorferi correlates with resistance to elimination by phagocytic cells. J Infect Dis 1991; 163:150–155.

97. Du Chateau BK, England DM, Callister SM, Lim LC, Lovrich SD, Schell RF. Macrophages exposed to Borrelia burgdorferi induce Lyme arthritis in hamsters. Infect Immun 1996; 64:2540–2547.

98. Boggemeyer E, Stehle T, Schaible UE, Hahne M, Vestweber D, Simon MM. Borrelia burgdorferi upregulates the adhesion molecules E-selectin, P- selectin, ICAM-1 and VCAM-1 on mouse endothelioma cells in vitro. Cell Adhes Commun 1994; 2:145–157.

99. Sellati TJ, Burns MJ, Ficazzola MA, Furie MB. Borrelia burgdorferi upregulates expression of adhesion molecules on endothelial cells and promotes transendothelial migration of neutrophils in vitro. Infect Immun 1995; 63:4439–4447.

100. Burns MJ, Sellati TJ, Teng EI, Furie MB. Production of interleukin-8 (IL-8) by cultured endothelial cells in response to Borrelia burgdorferi occurs independently of secreted IL-1 and tumor necrosis factor alpha and is required for subsequent transendothelial migration of neutrophils. Infect Immun 1997; 65:1217–1222.

101. Schaible UE, Vestweber D, Butcher EG, Stehle T, Simon MM. Expression of endothelial cell adhesion molecules in joints and heart during Borrelia burgdorferi infection of mice. Cell Adhes Commun 1994; 2:465–479.

102. Shamaei-Tousi A, Burns MJ, Benach JL, Furie MB, Gergel EI, Bergström S. The relapsing fever spirochaete, Borrelia crocidurae, activates human endothelial cells and promotes the transendothelial migration of neutrophils. Cell Microbiol 2000; 2:591–599.

103. Vidal V, Scragg IG, Cutler SJ, Rockett KA, Fekade D, Warrell DA, et al. Variable major lipoprotein is a principal TNF-inducing factor of louse- borne relapsing fever. Nat Med 1998; 4:1416–1420.

104. Gross DM, Forsthuber T, Tary-Lehmann M, Etling C, Ito K, Nagy ZA, et al. Identification of LFA-1 as a candidate autoantigen in treatment- resistant Lyme arthritis. Science 1998; 281:703–706.

105. Steere AC, Gross D, Meyer AL, Huber BT. Autoimmune mechanisms in antibiotic treatment-resistant Lyme arthritis. J Autoimmun 2001; 16:263–268.

106. Paster BJ, Dewhirst FE, Weisburg WG, Tordoff LA, Fraser GJ, Hespell RB, et al. Phylogenetic analysis of the spirochetes. J Bacteriol 1991; 173:6101–6109.

107. Cadavid D, Barbour AG. Neuroborreliosis during relapsing fever: review of the clinical manifestations, pathology, and treatment of infections in humans and experimental animals. Clin Infect Dis 1998; 26:151–164.

108. Southern P, Sanford J. Relapsing fever: a clinical and microbiological review. Medicine 1969; 48:129–149.

109. Cadavid D, Bundoc V, Barbour AG. Experimental infection of the mouse brain by a relapsing fever Borrelia species: a molecular analysis. J Infect Dis 1993; 168:143–151.

110. Cadavid D, Thomas DD, Crawley R, Barbour AG. Variability of a bacterial surface protein and disease expression in a possible mouse model of systemic Lyme borreliosis. J Exp Med 1994; 179:631–642.

111. Cadavid D, Pennington PM, Kerentseva TA, Bergström S, Barbour AG. Immunologic and genetic analyses of VmpA of a neurotropic strain of Borrelia turicatae. Infect Immun 1997; 65:3352–3360.

112. Pennington PM, Cadavid D, Barbour AG. Characterization of VspB of Borrelia turicatae, a major outer membrane protein expressed in blood and tissues of mice. Infect Immun 1999; 67:4637–4645.

113. Hinnebusch BJ, Barbour AG, Restrepo BI, Schwan TG. Population structure of the relapsing fever spirochete Borrelia hermsii as indicated by polymorphism of two multigene families that encode immunogenic outer surface lipoproteins. Infect Immun 1998; 66:432–440.

114. Shamaei-Tousi A, Martin P, Bergh A, Burman N, Brännström T, Bergström S. Erythrocyte-aggregating relapsing fever spirochete Borrelia crocidurae induces formation of microemboli. J Infect Dis 1999; 180:1929–1938.

115. Shamaei-Tousi A, Collin O, Bergh A, Bergström S. Testicular damage by microcirculatory disruption and colonization of an immune-privileged site during Borrelia crocidurae infection. J Exp Med 2001; 193:995–1004.

116. Udomsangpetch R, Wahlin B, Carlson J, Berzins K, Torii M, Aikawa M, et al. Plasmodium falciparum-infected erythrocytes form spontaneous erythrocyte rosettes. J Exp Med 1989; 169:1835–1840.

117. Carlson J, Wahlgren M. Plasmodium falciparum erythrocyte rosetting is mediated by promiscuous lectin-like interactions. J Exp Med 1992; 176:1311–1317.

118. Newbold C, Craig A, Kyes S, Rowe A, Fernandez-Reyes D, Fagan T. Cytoadherence, pathogenesis and the infected red cell surface in Plasmodium falciparum. Int J Parasitol 1999; 29:927–937.

119. Anda P, Sanchez-Yebra W, del Mar Vitutia M, Perez Pastrana E, Rodriguez I, Miller, NS, et al. A new Borrelia species isolated from patients with relapsing fever in Spain. Lancet 1996; 348:162–165.

120. Gebbia JA, Monco JC, Degen JL, Bugge TH, Benach JL. The plasminogen activation system enhances brain and heart invasion in murine relapsing fever borreliosis. J Clin Investing 1999; 103:81–87.

121. Barthold SW, Persing DH, Armstrong AL, Peeples RA. Kinetics of Borrelia burgdorferi dissemination and evolution of disease after intradermal inoculation of mice. Am J Pathol 1991; 139:263–273.

122. Steere AC, Sikand VK, Meurice F, Parenti DL, Fikrig E, Schoen RT, J, et al. Vaccination against Lyme disease with recombinant Borrelia burgdorferi outer-surface lipoprotein A with adjuvant. Lyme Disease Vaccine Study Group. N Engl J Med 1998; 339:209–215.

123. Sigal LH, Zahradnik JM, Lavin P, Patella SJ, Bryanti G, Haselby R, et al. A vaccine consisting of recombinant Borrelia burgdorferi outer-surface protein A to prevent Lyme disease. Recombinant Outer-Surface Protein A Lyme Disease Vaccine Study Consortium. N Engl J Med 1978; 339:216–222.

124. de Silva AM, Zeidner NS, Zhang Y, Dolan MC, Piesman J, Fikrig E. Influence of outer surface protein A antibody on Borrelia burgdorferi within feeding ticks. Infect Immun 1999; 67:30–35.

125. Wilske B, Busch U, Eiffert H, Fingerle V, Pfister HW, Rossler D, Preac-Mursic V. Diversity of OspA and OspC among cerebrospinal fluid isolates of Borrelia burgdorferi sensu lato from patients with neuroborreliosis in Germany. Med Microbiol Immunol (Berl) 1996; 184:195–201.

126. Trollmo C, Meyer AL, Steere AC, Hafler DA, Huber BT. Molecular mimicry in Lyme arthritis demonstrated at the single cell level: LFA-1 alpha L is a partial agonist for outer surface protein A- reactive T cells. J Immunol 2001; 166:5286–5291.

127. Wahlberg P. Vaccination against Lyme borreliosis. Ann Med 1999; 31:233–235.

128. Jauris-Heipke S, Liegl G, Preac-Mursic V, Rossler D, Schwab E, Soutschek E, et al. Molecular analysis of genes encoding outer surface protein C (OspC) of Borrelia burgdorferi sensu lato: relationship to ospA genotype and evidence of lateral gene exchange of ospC. J Clin Microbiol 1995; 33:1860–1866.

129. Livey I, Gibbs CP, Schuster R, Dorner F. Evidence for lateral transfer and recombination in OspC variation in Lyme disease Borrelia. Mol Microbiol 1995; 18:257–269.

130. Wang IN, Dykhuizen DE, Qiu W, Dunn JJ, Bosler EM, Luft BJ. Genetic diversity of ospC in a local population of Borrelia burgdorferi sensu stricto. Genetics 1999; 151:15–30.

131. Feng S, Hodzic E, Stevenson B, Barthold W. Humoral immunity to Borrelia burgdorferi N40 decorin binding proteins during infection of laboratory mice. Infect Immun 1998; 66:2827–2835.

132. Hagman KE, Lahdenn P, Popova TG, Porcella SF, Akins DR, Radolf JD, et al. Decorin-binding protein of Borrelia burgdorferi is encoded within a two-gene operon and is protective in the murine model of Lyme borreliosis. Infect Immun 1998; 66:2674–2683.

133. Brown EI, Wooten RM, Johnson BJ, Iozzo RV, Smith A, Dolan MC, et al. Resistance to Lyme disease in decorin-deficient mice. J Clin Investing 2001; 107:845–852.

134. Hanson MS, Patel NK, Cassatt, DR, Ulbrandt ND. Evidence for vaccine synergy between Borrelia burgdorferi decorin binding protein A and outer surface protein A in the mouse model of lyme borreliosis. Infect Immun 2000; 68:6457–6460.

135. Hagman KE, Yang X, Wikel SK, Schoelen GB, Caimano MJ, Radolf JD, et al. Decorin-binding protein A (DbpA) of Borrelia burgdorferi is not protective when immunized mice are challenged via tick infestation and correlates with the lack of DbpA expression by B. burgdorferi in ticks. Infect Immun 2000; 68:4759–4764.

136. Ulbrandt ND, Cassatt DR, Patel NK, Roberts WC, Bachy CM, Fazenbaker CA, et al. Conformational nature of the Borrelia burgdorferi decorin binding protein A epitopes that elicit protective antibodies. Infect Immun 2001; 69:4799–4807.

137. Grab DJ, Givens C, Kennedy R. Fibronectin-binding activity in Borrelia burgdorferi. Biochim Biophys Acta 1998; 1407:135–145.

138. Probert WS, Johnson BJ, Identification of a 47 kDa fibronectin-binding protein expressed by Borrelia burgdorferi isolate B31. Mol Microbiol 1998; 30:1003–1015.

139. Leong JM, Robbins D, Rosenfeld L, Lahiri B, Parveen N. Structural requirements for glycosaminoglycan recognition by the Lyme disease spirochete, Borrelia burgdorferi. Infect Immun 1998; 66:6045–6048.

140. Ntchobo H, Rothermel H, Chege W, Steere AC, Coburn J. Recognition of multiple antibody epitopes throughout Borrelia burgdorferi p66, a candidate adhesin, in patients with early or late manifestations of Lyme disease. Infect Immun 2001; 69:1953–1956.

141. Brandt ME, Riley BS, Radolf JD, and Norgard MV. Immunogenic integral membrane proteins of Borrelia burgdorferi are lipoproteins. Infect Immun 1990; 58:983–991.

142. Radolf JD, Bourell KW, Akins DR, Brusca JS, and Norgard MV. Analysis of Borrelia burgdorferi membrane architecture by freeze- fracture electron microscopy. J Bacteriol 1994; 176:21–31.

143. Walker EM, Borenstein LA, Blanco DR, Miller JN, Lovett MA. Analysis of outer membrane ultrastructure of pathogenic Treponema and Borrelia species by freeze-fracture electron microscopy. J Bacteriol 1991; 173:5585–5588.

144. Skare JT, Champion CI, Mirzabekov TA, Shang ES, Blanco DR. Erdjument-Bromage et al. Porin activity of the native and recombinant outer membrane protein Oms28 of Borrelia burgdorferi. J Bacteriol 1996; 178:4909–4918.

145. Skare JT, Mirzabekov TA, Shang ES, Blanco DR, Erdjument-Bromage H, Bunikis J, et al. The Oms66 (p66) protein is a Borrelia burgdorferi porin. Infect Immun 1997; 65:3654–3661.

146. Bunikis J, Noppa L, Bergström S. Molecular analysis of a 66-kDa protein associated with the outer membrane of Lyme disease Borrelia. FEMS Microbiol Lett 1995; 131:139–145.

147. Noppa L, Östberg Y, Lavrinovicha M, Bergström S. P13, an integral membrane protein of Borrelia burgdorferi, is C- terminally processed and contains surface-exposed domains. Infect Immun 2001; 69:3323–34.

148. Cowan SW, Schirmer T, Rummel G, Steiert M, Ghosh R, Pauptit RA, et al. Crystal structures explain functional properties of two E. coli porins. Nature 1992; 358:727–733.

149. Sadziene A, Thomas DD, Barbour AG. Borrelia burgdorferi mutant lacking Osp: biological and immunological characterization. Infect Immun 1995; 63:1573–1580.

150. Diehn M, Relman DA. Comparing functional genomic datasets: lessons from DNA microarray analyses of host-pathogen interactions. Curr Opin Microbiol 2001; 4:95–101.

III FUNGI

11

Antifungal Target Discovery and Evaluation

Lessons from Saccharomyces cerevisiae

Beth DiDomenico and Scott S. Walker

INTRODUCTION

Fungi are a diverse group of industrially and medically important eukaryotic organisms. Those that cause human disease are but a handful of the species that have been documented. During the latter part of the twentieth century, invasive fungal infections became one of the major causes of human suffering and morbidity, especially in immunocompromised patients. Fungal infections emerged as significant, difficult-to-treat pathogens as physicians began treating a wider variety of afflictions more aggressively with chemotherapeutic agents or implanted medical devices, immunosuppressive drugs reduced the rate of organ-transplant rejection, and retroviral infections became more prevalent.

Today, *Candida* species are a common cause of hospital-acquired bloodstream infections, and oral candidiasis is a leading indicator of opportunistic infection in HIV-infected patients. In addition, serious pulmonary aspergillosis has recently been recognized as a leading cause of mortality in bone-marrow transplant recipients. Less common but equally pernicious fungal pathogens include *Cryptococcus neoformans, Fusarium* spp., *Pneumocystis carinii,* and *Blastomyces dermatitidis.*

Treatment of this diverse group of microbes is limited to amphotericin B deoxycholate and its newer, less toxic formulations, as well as a number of azoles, both old and new. Amphotericin B and the azoles target ergosterol, the major sterol present in fungal cell membranes. In January 2001, a new compound was approved for the treatment of aspergillosis that represents a new class of molecule, the pneumocandins, with a unique mechanism of action. Recent studies of the mechanism of action of these and other antifungals in use or development are available *(1).* Also, the spectrum, uses, limitations, and targets of commonly prescribed antifungals are explored in Chapter 12.

ANTIFUNGAL DRUG DISCOVERY

Historically, antifungal drug discovery was based entirely on identifying and characterizing novel chemistries that are active against the cell. This approach has been fruitful, allowing the discovery and evaluation of an array of mechanistically distinct classes of potent antifungal agents *(2,3).* In light of the constraints on the

From: *Pathogen Genomics: Impact on Human Health*
Edited by: K. J. Shaw © Humana Press Inc., Totowa, NJ

clinical usefulness of these agents stemming from toxicity issues, fungistatic activity, and rising resistance levels, a new approach to antifungal drug discovery may be warranted. The application of genomics to antifungal drug discovery has the potential to turn the traditional antifungal compound-target relationship on its head.

Drug development has traditionally been based on the premise that a certain level of understanding of the biology of disease would lead to rational choices in terms of drug targets (i.e., proteins or enzymes gone awry), followed by the subsequent screening of libraries of compounds to search for inhibitors. But what is an effective drug target?

To define a good target, perhaps the first consideration should be the desired characteristics of the drug. Although the characteristics of an ideal antifungal drug are debatable, one clear choice would be broad-spectrum activity, primarily because of the limited diagnostic tests currently available to medical practitioners. Other characteristics such as fungicidal, rather than fungistatic activity, with very few side effects, (mechanism-based toxicity) would also be desirable. Taken together, these three broad factors are important considerations in light of the available diagnostics, immunologically debilitated patients burdened with more than one etiological agent, the extended courses of treatment required, drug resistance, cost of development, and the relatively (fortunately) small patient populations. However, with the growing knowledge of virulence and pathogenesis factors, there may be other choices for therapeutic intervention as well. In either case, whether a traditional drug or one aimed at a particular aspect of disease progression is desired, the growing availability of complete genome-sequence information means that for the first time, all potential targets within a pathogen are available for consideration. A combined approach, using sequence comparisons and classical genetics, holds the promise for antifungal target discovery.

An understanding of the life cycles of fungal pathogens has led to a limited range of rational targets for drug discovery. Included among these are proteins and enzymes that are unique to the fungal world, present in most fungal pathogens, and critical for growth (e.g., ergosterol, chitin synthase, or glucan synthase). Other fungal targets that have been explored, although present in mammalian cells, may be divergent enough to suggest that differential binding of inhibitors could be achieved such as, sphingolipids *(4)*, translation elongation factors *(5)*, DNA topoisomerases *(6)*, or N-myristoyltransferase *(7,8)*. Although none of these targets has yet been successful, the rationale behind their choice remains valid.

S. cerevisiae: **A MODEL FOR FUNGAL PATHOGENS**

Model organisms have always been the bricks and mortar upon which applied research has gained an advantage in understanding the life cycle and physiology of a pathogen. Nowhere is this more evident than in the contributions of the yeast *Saccharomyces cerevisiae* to the understanding of many aspects of fungal growth and differentiation. *S. cerevisiae* continues to play a key role in both the development of methodologies and the understanding of cell physiology, with broad applications to the field of antifungal drug discovery. With its tractable genetics, moderate genome size, and simple life cycle, yeast is a model system for genomics with few if any peers. Although the ramifications of physiological and technological studies in yeast reach far beyond the simple eukaryotes, this chapter focuses on the impact of this work on the growing knowledge of important fungal pathogens and target-based antifungal drug discovery. Thus, if *S. cerevisiae,* with its 50+ years of genetics, well-defined recombination, and molecular systems, and ability to grow as both a haploid and diploid organism, can reasonably substitute for fungal pathogens with much more recalcitrant physiologies and transformation systems, then it may continue to hasten the pace of research.

In 1996, a key milestone was reached with the completion of the *S. cerevisiae* genome by a consortium of laboratories across the world *(9).* This data has been made publicly available at Stanford University *(10).* *S. cerevisiae* has a haploid content of 16 chromosomes with approximately 12 million basepairs (bp) of sequence and about 6000 genes *(9).*

Comparative Genomics

Partial genomic sequence comparisons have identified potential orthologs between various fungal species and genera. The application of whole-genome comparisons is now possible. Choosing targets to screen that have significant homologues in other common fungi meets the consideration for a broad-spectrum drug. Of principal concern in applying this criterion is the choice of the metric by which a significant homologue is determined—is 30% similarity sufficient, or does one require 70% similarity? Is overall homology important, or just specific functional domains? With many of these methods, the stringency of relatedness between orthologs can easily be adjusted, thus affecting the potential number of genes to be further validated. Although *S. cerevisiae* leads the way, as more fungal organisms are added to the growing list of sequenced pathogens, this type of data mining becomes more sensitive and applicable to clinical pathogens such as *Candida albicans* (sequence-www.stanford.edu/group/candida/index.html).

Today, more than 50 bacterial organisms have a sequence that is publicly accessible, as well as the two completed fungal species (*S. cerevisiae* and *C. albicans*). Other projects in various stages of completion (although not always generally available) include *Aspergillus nidulans, Aspergillus fumigatus, Cryptococcus neoformans,* and *Pneumocystis carinii,* as well as a number of other important agricultural fungi (*see* www.tigr.org for a progress report).

To address the issue of possible mechanism-based toxicity, queries that exclude potential targets because of strong homology between pathogen and host protein sequences are of considerable importance, and may further narrow the field of potential genes for screening. With the completion of the Human Genome Project in 2000 *(11,12),* the comparator host genome became readily available.

Functional Genomics

Genomic-sequence comparisons can only provide clues to a limited number of biological questions concerning gene essentiality or function. There are still too many choices for massive parallel screening efforts from simply a subtractive and comparative *in silico* analysis. Furthermore, the bedrock of drug discovery lies in the specificity and selectivity of the screens used to sift through the thousands of small molecules available. Understanding the function and interaction among the proteins within the intracellular environment is thus a critical part of drug discovery. The publication of the complete genome sequence of *S. cerevisiae* in 1996 heralded the beginning of an ongoing systematic effort to understand the importance, expression pattern, interrelationship, and function of all the 6000 genes of yeast *(9)*. The tools and knowledge already generated from this work have and will impact the fields of fungal pathogenesis, diagnostics, and antifungal drug discovery, and will offer a roadmap to researchers in human genetics and other fields.

Tools for Gene Disruption

If one assumes that the inhibition of essential cellular functions will lead to the discovery of fungicidal drugs, then functional genomics begins with tools for disrupting and analyzing the entire complement of open reading frames (ORFs). Two different methodologies have been developed for *S. cerevisiae* that have proven useful in this regard: one-step gene disruptions *(13,14)* and genetic footprinting *(15)*.

Early studies with yeast provided the basic parameters for one-step, targeted gene disruption by homologous recombination with a selectable marker gene flanked by regions of chromosomal sequence, usually a few hundred bp in length *(13)*. Further studies in yeast and subsequently in a common human pathogen, *C. albicans,* showed that efficient gene disruption could be achieved with as few as 40–60 bp of homologous sequence flanking each side of a selectable marker gene *(16,17)*. Application of the minimal gene-disruption cassette on a genome-wide scale has resulted in gene knockouts for all 6000 ORFs of *S. cerevisiae,* and suggested that approximately 17% of these genes are essential for growth under laboratory conditions *(18,19)*. Targeted gene-disruption approaches, with some limitations *(20),* have also had broad application to a variety of yeasts and dimorphic and filamentous fungi (*see* refs. *21–25)*.

As an alternative to directed gene knockouts, genetic footprinting by transposon-mediated insertional mutagenesis can expose even the subtle contribution of a gene to competitive growth in a heterogeneous cell population *(15,26)*. Since natural transposons exist in fungi *(27),* the application of this approach to other fungi awaits the development of efficient transposable elements in those species.

Tools for Gene Expression

The other key resource in any molecular genetic examination of clinically relevant pathogens is a robust expression system. Again, many of the fundamental features of expression systems now used in a variety of pathogenic fungi were first identified in *S. cerevisiae.* Transcription promoters, perhaps derived from the gene of interest or from a conditionally expressed gene, (reviewed in ref. *28)* are well-documented in *S. cerevisiae,* and have found application in other fungi *(29–31)*. Delivery of expression systems can be simple (directed to the chromosome either through homologous recombination for yeasts) or complex (requiring ectopic integration, as has been necessary for many filamentous pathogens such as *A. fumigatus*). Alternatively, delivery of autonomously replicating plasmid-based expression requires harnessing the replication *(32),* segregation *(33),* and for linear plasmids, the telomeric functions of the cell *(34)*. Recently, a number of expression systems founded on the principals developed in *S. cerevisiae* have been successfully adapted to other fungi *(31,35–38)*. The growing availability of additional genome sequences and our increased understanding of chromosome dynamics and gene expression presage successes in harnessing these sophisticated expression systems for other fungal species.

Cell Biology and Physiology

The completion of the consortium deletion project has provided the knowledge of gene essentiality *(18,19),* and has produced a collection of mutants for genetic manipulation and functional studies that will further aid in the delineation and understanding of the functions of all 6000 genes of yeast (www.resgen.com). A recent report detailed the use of a collection of heterozygotes to identify drug targets resulting from increased drug sensitivity resulting from the induced haploinsufficiency *(39).* This approach may be particularly useful in obligate diploid fungi, such as *C. albicans.*

Perturbations in gene expression can have dramatic effects on the physiology of a microbe. For example, underexpression of a gene using an anti-sense approach to regulate gene expression in *C. albicans* can be used to assess essentiality and expose gene-dependent drug sensitivities *(40).* In contrast, it has been demonstrated in *S. cerevisiae* that overexpression of some genes can lead to phenotypes that have revealed functional roles for those proteins (*see* refs. *41–43*).

Whole-Genome Transcription and Translation Analysis

Analysis of global regulation of gene expression is an exciting new tool that has suggested gene functions and novel gene interactions. With the availability of the complete yeast genome and technologies to measure gene expression at the RNA and protein levels, a complete description of gene expression within a variety of environments is now achievable. Oligonucleotide or double-stranded DNA microarrays provide a format to simultaneously survey the expression patterns of all the identified genes in *S. cerevisiae (44,45).* Recently, microarray technology has been applied to the study of the clinically relevant fungal pathogen *C. albicans (46).*

Coordinately regulated changes in gene-expression patterns following an environmental insult, a genetic mutation, or the presence of a drug may indicate functional relations in the same or closely parallel biological pathways. Microarray platforms provide the means to follow each gene in a single experiment. By monitoring the expression patterns of all genes at once, unannotated genes are clustered with those having the most similar expression patterns, thus facilitating follow-up confirmatory experiments to validate a putative function. To date, the most comprehensive application of expression profiling in yeast used 300 mutants and chemical treatments to demonstrate coregulation of a large number of genes *(47).* This study hinted at the power of this approach by identifying a novel gene involved in ergosterol biosynthesis in response to an inhibitor of this pathway. However, a follow-up study suggested that aneuploidy within some of these strains, and presumably others, may complicate global expression studies *(48).* Nevertheless, the opposite analysis, in which the pattern of gene expression predicts a potential mechanism of action (MOA) for an unknown compound, may also be systematically applied. A recent microarray study of the related global responses to perturbations in ergosterol synthesis by novel and well-known azoles supports this theory *(49).* Since *S. cerevisiae* is a model eukaryotic organism with many mammalian homologues already identified, it is not inconceivable that a functional genomics approach may reveal novel MOA or potential toxicities (e.g., upregulation of DNA-repair enzymes or chaperonins) of candidate compounds. By the same reasoning, a molecular phenotype of genetic mutations compared with isogenic wild-type strains can reveal previously unknown effects on other pathways, or unknown genes in known pathways.

The application of microarray technology does not require a complete genome sequence. A normalized cDNA sequence collection is an appropriate starting point, making this approach particularly useful in characterizing even an incompletely sequenced fungal pathogen. Another method of expression profiling that does not require complete genomic sequencing, serial analysis of gene expression (SAGE) presents a comprehensive picture of the expressed genes in *S. cerevisiae* (transcriptome) and elucidates the expression of previously unannotated ORFs *(50)*.

The burgeoning field of proteomics also warrants attention as an analytical profiling tool (reviewed in ref. *51*). As a complementary approach to transcript analysis, proteomics—by traditional 2-dimensional gels or by newer chromatographic means—provides insight into gene expression at the protein level, and has been applied to studies of post-translational modifications and protein-function determination *(52)*. Even in the absence of extensive genomic sequence, two-dimensional gels and fluorescent dyes, coupled with peptide sequencing by mass spectrometry, can be used to provide at least a hint about the identity of up- or downregulated gene products in an experimental scenario.

Tools for Protein Localization, Protein-Protein Interaction, and Functional Analysis

Protein localization, interaction, and other functional studies, when applied on a large scale, have begun to broaden our understanding of the complex regulatory and structural relationships that exist within a yeast cell. For example, as an adjunct to a large-scale gene-disruption effort, Snyder and colleagues have produced a substantial number of epitope-tagged proteins expressed from their native promoters, and have described their intracellular localization and possible function *(53)*.

Although the localization of some proteins may provide clues to their function or suitability for immunodiagnostics or vaccine development, a fuller understanding of protein-protein interactions will contribute much more to our knowledge of function and regulation. A now classic and still elegant method to identify interacting proteins is the yeast two-hybrid system *(54)*. Three separate efforts at genome-scale application of this technique have produced a wealth of potential interactions, suggesting some new and intriguing relationships in *S. cerevisiae (55–57)*.

The lofty goal of any genome-wide study is to understand the function of a large number of previously uncharacterized proteins. Traditional methods of protein purification and enzyme or interaction assays are at best impractical on a large scale. However, recent developments in applying microarray technology to proteins are likely to prove useful on a functional genomics scale. To demonstrate this notion, Zhu et al. *(58)* prepared a protein array containing 119 of the 122 predicted protein kinases of yeast, and subjected them to 17 different substrates exhibiting a variety of novel activities. The protein microarray or proteome array has been subsequently extended to cover nearly the entire genomic complement of yeast *(59)*. Although this study detailed a limited number of probes for the array, the broad use of this approach is likely to fuel significant progress in our efforts at functional genomics.

IN VIVO TARGET VALIDATION

One of the critical observations in antifungal drug development has been that traditional in vitro MIC data does not always correlate well with in vivo efficacy. Possible reasons for this discrepancy include: inhibition of non-cidal protein targets, the importance of pharmacokinetics in the efficacy of drugs, and differences between the microbial environment in tissues and in the test tube. One way to eliminate some of the variability is to utilize new technologies to validate targets directly in animal model systems. Which of the so-called essential genes identified from in vitro testing in ideal growth media are necessary for survival and growth in vivo can be systematically tested with available tools.

One approach with the potential for widespread application has been utilized systematically to test potential target genes for their contribution to growth or pathogenesis in vivo, in an animal model. Nagahashi and colleagues reported the use of regulated gene expression under the control of a tetracycline-responsive promoter and an ectopically expressed tetracycline repressor (*tet*R), fused to a eukaryotic transcription activation domain *(60)*. In this instance, expression of a gene was induced by the removal of tetracycline or repressed in its presence. In the genetic background of a deletion of the wild-type locus of the target gene, the contribution of the tetracycline-regulated gene to infection was determined. Nakayama et al. constructed a pathogenic *C. glabrata* strain with either a *tet*O/*tet*R-dependent *TEF3* (peptide elongation factor 3) or a *TOP2* (topoisomerase II) gene, and showed that these strains could not establish or maintain an infection in the presence of tetracycline *(61)*. For target evaluation, this type of experiment would ensure that the impact of target depletion in an established infection could be assessed. The most desired targets would be those that cause the infection to abate in the absence of target expression in an animal model of immunocompromised host infection.

The interaction between host and pathogen is a complex and poorly understood process. The virulence of closely related fungal isolates can vary widely. Similarly, protein-expression patterns of related but distinct isolates of *S. cerevisiae* can also vary widely *(52)*. Signature-tagged mutagenesis, a random screening approach originally described for bacteria *(62)*, has now been applied on a limited scale to *A. fumigatus* and *C. neoformans (63,64)*. This technology consists of infecting a host with a collection of uniquely marked mutants made by site-directed mutagenesis. Following competitive growth in the host, the presence or absence of each mutant is determined by polymerase chain reaction (PCR) of the unique sequence tag. It is important to note that only nonessential genes (as defined by the ability to grow in vitro in complex medium in the absence of a particular gene) can be analyzed in this way. However, they provide a subset of targets of potential clinical relevance, which may otherwise be overlooked using other criteria.

VIRULENCE FACTORS

One of the arguments against using *S. cerevisiae* and its tools for drug discovery has been its limited pathogenic potential. However, *S. cerevisiae* has been isolated from severely immunocompromised patients *(65),* and it does mimic an important physiological trait exhibited by genuine clinical pathogens. In response to nutrient limitation, certain strains of *S. cerevisiae* undergo a switch similar to the transition from the yeast to the filamentous form seen in *C. albicans* and known to be critical to pathogenesis (reviewed in ref. *66*). Similar morphological changes are observed in other dimorphic fungal pathogens *(67)*. However, it was in *S. cerevisiae* that the key features and modulators of this process were initially characterized *(68,69)*. This work indicated that homologues of members of the mitogen-activated protein (MAP) kinase cascade play critical roles in the yeast-to-pseudohyphal switch in *S. cerevisiae*. Subsequent studies with other fungi confirmed this concept and further suggested that these factors are required at least in part for the critical phase transition event *(70)*. Although *S. cerevisiae* may not be well suited to animal model testing of many of the other documented virulence factors *(71)*, it can provide a robust in vitro system for hypothesis testing. For example, an integrin-like factor—*CaINT1* from *C. albicans,* tested using *S. cerevisiae* as a genetically tractable surrogate—suggested that *CaINT1* plays a role in cellular adhesion, filamentous growth, and virulence in the pathogen *(72,73)*.

The growing understanding of pathogenic factors and their appearance in clinical isolates may be a source for antifungal intervention targets. A recent study indicated that microarray technology could be used to compare the allelic differences that exist between *S. cerevisiae* laboratory strains on a genome-wide scale *(74)*. A related approach has recently been used in bacteria to identify potential virulence factors *(75)*, and could conceivably be applied to fungi as well to provide insight on a genomic scale on important virulence targets.

DRUG DISCOVERY ON A GENOMIC SCALE

What do all these new technologies, founded in a model organism and applied to pathogens, mean for drug development? First, the effort shifts away from traditional, mechanism-based screening of selected single gene targets to multiple, parallel protein-specific screening efforts. Second, target validation and ultra high-throughput screening efforts move forward as essential components of the discovery process. Third, in vivo disease model systems and methods for evaluating potential interactions in human tissue-culture systems become critical parameters in eliminating and predicting drug failures prior to clinical evaluation. As technologies that can identify the potential interactions between a drug and intracellular components (of either the pathogen or host cells) become more readily available, preclinical evaluation will become a much more critical factor in bringing a compound to the clinic. Instead of choosing the compound that exhibits the best interaction between inhibitor and a single target, high-throughput parallel robotics systems will permit scientists to choose among compounds that exhibit a suitable interaction concomitant with poor binding to other host components.

Ultimately, genomics—in conjunction with all the other recent developments in chemistry, robotics, miniaturization, and parallel processing—offers the promise of newer medicines, developed more rapidly and thus more cost-effectively than traditional methods of discovery *(76)*. How soon we will realize these goals depends on how far in the future one is willing to look. Realistically, fungal genomics does little more than place pre-existing genetics capabilities on a logarithmic scale. Prior to 1998, only a few hundred phenotypes were known from knockouts or disruption experiments.

Genomics and footprinting/knockout experiments have now identified all the essential genes in yeast. Have potential new targets been identified? Have they been validated? Genomics has led us inside the candy store—like a child, one's eyes are wide with wonder, and as an adult we need to make choices.

CONCLUSION

Where do we stand, six years after the first fungal organism was sequenced to completion and one year after the human genome was mapped? Are we any closer to eradicating the pathogens of the microbial world? How many complete genomes must be sequenced before a new product, derived solely on the basis of genomic research, reaches the pharmacy shelves? We can assay many more targets, screen millions of compounds in ever smaller micro-volumes, and predict the binding pockets of related chemical structures. But where are the drugs? More importantly, how many of them will actually make it out of industry pipelines and into the marketplace?

Clearly, the opportunities for new research and new directions that have been afforded to the scientific community cannot be easily quantified. And the slow, careful pace of systematic research into human disease can often appear agonizingly glacial to anyone touched by disease. Yet it can hardly be argued that genomic research, and more importantly, the post-genomic era, will ultimately yield breakthrough products to benefit humankind.

ACKNOWLEDGMENTS

The authors wish to thank Roberta S. Hare for her support and Todd A. Black for his critical review of the manuscript.

REFERENCES

1. Tkacz J, DiDomenico B. Antifungals: what's in the pipeline? Curr Opin Microbiol 2001;4:540–545.
2. Georgopapdakou NH. Antifungals: mechanism of action and resistance, established and novel drugs. Curr Opin Microbiol 1998;1:547–557.
3. DiDomenico B. Novel antifungal drugs. Curr Opin Microbiol 1999;2:509–515.
4. Nagiec M, Nagiec E, Baltisberger J, Wells G, Lester R, Dickson R. Sphingolipid synthesis as a target for antifungal drugs. Complementation of the inositol phosphorylceramide synthase defect in a mutant strain of Saccharomyces cerevisiae by the AUR1 gene. J Biol Chem 1997;272:9809–9817.
5. Sandbaken M, Lupisella J, DiDomenico B, Chakraburtty K. Protein synthesis in yeast. Structural and functional analysis of the gene encoding elongation factor 3. J Biol Chem 1990;265:15,838–15,844.
6. Fostel J, Montgomery D, Shen L. Characterization of DNA topoisomerase I from Candida albicans as a target for drug discovery. Antimicrob Agents Chemother 1992;36:2131–2138.
7. Kishore N, Lu T, Knoll L, Katoh A, Rudnick D, Mehta P, et al. The substrate specificity of Saccharomyces cerevisiae myristoyl-CoA:protein N-myristoyltransferase. Analysis of myristic acid analogs containing oxygen, sulfur, double bonds, triple bonds, and/or an aromatic residue. J Biol Chem 1991;266:8835–8855.
8. Lodge J, Jackson-Machelski E, Toffaletti D, Perfect J, Gordon J. Targeted gene replacement demonstrates that myristoyl-CoA: protein N-myristoyltransferase is essential for viability of Cryptococcus neoformans. Proc Natl Acad Sci USA 1994;91:12,008–12,012.
9. Goffeau A, Barrell B, Bussey H, Davis R, Dujon B, Feldmann H, et al. Life with 6000 genes. Science 1996;274:563–567.

10. Ball C, Jin H, Sherlock G, Weng S, Matese J, Andrada R, et al. Saccharomyces Genome Database provides tools to survey gene expression and functional analysis data. Nucleic Acids Res 2001;29:80–81.

11. International Human Genome Sequencing Consortium. Initial sequencing and analysis of the human genome. Nature 2001;409:860–921.

12. Venter JC, et al. The sequence of the human genome. Science 2001;291:1304–1351.

13. Rothstein R. One-step gene disruption in yeast. Meth Enz 1983;101:202–211.

14. Wach A, Brachat A, Pohlmann R, Philippsen P. New heterologous modules for classical or PCR-based gene disruptions in Saccharomyces cerevisiae. Yeast 1994;10:1793–1808.

15. Smith V, Botstein D, Brown P. Genetic footprinting: a genomic strategy for determining a gene's function given its sequence. Proc Natl Acad Sci USA 1995;92:6479–6483.

16. Baudin A, Ozier-Kalogeropoulos O, Denouel A, Lacroute F, Cullin C. A simple and efficient method for direct gene deletion in Saccharomyces cerevisiae. Nucleic Acids Res 1993;21:3329–3330.

17. Wilson R, Davis D, Mitchell A. Rapid hypothesis testing with Candida albicans through gene disruption with short homology regions. J Bacteriol 1999;181:1868–1874.

18. Winzeler E, Shoemaker D, Astromoff A, Liang H, Anderson K, Andre B, et al. Functional characterization of the S. cerevisiae genome by gene deletion and parallel analysis. Science 1999;285:901–906.

19. Kelly DE, Lamb DC, Kelly SL. Genome-wide generation of yeast gene deletion strains. Comp Funct Genomics 2001;2:236–242.

20. Asch D, Kinsey J. Relationship of vector insert size to homologous integration during transformation of Neurospora crassa with the cloned am (GDH) gene. Mol Gen Genet 1990;221:37–43.

21. Kelly R, Miller S, Kurtz M, Kirsch D. Directed mutagenesis in Candida albicans: one-step gene disruption to isolate ura3 mutants. Mol Cell Biol 1987;7:199–208.

22. Kwon-Chung K. Gene disruption to evaluate the role of fungal candidate virulence genes. Curr Opin Microbiol 1998;1:381–389.

23. Gonzalez C, Perdomo G, Tejera P, Brito N, Sivero J. One-step, PCR-mediated, gene disruption in the yeast Hansenula polymorpha. Yeast 1999;15:1323–1329.

24. Wendland J, Ayad-Durieux Y, Knechtle P, Rebischung C, Philippsen P. PCR-based gene targeting in the filamentous fungus Ashbya gossypii. Gene 2000;242:381–391.

25. Reichard U, Cole G, Hill T, Ruchel R, Monod M. Molecular characterization and influence on fungal development of ALP2, a novel serine proteinase from Aspergillus fumigatus. Int J Med Microbiol 2000;290:549–558.

26. Smith V, Chou K, Lashkari D, Botstein D, Brown P. Functional analysis of the genes of yeast chromosome V by genetic footprinting. Science 1996;274:2069–2074.

27. Brown J, Holden D. Insertional mutagenesis of pathogenic fungi. Curr Opin Microbiol 1998;1:390–394.

28. Schneider J, Guarente L. Vectors for expression of cloned genes in yeast: regulation, overproduction, and underproduction. Meth Enzymol 1991;194:373–388.

29. Zhou P, Thiele D. Isolation of a metal-activated transcription factor gene from Candida glabrata by complementation in Saccharomyces cerevisiae. Proc Natl Acad Sci USA 1991;88:6112–6116.

30. Wickes B, Edman J. The Cryptococcus neoformans GAL7 gene and its use as an inducible promoter. Mol Microbiol 1995;16:1099–1109.

31. Backen A, Broadbent I, Fetherston R, Rosamond J, Schnell N, Stark M. Evaluation of the CaMAL2 promoter for regulated expression of genes in Candida albicans. Yeast 2000;16:1121–1129.

32. Struhl K, Stinchcomb D, Scherer S, Davis R. High-frequency transformation of yeast: autonomous replication of hybrid DNA molecules. Proc Natl Acad Sci USA 1979;76:1035–1039.

33. Clarke L, Carbon J. Isolation of a yeast centromere and construction of functional small circular chromosomes. Nature 1980;287:504–509.
34. Szostak J, Blackburn E. Cloning yeast telomeres on linear plasmid vectors. Cell 1982;29:245–255.
35. Thorvaldsen J, Mehra R, Yu W, Sewell A, Winge D. Analysis of copper-induced metallothionein expression using autonomously replicating plasmids in Candida glabrata. Yeast 1995;11:1501–1511.
36. Pla J, Perez-Diaz R, Navarro-Garcia F, Sanchez M, Nombela C. Cloning of the Candida albicans HIS1 gene by direct complementation of a C. albicans histidine auxotroph using an improved double-ARS shuttle vector. Gene 1995;165:115–120.
37. Aleksenko A, Nikolaev I, Vinetski Y, Clutterbuck A. Gene expression from replicating plasmids in Aspergillus nidulans. Mol Gen Genet 1996;253:242–246.
38. d'Enfert C, Weidner G, Mol P, Brakhage A. Transformation systems of Aspergillus fumigatus. In: (Brakhage A, Jahn B, Schmidt A, eds.) Aspergillus fumigatus. 1999, Kager: Basel, pp. 149–166.
39. Giaever G, Shoemaker D, Jones T, Liang H, Winzeler E, Astromoff A, et al. Genomic profiling of drug sensitivities via induced haploinsufficiency. Nat Genet 1999;21:278–283.
40. De Backer M, Nelissen B, Logghe M, Viaene J, Loonen I, Vandoninck S, et al. An antisense-based functional genomics approach for identification of genes critical for growth of Candida albicans. Nat Biotechnol 2001;19:235–241.
41. Song S, Lee K. A novel function of Saccharomyces cerevisiae CDC5 in cytokinesis. J Cell Biol 2001;152:451–469.
42. Anthony C, Zong Q, De Benedetti A. Overexpression of eIF4E in S. cerevisiae causes slow growth and decreased alpha-factor response through alterations in Cln3 expression. J Biol Chem 2001;276:39645–39652.
43. Grandin N, Charbonneau M. Hsp90 levels affect telomere length in yeast. Mol Genet Genomics 2001;265:126–134.
44. Chee M, Yang R, Hubbell E, Berno A, Huang X, Stern D, et al. Accessing genomic information with high-density arrays. Science 1996;274:610–614.
45. Lashkari D, DeRisi J, McCusker J, Namath A, Gentile C, Hwang S, et al. Yeast microarrays for genome wide parallel genetic and gene expression analysis. Proc Natl Acad Sci USA 1997;94:13,057–13,062.
46. De Backer M, Ilyina T, Ma X, Vandoninck S, Luyten W, Vanden Bossche H. Genomic profiling of the response of Candida albicans to Itraconazole treatment using a DNA microarray. Antimicrob Agents Chemother 2001;45:1660–1670.
47. Hughes T, Marton M, Jones A, Roberts C, Stoughton R, Armour C, et al. Functional discovery via a compendium of expression profiles. Cell 2000;102:109–126.
48. Hughes T, Roberts C, Dai H, Jones A, Meyer M, Slade D, et al. Widespread aneuploidy revealed by DNA microarray expression profiling. Nat Genet 2000;25:333–337.
49. Bammert G, Fostel J. Genome-wide expression patterns in Saccharomyces cerevisiae: Comparison of drug treatments and genetic alterations affecting biosynthesis of ergosterol. Antimicrob Agents Chemother 2000;44:1255–1265.
50. Velculescu V, Zhang L, Zhou W, Vogelstein J, Basrai M, Bassett D, et al. Characterization of the yeast transcriptome. Cell 1997;88:243–251.
51. Padney A, Mann M. Proteomics to study genes and genomes. Nature 2000;405:837–846.
52. Rogowska-Wrzesinska P, Mose Larsen P, Blomberg A, Gorg A, Roepstorff P, Norbeck J, et al. Comparison of the proteomes of three yeast wild type strains: CEN.PK2, FY1679 and W303. Comp Funct Genomics 2001;2:207–225.
53. Ross-Macdonald P, Coelho P, Roemer T, Agarwal S, Kumar A, Jansen R, et al. Large-scale analysis of the yeast genome by transposon tagging and gene disruption. Nature 1999;402:413–418.
54. Fields S, Song O. A novel genetic system to detect protein-protein interactions. Nature 1989;340:245–246.

55. Uetz P, Giot L, Cagney G, Mansfield T, Judson R, Knight J, et al. A comprehensive analysis of protein-protein interactions in Saccharomyces cerevisiae. Nature 2000;403:623–627.

56. Schwikowski B, Uetz P, Fields S. A network of protein-protein interactions in yeast. Nat Biotechnol 2000;18:1257–1261.

57. Ito T, Chiba T, Ozawa R, Yoshida M, Hattori M, Sakaki Y. A comprehensive two-hybrid analysis to explore the yeast protein interactome. Proc Natl Acad Sci USA 2001;98:4569–4574.

58. Zhu H, Klemic J, Chang S, Bertone P, Casamayor A, Klemic K, et al. Analysis of yeast protein kinases using protein chips. Nat Genet 2000;26:283–289.

59. Zhu H, Bilgin M, Bangham R, Hall D, Casamayor A, Bertone P, et al. Global analysis of protein activities using proteome chips. Science 2001;293:2101–2105.

60. Nagahashi S, Nakayama H, Hamada K, Yang H, Ariwasa M, Kitada K. Regulation by tetracycline of gene expression in Saccharomyces cerevisiae. Mol Gen Genet 1997;255:372–375.

61. Nakayama H, Izuta M, Nagahashi S, Sihta E, Sato Y, Yamazaki T, et al. A controllable gene-expression system for the pathogenic fungus Candida glabrata. Microbiology 1998;144:2407–2415.

62. Unsworth K, Holden D. Identification and analysis of bacterial virulence genes in vivo. Philos Trans R Soc Lond B Biol Sci 2000;355:613–622.

63. Brown J, Aufauvre-Brown A, Brown J, Jennings J, Arst Jr. H, Holden D. Signature-tagged and directed mutagenesis identify PABA synthetase as essential for Aspergillus fumigatus pathogenicity. Mol Microbiol 2000;36:1371–1380.

64. Nelson R, Hua J, Pryor B, Lodge J. Identification of virulence mutants of the fungal pathogen Cryptococcus neoformans using signature-tagged mutagenesis. Genetics 2001;157:935–947.

65. Zerva L, Hollis R, Pfaller M. In vitro susceptibility testing and DNA typing of Saccharomyces clinical isolates. J Clin Microbiol 1996;34:3031–3034.

66. Gow N. Germ tube growth of Candida albicans. Curr Top Med Mycol 1997;8:43–55.

67. Larone D. Medically important fungi: a guide to identification, 3rd ed. Washington, DC: ASM Press, 1995; 1–78.

68. Gimeno C, Ljungdahl P, Styles C, Fink G. Unipolar cell divisions in the yeast S. cerevisiae lead to filamentous growth: regulation by starvation and RAS. Cell 1992;68:1077–1090.

69. Pan X, Harashima T, Heitman J. Signal transduction cascades regulating pseudohyphal differentiation of Saccharomyces cerevisiae. Curr Opin Microbiol 2000;3:567–572.

70. Lengeler K, Davidson R, D'souza C, Harashima T, Shen W, Wang P, et al. Signal transduction cascades regulating fungal development and virulence. Microbiol Molec Biol Rev 2000;64:746–785.

71. Perfect J. Fungal virulence genes as targets for antifungal chemotherapy. Antimicrob Agents Chemother 1996;40:1577–1583.

72. Gale C, Finkel D, Tao N, Meinke M, McClellan M, Olson J, et al. Cloning and expression of a gene encoding an integrin-like protein in Candida albicans. Proc Natl Acad Sci USA 1996;93:357–361.

73. Gale C, Bendel C, McClellan M, Hauser M, Becker J, Berman J, et al. Linkage of adhesion, filamentous growth, and virulence in Candida albicans to a single gene, INT1. Science 1998;279:1355–1358.

74. Winzeler E, Richards D, Conway A, Goldstein A, Kalman S, McCullough M, et al. Direct allelic variation scanning of the yeast genome. Science 1998;281:1194–1197.

75. Chizhikov V, Rasooly A, Chumakov K, Levy D. Microarray analysis of microbial virulence factors. Appl Environ Microbiol 2001;67:3258–3263.

76. Black T, Hare R. Will genomics revolutionize antimicrobial drug discovery? Curr Opin Microbiol 2000;3:522–527.

12

Antifungal Drug Discovery: Old Drugs, New Tools

Marianne D. De Backer, Walter H. M. L. Luyten, and Hugo F. Vanden Bossche

MYCOSES

In the first part of the twentieth century, medical mycology focused on the identification of fungal species that affect the skin, nails and mucous membranes *(1)*. Although superficial infections, such as athlete's foot and vaginal thrush, occur in every climatic zone and afflict all strata of society, these infections are mostly mild in nature and mainly of cosmetic importance. However, over the past twenty years, the actual incidence of invasive fungal infections has increased as well as the clinical awareness that fungal infections are a serious risk to health and can be life-threatening *(1,2)*. The increasing frequency at which pathogenic fungi are identified is related to the heightened use of powerful and broad-spectrum antibacterial agents, cancer chemotherapy, transplantations, and more aggressive immunosuppression, the increased survival of premature infants in neonatal intensive care units, the growing population of the elderly, and finally the emergence of AIDS *(1,3–5)*.

The increasing incidence of fungal infections is largely caused by opportunistic pathogens such as the *Candida* species. Until the 1970s, *Candida* species were generally regarded as little more than culture contaminants *(6)*. However, more recently, Pfaller et al. reported that *Candida albicans* has become the fourth leading cause of nocosomial bloodstream infections in the United States *(6,7)*. In a surveillance study of candidemia in cancer patients that was conducted by the European Organization for Research and Treatment of Cancer, 249 episodes were noted. *C. albicans* was isolated in 70% of the 90 cases involving patients with solid tumors and in 36% of the 159 involving those with hematologic disease *(8)*. In the same study, it was shown that neutropenia in tumor patients and acute leukemia and antifungal prophylaxis in hematology patients were significantly associated with non-albicans candidemia, and *C. glabrata* was associated with the highest mortality rate *(8)*. The role of *C. dubliniensis* as a pathogen has been limited to oral candidiasis, but recently cases of *C. dubliniensis* fungemia have been reported in bone-marrow transplant recipients with chemotherapy-induced neutropenia *(9)*, in two patients with end-stage liver disease, and also in a HIV-infected person *(10)*. Another non-*albicans* species of clinical importance is *C. tropicalis*. Unlike *C. albicans*, which can be

From: *Pathogen Genomics: Impact on Human Health*
Edited by: K. J. Shaw © Humana Press Inc., Totowa, NJ

found as a commensal, *C. tropicalis* is almost invariably associated with the development of fungal infections.

In addition to candidemia, aspergillosis and cryptococcosis have become increasingly prevalent in immunocompromised or seriously ill patients. Recently the *Aspergillus* Study Group *(11)* collected data from 595 patients with proven or probable invasive aspergillosis. The major risk factors for aspergillosis were bone-marrow transplantation (36%) and hematologic malignancy (29%), but patients had a variety of underlying conditions including solid-organ transplants (9%), AIDS (8%), and pulmonary diseases (9%) *(11)*.

Cryptococcosis was a rare disease before the HIV epidemic *(5)*. Indeed, patients with T-cell deficiencies are most susceptible to infection with *Cryptococcus neoformans*. Subacute meningitis and meningoencephalitis are clinically typical *(12)*. If untreated, meningo-encephalitis is 100% fatal, and even when treated with the presently available antifungal agents, infections with *C. neoformans* can be fatal in patients with T-cell deficiencies *(13)*.

Pneumocystis carinii pneumonia (PCP) is a major opportunistic infection in HIV-positive individuals, yet PCP may also be the cause of pneumonia in 10–40% of HIV-negative immunocompromised patients, with mortality rates of 20–50% *(14,15)*. Other fungi once believed to be nonpathogenic are now routinely encountered in the clinical setting, among them the well-known baker's or brewer's yeast, *Saccharomyces cerevisiae,* and *S. boulardii (16)*. *S. boulardii* is an increasing cause of fungemia in hospitalized patients *(16)*.

In addition to these opportunistic fungi, a number of fungi exist with a true pathogenic potential for healthy hosts, and causing life-threatening infections restricted to their geographical areas. During the last 10–15 years, they are evolving into opportunistic infections that may be encountered elsewhere *(17)*.

Histoplasmosis caused by *Histoplasma capsulatum* var. *capsulatum* is the most commonly diagnosed endemic mycosis in patients with AIDS *(18);* it is also the most common endemic fungal infection among organ-transplant recipients *(19)*. Infection is concentrated in the eastern United States, but is also found in Central and parts of South America, such as Argentina, Paraguay, and Venezuela. For example, approximately 4–5% of AIDS patients are afflicted with disseminated histoplasmosis in Buenos Aires *(20)*. Disseminated histoplasmosis has also been found in immunocompromised patients in non-endemic areas *(21)*.

Coccidioidomycosis, a systemic disease caused by the dimorphic fungus *Coccidioides immitis,* is endemic in the southwestern United States, Northern Mexico, Central America and parts of Southern America *(18,22)*. Coccidioidomycosis has also been reported in areas where the disease is not endemic, such as New York State, although most cases involved patients who had visited endemic areas *(23)*. In most healthy individuals, *C. immitis* causes asymptomatic or mild respiratory illness. However, severe and often fatal disease occurs in profoundly immunodeficient patients infected with HIV, or treated for cancer *(18,23)*. Disseminated infections caused by the dimorphic fungus *Penicillium marneffei* were rarely reported prior to 1985 *(24)*. The subsequent rapid rise in the number of the reported cases of penicilliosis paralleled the explosive epidemic of AIDS in Thailand. In this country, approximately 1200 cases were observed in a single hospital in a 7-yr period *(20)*.

It should be noted that changes are occurring in the epidemiology of opportunistic infections in patients with AIDS and treated with highly active antiretroviral therapy (HAART). However, the situation is less clear for cryptococcosis or endemic mycoses, and the epidemiology is dramatically different in the countries that cannot afford the cost of HAART (reviewed in ref. *25*).

ANTIFUNGAL DRUG THERAPIES

Introduction

The development of antifungal drug therapies has not evolved as rapidly as the development of antibacterial drug therapies, in part because the human or animal host and the fungal pathogen are all eukaryotes and have many genes and proteins in common. Agents that inhibit protein, RNA, and DNA synthesis have a great potential for toxicity. Compounds that exist for treating fungal disorders are therefore generally limited in their treatment because of their toxicity and side effects. Furthermore, the currently available antifungals are small in number and belong to only a limited number of different chemical classes. Indeed, on the basis of their molecular mechanism of action (MOA) the presently available compounds can be classified in only five classes (Table 1). Amphotericin B, still considered the gold standard for the treatment of most life-threatening fungal infections, was discovered in the early 1950s, and flucytosine in the early 1960s. In the late 1970s, the number of available agents doubled with the addition of intravenous (iv) miconazole and oral ketoconazole, and it was not until the late 1980s that options for systemic treatment substantially expanded through the clinical development of fluconazole and itraconazole. Some of the antifungals listed in Table 1, such as flucytosine (5FC), griseofulvin, the allylamines, naftifine and terbinafine, and the topical polyene nystatin have relatively narrow spectrums of activity that restrict their use to either yeasts or dermatophyte infections *(50)*.

The characteristics of therapeutics currently used to combat fungal infections are discussed in the following section.

Flucytosine

The synthetic fluorinated pyrimidine 5-FC inhibits growth of *Candida* spp and *C. neoformans* at low concentrations; dematiaceous fungi such as *Fonsecaea pedrosoi* are moderately sensitive *(35)*. Although 5-FC inhibits growth of many *Aspergillus* isolates, its clinical efficacy in aspergillosis is equivocal. This difference in sensitivity may result from the fact that in *Aspergillus* 5-FC exerts only fungistatic activity, whereas a fungicidal effect is seen in yeast and dematiaceae after prolonged contact (reviewed in refs. *35,51*). Monotherapy with 5-FC is limited because of the frequent development of resistance *(51)*. Indeed, the incidence of primary resistance and the selection of secondary resistance during monotherapy with 5-FC is a major problem *(52)*. In *Candida,* the incidence of resistance is dependent on variables such as the country, between 10% and 40%. *(50)*. In *C. neoformans,* 1.8% of strains tested were found to be naturally resistant, but during treatment resistant mutants are easily selected *(52)*. The main side-effects are nausea and vomiting. A more serious, but rare, adverse reaction is hepatotoxicity, and the most serious side effect is bone-marrow depression *(51)*. At present, flucytosine is mainly used in combination with amphotericin B.

Table 1
Antifungal drugs

Status	Chemical classes	Drugs*	Targets	References
Registered	Pyrimidine	Flucytosine (o, iv)	DNA & RNA synthesis	26,27
	Polyenes	Amphotericin B (iv, t, o)	Membrane barrier function	27,28
		Nystatin (t,o)		
	Azoles	Bifonazole (t)	Ergosterol biosynthesis 14α-demethylase CYP51	27,29,30
	Imidazoles	Clotrimazole (t)		
		Econazole (t)		
		Ketoconazole (t, o)		
		Miconazole (t)		
	Triazoles	Fluconazole (o, iv)		
		Itraconazole (o, iv)		
		Terconazole (t)		
	Allylamines	Naftifine (t)	Squalene epoxidase	31,32
		Terbinafine (t, o)		
	Morpholines	Amorolfine (t)	Δ^{14}-Reductase + Δ^8-Δ^7-isomerase	26
	Echinocandins	Caspofungin (MK-0991) (iv)	1,3 β-D-glucan synthase	33,34
	Antibiotic	Griseofulvin (o)	inhibits microtubule sliding	35
Clinical development	Triazoles	Voriconazole (UK-109496) (o, iv)	14α-Demethylase	17,33,36,37
		Posaconazole (Sch-56592) (o)		33,38
		Ravuconazole (BMS-207147) (o)		33,39
		UR-9825 (o)		40
	Echinocandins	VER-002 (LY303366) (iv)	1,3 β-D-glucan synthase	33,41,42
		FK 463 (iv)		33
Preclinical	Nikkomycins	Nikkomycin Z**	Chitin synthases	40,43
	Sordarins	GM-237354	Elongation factor 2	44,45
	Cyclic depsipeptides (Aureobasidins)	Aureobasidin A	Inositolphosphoryl-ceramide synthase	46–49

* o, oral; t, topical; iv, intravenous.

** Nikkomycin Z is not currently under active development (43)

Polyenes

Polyenes are effective in the treatment of many mycoses. The most widely used member of the group is amphotericin B (AmB). AmB-deoxycholate (AmB-d) is not absorbed from the gastrointestinal tract or from sites of muscular injection, and is thus administered intravenously almost exclusively. Since AmB is a fungicidal, broad-spectrum antifungal agent with a rapid onset of action, it is still indicated for treatment of life-threatening fungal infections. However, adverse effects are common, and nephrotoxicity is the most serious, occurring early in the course of treatment *(53)*. Renal toxicity is mostly reversible, but, permanent changes in renal function and histology have been demonstrated *(54)*. To overcome the problem of nephrotoxicity, AmB has been formulated in liposomes and other lipid complexes. At present, three different formulations are commercially available: liposomal amphotericin B (AmBisome), amphotericin B lipid complex (ABLC), and amphotericin B colloidal dispersion (ABCD) *(55)*. Most studies indicate that the lipid formulations have reduced glomerular toxicities compared to AmB-d *(55)*. However, all the lipid preparations are relatively expensive *(55)*.

Griseofulvin

The use of griseofulvin as an orally active antifungal against ringworm in man was first described in 1958 *(56)*. The spectrum of activity of this fungicidal treatment is limited to dermatophytes. This is because dermatophytes possess a prolonged energy-dependent transport system for this antibiotic, whereas in insensitive cells, such as *C. albicans,* this is replaced by a short energy-independent transport system (reviewed in ref. *26*). Griseofulvin has become a standard treatment for onychomycosis caused by dermatophytes *(57)*. Fingernails usually must be treated for 5–6 mo, and toenails for 8–18 mo. Side effects include leukopenia *(57)*. Whereas griseofulvin is considered by many as the mainstay of treatment in tinea capitis, newer oral antifungal agents—including azole antifungal agents such as itraconazole, and the allylamine, terbinafine—have demonstrated higher efficacy, allowing shorter duration of treatment *(58)*.

Azoles

The imidazole and triazole derivatives (Table 1) are the agents most often used in the clinic against a wide range of fungal pathogens *(50)*. The antifungal activity of azole derivatives such as miconazole *(59)*, econazole, bifonazole, clotrimazole *(60)*, ketoconazole *(60,61)*, itraconazole *(30,60,62)* and fluconazole *(63)*, arises from a complex multi-mechanistic process initiated by the inhibition of two cytochromes P450 involved in the biosynthesis of ergosterol, namely the P450 that catalyzes the 14α-demethylation step encoded by *ERG11 (CYP51),* and the Δ22-desaturase, encoded by *ERG5 (CYP61)* (30). The sterol-14α-demethylase is the major fungal target for all azole derivatives studied thus far. Interaction with CYP51 results in a decreased availability of ergosterol and an accumulation of 14-methylsterols and 3-ketosteroids *(30,35,60,64–66)*.

The in vitro and in vivo activities of the azole antifungal agents have been examined in multiple studies (*see* refs. *17,35,37,50*). Most of the imidazole derivatives (e.g., miconazole, clotrimazole, and econazole) are available for topical application only, but

ketoconazole is the exception. This dioxolane imidazole derivative was the first compound of the azole class to be systemically absorbed after oral administration *(67,68)*,
and is used both orally and topically. Ketoconazole's activity spectrum in clinical use
includes superficial mycoses (such as dermatophytosis, *Candida* infections, pityriasis
versicolor), chronic *Candida* infections, forms of blastomycosis, coccidioidomycosis,
histoplasmosis, and paracoccidioidomycosis *(50,69)*. In immunocompetent parients,
ketoconazole has been described as a reasonable alternative to amphotericin B, with
comparable response and no nephrotoxicity *(69)*. Yet HIV-infected patients with histoplasmosis respond poorly to ketoconazole, and it is not effective for long-term suppres-
sive therapy in immunocompromised patients *(17)*.

When used at higher concentrations, ketoconazole affects other cytochrome P450s
in addition to CYP51. For example, at concentrations >100 nm, it inhibits not only the
mammalian CYP51, but also 17-hydroxylase-17,20-lyase (CYP17), the cholesterol
side-chain cleavage (CYP11A1) and the 11β-hydroxyalse (CYP11B1) *(70)*. Ketoconazole is also an inhibitor of CYP3A4, a major drug-metabolizing P450 isoform in
humans. Co-administration of ketoconazole with CYP3A4 substrates such as
cyclosporine, tacrolimus, lovastatin, terfenadine, and astemisole can result in clinically
significant drug interactions *(71)*. Ketoconazole should not be used in patients with
abnormal liver-function tests.

It took almost ten years before the triazole derivatives, itraconazole *(72)* and fluconazole *(73)*, became available for treatment of systemic mycoses. Itraconazole is
indicated for the oral treatment of superficial mycoses, including *Candida* infections,
dermatophytosis, and pityriasis versicolor *(35,74)*. It has a broad range of indications
for oral therapy in systemic mycoses such as blastomycosis, histoplasmosis, paracoccidioidomycosis, phaeohyphomycosis, and sporotrichosis. It can also be used to treat
disseminated *Candida* infections and some forms of coccidioidomycosis. Itraconazole
is also indicated for maintenance therapy of cryptococcosis in AIDS *(17,50,74)*, and
has been approved by the FDA as a second-line agent for the treatment of aspergillosis
(75,76). This triazole derivative is almost devoid of effects on P450-dependent steroid
biosynthesis and catabolism *(62)*. However, like ketoconazole, itraconazole also
inhibits CYP3A4 *(71)*. Asymptomatic elevation of liver enzymes has been reported in
some patients *(74)*.

The fluorinated *bis*-triazole known as fluconazole is indicated for the treatment of
superficial and disseminated *C. albicans* infections, and for primary and maintenance
treatment of cryptococcosis *(17,50)*. It is not indicated for aspergillosis or zygomy-
coses, and is not active against *C. krusei* and many isolates of *C. glabrata* *(50)*. Fluconazole is a potent inhibitor of CYP2C9 *(71)*. Co-administration of phenytoin,
warfarin, sulfamethoxazole, and losartan with fluconazole also results in clinically significant drug interactions *(71)*.

Until the late 1980s, resistance of pathogens to azole antifungals was rarely
reported, and invariably occurred in immunocompromised patients. It was the increase
in the number of these patients, partially as a result of the AIDS pandemic, that preceded the sudden increase of reports of clinical failure to fluconazole therapy (see refs.
6,27,77,78). The importance of a normal immune system can be related to the fungistatic mode of action of the azoles, which implies that part of the clearance of the fungal
infection must be accomplished by host-related factors *(79)*. The development of azole

resistance in *C. albicans* is most problematic in patients with AIDS who receive long courses of drug treatment for therapy or prevention of oral candidiasis, but a rapid development of resistance has been noted in other immunosuppressed patients who developed disseminated candidiasis despite fluconazole prophylaxis *(80)*. Of great concern is the multi-azole resistance among patients with oropharyngeal candidiasis *(78)*. Long-term itraconazole prophylaxis in patients with AIDS is associated with a reduction in susceptibility to itraconazole and cross-resistance to fluconazole *(81)*. Cross-resistance is not limited to the presently available azole derivative. Weig and Muller recently studied 39 clinical *C. albicans* isolates that were cross-resistant to fluconazole and voriconazole *(82)*.

Terbinafine

Terbinafine is an allylanine that affects ergosterol biosynthesis by inhibiting squalene epoxidase. The present clinical use of this fungicidal agent *(31,32,50)* is restricted to dermatophyte infections. Recent clinical studies have shown that terbinafine is also active in the treatment of sporotrichosis and disseminated aspergillosis *(83)*. A number of in vitro studies with combinations of fluconazole-terbinafine, itraconazole-terbinafine (reviewed in ref. *17*) or voriconazole-terbinafine *(82)* have shown synergy in vitro against *C. albicans,* including even fluconazole-resistant strains. These findings may broaden the clinical usage of terbinafine.

Caspofungin

Unlike the azole antifungal agents, the echinocandins attack the cell wall by inhibiting the β-1,3-glucan synthase *(33,34)*. Recently, the FDA granted marketing clearance for the echinocandin from Merck known as caspofungin acetate (Cancidas®). Caspofungin, a fungicidal, is indicated for the treatment of invasive aspergillosis in patients who do not respond to or cannot tolerate other antifungal therapies (PRNewswire Jan. 29, 2001). A major problem is the low oral bio-availability, limiting it to iv administration *(33,34)*.

IN SEARCH OF NEW ANTIFUNGAL DRUGS

Introduction

The challenge of resistance drives the pharmaceutical industry as well as some biotechnology companies to search for antifungal compounds with a novel mode of action. Ideally, a new antifungal drug should be characterized by broad-spectrum (non-pathogen-specific) activity, no toxicity, oral activity, and minimal resistance. The design of the screens should incorporate as much knowledge as possible to detect compounds that are less likely to develop resistance. One could assume that if a novel compound had a fast-acting fungicidal mode of action, such a compound would give less opportunity for the pathogen to develop resistance. In terms of target selection, fast-acting fungicidal inhibitors should target essential, and preferably fungal-specific, pathways for survival of the pathogen. Strategies for finding new antifungal agents fall into a few general categories:

(1) Classical approaches for identifying antifungal compounds have relied almost exclusively on the inhibition of fungal or yeast growth as an end point. Libraries of

natural products, semi-synthetic, or synthetic chemicals are screened for their ability to kill or arrest growth of the target pathogen or a related nonpathogenic model organism. The promising lead compounds that emerge from such screens are then tested for possible host-toxicity, and detailed MOA studies must subsequently be conducted to identify the affected molecular target. Although this approach has clearly proven useful in the past, it has yielded very little success for the last 10–15 years.

(2) A second approach relies on the creation of analogs of existing antifungal agents. For example, upon development of the antifungals miconazole and clotrimazole (by Janssen Pharmaceutica and Bayer, respectively), many imidazole and triazole derivatives have been synthesized and developed. Working with known classes of compounds provides some predictability concerning, for example, potential side effects, bio-availability, metabolism, and effects on P450-mediated processes. Another important advantage is that this approach requires a limited research investment. One disadvantage is the potential for rapid development of resistance.

(3) The decline in success of the more classical strategies clearly highlights the need for alternative approaches. One such approach relies on the identification of novel targets (i.e., gene products) as a means to find new drugs against fungal pathogens. Drug targets can be specific for either a particular pathogen or for a subset of different pathogens, even when not present in the (human) host. Purified target macromolecules can be used in in vitro assays to screen large compound libraries for inhibitory drugs. This last approach strongly capitalizes on the advances in the molecular biology and biotechnology field *(84,85)*. Examples of how a combination of both biochemical and molecular biology-based approaches can provide us with important targets for new classes of antifungal drugs (e.g., IPC synthase) or can help us to elucidate the molecular basis of resistance (e.g., azole resistance of *Candida*), are outlined in the following section.

IPC Synthase, an Important Target for a New Class of Antifungal Drugs

The discovery of IPC-synthase as a novel antifungal drug target resulted from studies on the mechanism of action of aureobasidin A. The aureobasidins are highly lipophilic, cyclic depsipeptide antibiotics derived from fermentation broths of *Aureobasidium pullulans* R106. In vitro and in vivo studies showed that the lead compound, aureobasidin A, has fungicidal activity against several clinical relevant fungi *(46,85)*. Molecular biological studies of an aureobasidin A-resistant *S. cerevisiae* mutant revealed that resistance resided in a dominant mutation of a single gene known as *AUR1 (86)*. Deletion of *AUR1*, accomplished in a diploid *S. cerevisiae* strain, indicated that the product of *AUR1* is essential for viability *(86)*. As aureobasidin A is fungicidal and deletion of *AUR1* is lethal, it has been suggested that the gene product of *AUR1* is the molecular target for aureobasidin A. More recent experiments in a mutant *S. cerevisiae* clone resistant to aureobasidin A and defective in inositolphosphorylceramide (IPC) synthase, have demonstrated that *AUR1* can fully restore the activity of IPC synthase *(87)*. These studies also showed that the cyclic depsipeptide antibiotic is a potent inhibitor of IPC synthase, with an IC50 of approximately 0.2 nm. IPC synthase is an enzyme involved in fungal, but not mammalian, sphingolipid biosynthesis. The inhibition of this essential biosynthetic step leads to the accumulation of ceramide in growing cells. Cytological studies of aureobasidin's fungicidal action against *S. cerevisiae* indicate that the ultimate effect of the compound is disturbance of the assembly of actin—a first step in the budding process—destruction of the cell membrane, and cell death *(88)*. If Aurlp (now also called the Ipclp) proves to be present in many other clinically relevant fungi, it may be a long sought-for and ideal antifungal target. The *AUR1* gene has been isolated from *Schizosaccaromyces pombe (89)*, *C. albicans (90)*, *C. glabrata*, *C. krusei*, *C. parapsilosis*, *C. tropicalis*, and *C. neoformans (47)*. Kuroda et al. *(91)* cloned and characterized the *AUR1* gene of *Aspergillus nidulans* and used this gene to identify homologs in *A. fumigatus*. The AurA protein of *A. fumigatus* showed some common characteristics with its *S. cerevisiae*, *S. pombe*, and *C. albicans* counterparts *(91)*. It is interesting to note that one amino-acid substitution of glycine with cysteine at residue 240 is solely responsible for the acquisition of aureobasidin A resistance in *S. pombe (89)*.

Zhong et al. *(48)* studied the sensitivity of IPC synthase to aureobasidin A in membrane preparations of *Candida* and *Aspergillus* species. As expected, preparations from the five *Candida* species, all sensitive to aureobasidin A (MICs < 2000 ng/mL), had a IPC synthase activity sensitive to aureobasidin A with IC50 values of 2–4 ng/mL. Surprisingly, preparations from the four *Aspergillus* species, including *A. fumigatus* and *A. flavus*, which are intrinsically resistant to aureobasidin A (MICs > 50 µg/mL), had IPC synthase activity also sensitive to aureobasidin A (IC50s: 3–5 ng/mL). The mammalian multidrug resistance modulators verapamil, chlorpromazine, and trifluoperazine lowered the minimum inhibitory concentration (MIC) of aureobasidin A for *A. fumigatus* from > 50 µg/mL to 2–3 µg/mL, suggesting that the resistance of this fungal pathogen is the result of increased efflux.

Studies on the mechanism of resistance proved that at least in *S. cerevisiae* and *C. albicans*, aureobasidin A interacts with ATP-binding cassette (ABC) transporters, especially the product of the *YOR1* gene *(92)*. Similar transporters are also found in *A. fumigatus* and *A. flavus (93)* and, therefore may be involved in aureobasidin resistance.

Several companies are now using high-throughput drug screening to find novel inhibitors of sphingolipid synthesis. In addition to aureobasidin A, three new compounds—galbonolide A (rustmicin), galbonolide B, and khafrefungin—have already been reported *(94,95)*.

The Molecular Basis of Antifungal Drug Resistance

Resistance of yeast pathogens to antifungal drugs in the clinic was once a rare occurrence, but by the early 1990s clinicians began to see an increasing number of reports on resistance to antifungal drugs all over the world. Outlined here are some of the efforts to elucidate the molecular basis of azole drug resistance in *Candida*.

Alterations of the CYP51 Gene

In an azole-resistant *C. albicans* strain isolated from a patient with chronic mucocutaneous candidiasis (strain NCPF 3363), we observed a diminished affinity of the cytochromes P450 for azole antifungals and a red shift in the maximum of the CO absorption spectrum from 448 to 450 nm *(96)*. We suggested that these changes resulted from a mutation in the gene coding for the 14α-demethylase. However, at that time no gene encoding *CYP51* had been cloned from an azole-resistant organism. With the cloning of the *C. albicans CYP51* gene and the acquisition of its nucleotide sequence *(97,98),* the study of *CYP51* genes from azole-resistant isolates became possible. Recently, we found that strain NCPF 3363 contained a Y132H mutation on both of its *CYP51* alleles *(99).* The importance of this Y132H mutation for azole susceptibility had previously been demonstrated by Sanglard et al. *(100).* They analyzed changes in the affinity of *CYP51* for azole antifungal agents by functionally expressing the *C. albicans CYP51* genes of sequential clinical isolates in *S. cerevisiae (100).* This selection, coupled with a susceptibility test, facilitated the detection of five different mutations in the cloned *CYP51* genes, which correlated with the occurrence of azole resistance in clinical *C. albicans* isolates. The mutations included replacement of the glycine at position 129 with alanine (G129A), Y132H, S405F, G464S, and R467K. The S405F mutation was found as a single amino-acid substitution, and other mutations were simultaneously found in individual *CYP51* genes, namely, R467K with G464S, S405F with Y132H, G129A with G464S, and R467K with G464S and Y132H. The investigators reintroduced each identified mutation by site-directed mutagenesis into a *CYP51* gene from a susceptible *C. albicans* isolate. Each of the *S. cerevisiae* strains expressing the mutated *CYP51* genes were then subjected to a MIC assay with fluconazole, ketoconazole, and itraconazole. Four (Y132H, S405F, G464S, and R467K) of the five single mutations increased the relative MICs of azole derivatives when the corresponding genes were expressed in *S. cerevisiae.* Only the G129A mutation did not. When two mutations were introduced sequentially by site-directed mutagenesis, the relative MICs of azole derivatives increased to levels similar to those observed when these mutations were combined in the genes from the clinical isolates. When the G129A mutation, which by itself has no effect on the MIC-value, was added to the G464S mutation, the relative increases in the MICs of fluconazole and ketoconazole rose compared to the values obtained when only the G464S mutation was introduced. The MIC-value of itraconazole was not affected. These results suggest that some mutations can exert an effect only when they are combined with other mutations, and that the affinity of itraconazole is much less affected by these mutations *(100).* The latter was further proven by measuring the effects of these mutations on subcellular ergosterol biosynthesis. For example, *C. albicans* isolate C26 *(see* ref. *100)* contained, next to a mutation also found in some azole-sensitive isolates (D116E), two mutations—S405F and Y132H *(99).* For subcellular fractions of sensitive *C. albicans* isolates, 50% inhibition of ergosterol synthesis was found at approx 40 nM fluconazole, whereas for the C26 isolate 48880 nM fluconazole was needed *(99).* With itraconazole, 50% inhibition of ergosterol synthesis by subcellular fractions of azole-sensitive *C. albicans* isolates was 33–44 nM, whereas 20 nM was required to reach 50% inhibition of ergosterol synthesis by the subcellular fraction of the C26 isolate *(99).* The smaller, hydrophilic fluconazole molecule has fewer stabilization sites in the active pocket compared to the lipophilic itraconazole molecule, which may explain this difference in activity *(30).*

An alteration of Y132 was found to be common among fluconazole-resistant isolates. The importance of this residue to the fluconazole resistance of the target enzyme was further proven by Kelly et al. *(101)* and Asai et al. *(102).* The results obtained by Kelly et al. showed that fluconazole binding to the mutant protein [*CYP51*(Y132H)] did not involve normal interaction with heme, as shown by inducing a Type I spectral change. This contrasted to the wild-type protein, for which fluconazole inhibition was

Table 2
Amino-acid sequences of P450s heme-binding region

Species	P450	Sequence
C. albicans	CYP51	FGGGRHRCIGEQF
C. glabrata	CYP51	FGGGRHRCIGELF
C. tropicalis	CYP51	FGGGRHRCIGEQF
S. cerevisiae	CYP51	FGGGRHRCIGEHF
M. tuberculosis	CYP51	FGAGRHRCVGAAF
Human	CYP51	FGAGRHRCIGENF
C. albicans	CYP51**G464S**	FSGGRHRCIGEQF
C. albicans	CYP51**R467K**	FGGGKHRCIGEQF
C. albicans	CYP61	FGTGPHVCLGKNY
Human	CYP3A4	FGSGPRNCIGMRF
Human	CYP2C9	FSAGKRICVGEAL
Human	CYP2E1	FSTGKRVCAGEGL
Rat	CYP2B1	FSTGKRICLGEGI
Human	CYP1A1	FGMGKRKCIGETI

reflected in coordination to heme as a sixth ligand and where the typical Type II spectrum was obtained. Of interest is that the Y132H substitution occurred without drastic perturbation of the heme environment or 14α-demethylase activity, allowing mutants to produce ergosterol and retain viability, an efficient strategy for resistance *(101)*. Asai et al. also found that strains with a *CYP51* altered at Y132 exhibited a low affinity for fluconazole but normal sterol 14α-demethylase activity *(102)*.

Other mutations substantially reduce the inhibitory effect of fluconazole, and also result in a reduced catalytic activity of the sterol 14α-demethylase. Examples are T315A *(103)*, G464S *(104)*, and the R467K *(105,106)* amino-acid substitutions. The change in T315A reduced enzyme activity two fold—as predicted for the removal of the residue that formed a hydrogen bond with the 3-OH oflanosterol or obtusifoliol—and helped to locate the substrate in the active site *(103)*. The substitutions G464S and R467K occur in a highly conserved heme-binding region. In a number of azole-binding *CYP51s*, such as those present in *C. glabrata, C. tropicalis, S. cerevisiae, S. pombe, Mycobacterium tuberculosis* and human, and in human CYP3A4 and CYPIAL, glycine aligns with G464 of the *C. albicans CYP51* (Table 2). In less sensitive P450s, serine and/or lysine instead of the glycine and arginine residues were found. Examples other than *C. albicans CYP51* (G464S) and *CYP51* (R467K) are rat CYP2B1, human CYP2C9, CYP2E1, and CYP1A1. Notably, for *CYP61* (sterol Δ²²-desaturase), a glycine residue aligns with G464 of the *C. albicans CYP51;* the product of the *CYP61 (ERG5)* gene has been claimed to be a second target for azole antifungal agents *(30,107–109)*. These results at least suggest that this glycine residue plays a role in the affinity of azole antifungals for *CYP51, CYP61,* and *CYP3A4*. Whereas *CYP51* and *CYP61* have a similar affinity for azole drugs *(108)*, the inhibition *CYP3A4* requires higher concentrations. Lamb et al. *(110)* compared the inhibition by azole antifungals of human *CYP3A4* and *C. albicans CYP51* following heterologous expression in *S. cerevisiae*. IC50-values for ketoconazole and itraconazole *CYP3A4* inhibition were 250 nM and 200 nM. These values compared with the much lower concentrations needed to obtain 50% inhibition of CYP51, for which IC50-values of 8 nM and 7.6 nM were observed for ketoconazole and itraconazole, respectively *(110)*.

Resistance to azole antifungals is not only caused by mutations in the *CYP51* gene. In a subcellular fraction of a fluconazole-resistant clinical isolate of *C. glabrata*, ergosterol synthesis was 8.2-fold higher than that from the pretreatment isolate; the increased synthesis coincided with an increase in microsomal P450 content *(111)*. This increased level of protein was associated with *CYP51 (ERG11)* gene amplification *(112,113)*. The *CYP51* mRNA transcript in the resistant isolate was 8 × greater than it was in the susceptible isolate *(113)*. This increase in copy number is caused by duplication of the chromosome containing the *CYP51* gene *(113)*. As expected, the amplification of an entire chromosome has a major impact on the protein expression in the cells: from 1377 proteins which were identified, 25 were upregulated by more than a factor of three, and 76 were downregulated by the same factor *(113)*. Further studies are needed to identify the up- and downregulated products. For example, it would be of interest to know whether one of the products is involved in drug efflux. In fact, changes in drug accumulation were also observed in this fluconazole-resistant *C. glabrata* isolate *(111)*.

Decreased Accumulation of Drug

In recent years, several studies have investigated the accumulation of azole antifungals in cells for which the azole MIC is high. Failure to accumulate azole antifungals has been identified as a major cause of resistance in several post-treatment fungal isolates and species that are less sensitive to azole antifungal agents and other ergosterol biosynthesis inhibitors (for review articles see refs. *27,77,79,114–117*). These isolates include *C. albicans (118–120)*, *C. krusei (121,122)*, *C. glabrata (110,123,124)*, *C. dubliniensis (125)*, *C. neoformans (126)*, *A. nidulans (127)*, *A. flavus*, and *A. fumigatus (92)*. Failure to accumulate antifungal agents can be the result of impaired drug influx or enhanced drug efflux. Drug import can be affected by changes in—for example,—membrane fluidity, which depends on the nature of the sterols present in the plasma membrane *(128)*. Jensen-Pergakes et al. *(129)* showed that a *C. albicans* sterol methyltransferase *(ERG6)* mutant was hypersusceptible to a number of sterol synthesis and metabolic inhibitors. Terbinafine susceptibility was increased about 50-fold, and the greatest increases in susceptibility were shown for the morpholines fenpropimorph (100–fold) and tridemorph (several thousandfold). However, the *erg6* strains showed nearly identical sensitivities to the azole antifungal agents clotrimazole and ketoconazole *(129)*. Apparently, the permeability changes are unrelated to the entry mechanism for the latter compounds. The availability of *erg6* strains allows characterization of potential antifungal agents that normally fail to reach intracellular targets because of a lack of permeability. The entry mechanism(s) for the various azole antifungal agents is still unknown. Our understanding of the molecular mechanisms responsible for the failure of antifungal agents to accumulate in resistant fungal isolates has progressed much more rapidly. Efflux pumps are now recognized as a common cause of the decreased intracellular content of ergosterol biosynthesis inhibitors. More than two decades ago, de Waard and Van Nistelrooy reported that resistance of *A. nidulans* mutants to the pyrimidine derivative fenarimol is the result of a high-energy-dependent efflux activity *(127,130,131)*.

Two types of efflux pumps are presently known: membrane-transport proteins belonging either to the major facilitators superfamily (MFS) or to the ABC superfamily. The MFS are energized by the proton-motive force *(132)*. The ABC-type transporters utilize ATP as a source of energy *(133)*. The complete sequence of the *S. cerevisiae* genome predicts the existence of 29 proteins belonging to the ubiquitous *ABC* superfamily *(132)* and 28 open reading frames (ORFs) are homologous to each other and to established bacterial members of the drug-resistant subfamily of the MFS *(132)*.

In *C. albicans,* more than 10 different ABC-type transporters have been reported *(134)*, but only the pumps encoded by *CDR1* and *CDR2* are known to be involved in the mechanisms of azole resistance *(77,135,136)*. Involvement of the *CDR1* gene in resistance to azole derivatives and other antifungal agents was confirmed by deletion of this gene in *C. albicans. CDR1*-null mutants were hypersusceptible not only to the azole antifungal agents, but also to terbinafine and amorolfine, and fluconazole accumulated to higher concentrations in these mutants than in wild-type cells *(77,137)*. *CDR1* or *CDR2* overexpression in *S. cerevisiae* was found to confer cross-resistance to several antifungal agents, such as fluconazole, ketoconazole, itraconazole, terbinafine, and amorolfine *(77,117,119,136)*.

In fluconazole-resistant *C. albicans* isolates from patients with oropharyngeal candidiasis, a multidrug efflux transporter of the class of major facilitators has been shown to be responsible for the low level of accumulation of fluconazole *(119)*. The MF gene *BEN^R* (now better known as *CaMDR1*) was found to be overexpressed in resistant isolates *(119)*. The product of the *CaMDR1*gene, CaMdr1p, expels terbinafine and fluconazole, but not itraconazole. This finding correlates with the observation by Albertson et al. *(138)* that a *C. albicans* mutant in which the *CaMDR1* gene is overexpressed is specifically resistant to fluconazole, but not to other azole antifungal agents. Examples of both types of pumps have been found in other human pathogenic fungi, and are shown in Table 3. Pumps involved in antifungal resistance have 12-membrane-spanning helices, or transmembrane domains (TMD) in their protein structure *(135,136,141)*. The fungal ABC-type transporters have two homologous halves, each with an ATP-binding domain (BD) followed by six transmembrane (TM) helices (BD-TM-BD-TM). ABC transporters of this type have only been reported in fungi and plants thus far, including AtrA and AtrB of the model filamentous fungus, *A. nidulans (147,148)*. They are mirror images of mammalian P-glycoproteins *(148):* the primary structure of mammalian P-glycoproteins can be abbreviated as TM-BD-TM-BD *(132,148)*. The actual cellular function of the ABC- and MFS-type proteins is not clear. However, great progress has been made by using the previously described mutants. Studies by Dogra et al. *(149)* showed that, as in mammalian cells, membrane phospholipids are asymmetrically distributed across the plasma membrane of *C. albicans.* They showed that phosphatidylethanolamine is predominantly present in the cytoplasmic leaflet, and that the movement of phosphatidylethanolamine across the plasma membrane of *C. albicans* could be prevented if cells were preincubated with energy inhibitors *(150)*. They also showed that, similar to human MDRs *(148)*, the product of the *CDR1* gene, Cdr1p, could be involved in phospholipid translocation *(149,150)*.

Table 3
Multidrug transporters identified in human pathogenic fungi

Species	Gene	Type*	References
C. albicans	CaCDR1	ABC	135
C. albicans	CaCDR2	ABC	136
C. albicans	CaCDR3	ABC	139
C. albicans	CaCDR4	ABC	140
C. albicans	CaCDR5	ABC	117
C. albicans	CaYOR1	ABC	92
C. albicans	CaMDR1	MFS	137,141
C. albicans	Flu1	MFS	117
C. dubliniensis	CdCDR1	ABC	125
C. dubliniensis	CdCDR2	ABC	125
C. dubliniensis	CdMDR1	MFS	125
C. glabrata	CgCDR1	ABC	124
C. glabrata	CgCDR2	ABC	124
C. glabrata	PDH1	ABC	123
C. glabrata	CgMDR1	MFS	124
C. krusei	ABC1	ABC	142
C. krusei	ABC2	ABC	142
C. tropicalis	CDR1	ABC	143
C. tropicalis	MDR1	MFS	143
Cr. neoformans	CneMDR1	ABC	144
Cr. neoformans	CneMDR2	ABC	144
Cr. neoformans	HTL1	MFS	145
A. fumigatus	AfuMDR1	ABC	93
A. fumigatus	AfuMDR2	ABC	93
A. fumigatus	Adr1	ABC	146
A. flavus	AflMDR1	ABC	93

* ABC, ATP-binding cassette type of efflux pump; MFS, Major facilitator superfamily.

Another ABC transporter protein, encoded by the gene *CDR4* in *C. albicans,* has also been suggested to be involved in phospholipid translocation *(151).* The *CaMDR1* gene of *C. albicans* expressed in *S. cerevisiae* did not affect the phosphatidylethanolamine distribution pattern between the inner and outer leaflet *(149).* Yet overexpression of the *CaMDR1* gene correlated with an enhanced production of the extracellularly secreted aspartyl proteinase (Sap) by *C. albicans* cells exposed to subinhibitory concentrations of fluconazole. Several lines of evidence indicate that Sap is a pathogenic factor of *C. albicans (152).* The results obtained by Wu et al. imply that patients infected with isolates with the capacity to overexpress *CaMDR1* and subsequently treated with suboptimal doses of fluconazole may experience enhanced *C. albicans* virulence *(152).*

C. albicans multidrug efflux transporter mutants *(137,153),* and *S. cerevisiae* strains expressing specific multidrug efflux transporter genes *(148)* may help to pinpoint substances that inhibit multidrug efflux transporters. Inhibition of P-glycoproteins is one of the strategies used to overcome the problem of resistance in cancer cells. Inhibitors of efflux pumps may also enhance the clinical efficacy of azoles against fungal pathogens. Using a Cdr1p-expressing azole-resistant *C. albicans* strain, we were able to show that tracrolimus (FK506) increased the intracellular itraconazole content and reduced the MIC-value from 8 mg/L to 0.5 mg/mL *(153)*. The studies of Egner et al. *(154)* showed that FK506 is also a potent inhibitor of the ABC-transporter Pdr5p in *S. cerevisiae.* They showed that a S1360F substitution in TMD 10 of Pdr5p abolished its susceptibility to inhibition by the immunosuppressant FK506. Their findings suggest that FK506 may interact directly with Pdr5, and that the S1360F mutation somehow prevents Pdr5-FK506 interaction. The mutant Pdr5-127 with the S1360F exchange in TMD10 showed an interesting pattern of substrate recognition. It confers resistance to ketoconazole (MIC = 16x that found for the sensitive strain), but showed a reduced ability to confer resistance to itraconazole. Pdr5-127 was completely deficient in reducing dexamethasone response, and was comparable to the complete lack of Pdr5. In a more recent study, Egner et al. *(155)* found that, as for the S1360F mutant, T1364F and T1364A mutants were nearly nonresponsive to FK506 inhibition. A T1364F mutation leads to the reduction in Pdr5p-mediated azole and rhodamine 6G resistance. Most remarkably, however, the S1360A mutation increased FK506 inhibitor susceptibility, because Pdr5p–S1360A is hypersensitive to FK506 inhibition when compared with either wild-type Pdr5p or the nonresponsive S1360F variant. Thus, the Pdr5p TMD10 determines both azole-substrate specificity and susceptibility to reversal agents. A single residue change in a eukaryotic ABC transporter causes either a loss or a gain in inhibitor susceptibility, depending on the nature of the mutational change. These results may be of great help in the design of effective reversal agents that could be used to overcome multidrug resistance mediated by ABC-transporter overexpression.

Although the usefulness of inhibitors of efflux transporters in the clinic requires further investigation, the studies on the molecular mechanisms of drug resistance have contributed to a major expansion of our knowledge in the field of mycology.

GENOMICS-BASED ANTIFUNGAL DRUG DISCOVERY

Introduction

A new era in antimicrobial drug discovery was ushered in by the availability of a wealth of genomic sequence information (*see* refs. *156–158*). Over the past few years, more than 36 microbial genomes have been sequenced to completion (http://www.tigr.org/tdb/mdb/mdbcomplete.html), and an additional ~120 are still in progress (http://www.tigr.org/tdb/mdb/mdbinprogress.html). These recent advances in genomics *(159)* have provided an opportunity to greatly expand the range of potential drug targets, and have clearly accelerated the shift from direct antimicrobial screening toward more target-based strategies *(160,161)*. The availability of the entire sequence of the gene target of interest permits rapid development of gene knockouts to validate the utility of the target, and facilitates construction of expression plasmids for production of protein and development of assays.

Comparative Genome Analysis

New sequence data from various organisms permits the use of a comparative genomic analysis to identify potential new targets that are shared across several species or particular to a single species. In this manner, it is possible to generate lists of genes that represent potential targets for either broad-spectrum or highly specific narrow-spectrum antimicrobials. Sequence comparisons can also provide some assurance against mammalian toxicity if proteins of similar sequence do not exist in mammalian-sequence databases. Especially now, with the complete sequence of the human genome in hand *(162),* this can be done accurately with the potential of discovering true pathogen-specific drug targets. Secondly, sequence similarity can provide some insights into the putative functions of unknown genes. Although the ideal antifungal compound would be broad-spectrum, the alarming paucity of new types of antifungals have led to the suggestion to maintain pathogen-specific therapy *(163).* Data from several genome-sequencing projects suggest that 10–20% of the predicted ORFs are putatively species-specific.

Gene-Expression Profiling Using DNA Micro-Arrays

Gene-expression profiling using DNA microarrays (reviewed in refs. *164–167*) has provided the pharmaceutical industry with an exciting new tool to discover novel drug targets as well as to determine how drugs work. The study of gene expression by DNA microarray technology is based on hybridization of mRNA to a high-density array of immobilized target sequences, each corresponding to a specific gene. Sample RNAs are labeled, usually by incorporation of a fluorescent nucleotide by oligo(dT)-primed reverse transcription. The labeled pool of mRNAs is then hybridized to the array, where each mRNA will quantitatively hybridize to its complementary target sequence. The level of fluorescence of each spot on the array is a quantitative measure corresponding to the expression level of the particular gene. Although DNA arrays have been used for biological experiments for many years *(168–170),* it is relatively recently that, thanks to minituarization, automation, and bioinformatics, the information content of these experiments has both increased and become more reliable *(171).* These advances in the post-genomics field are clearly rapidly changing our views of how we can approach antimicrobial research.

Target Identification

From a drug discovery point of view, the expression patterns generated from the parallel analysis of all genes in a microorganism can provide clues to the function of previously uncharacterized genes (target identification). Even in one of the smallest genomes sequenced, *Mycoplasma genitalium,* approximately 35% of the genes encode proteins of unknown function. A frequently used approach involves clustering of expression patterns from genes over multiple experiments by statistical means (*see* refs. *172,173*). The idea is that genes which behave similarly under similar circumstances are likely to be functionally related. This approach has been proven valid for many organisms, including *Saccharomyces cerevisiae (173,174).* Although expression behavior by itself is still insufficient evidence for functional assignment, it allows the researcher to focus on a smaller subset of candidate target genes, as such putatively accelerating the drug-target discovery process. First hints of possible functions of unknown genes may also come from their response to disturbances in other gene functions (e.g., strong up- or downregulation in response to knocking-out another gene), or upon treatment with compounds. In one of our studies, which examined the effect of the antifungal itraconazole on the *Candida albicans* transcriptome, we found over 140 proteins of unknown function that were responsive to treatment with itraconazole in the test conditions used *(175)*. One ORF encoding a hypothetical 25.3-Kd protein in the *TIM23-ARE2* intergenic region and showing similarity to *S. cerevisiae* ORF *YNR018w* was over 37-fold upregulated. Two genes that did not show homology to any gene in the sequence databases (i.e., putatively *C. albicans*-specific) were 24- and 17-fold upregulated, respectively. These genes may thus be strongly linked to either azole or ergosterol function. In addition to providing novel potential drug targets, the transcriptome can provide information on how drugs or drug candidates achieve their therapeutic effect through mechanism of action (MOA) studies.

Mechanism of Action Studies

It is now generally accepted that the antifungal activity of azole derivatives arises from a complex multi-mechanistic process initiated by the inhibition of two P450 cytochromes involved in the biosynthesis of ergosterol *(30,59–66)*. Ergosterol is an essential component of fungal plasma membranes, which affects membrane permeability and the activity of membrane-bound enzymes. This sterol is a major component of secretory vescicles, and plays an important role in mitochondrial respiration and oxidative phosphorylation. The elucidation of the *MOA* of azoles resulted from "traditional" biochemical research. The publication of the complete sequence of the *S. cerevisiae* genome and the availability of DNA microarrays made it possible to explore drug-induced alterations in gene expression on a genome-wide scale. In order to better understand the response of *S. cerevisiae* to perturbations in the ergosterol pathway, Bammert and Fostel *(176)* determined genome-wide transcript profiles following exposure of *S. cerevisiae* to clotrimazole, ketoconazole, fluconazole, itraconazole, voriconazole (14α-demethylase inhibitors), terbinafine (squalene epoxidase inhibitor), and amorolfine (inhibits the sterol C-14 reductase and C-8 isomerase). A total of 156 genes showed significant increases in transcript levels in five or more treatments, and 78 showed significantly decreased transcript levels in five or more treatments. Twenty-two responsive genes involved in the biosynthesis of sphingolipids, sterol metabolism, and the elongation of fatty acids were identified, suggesting those as a putative site of action. More specifically, we studied the effect of itraconazole on the pathogenic fungus *C. albicans (175)*. Simultaneous examination of over 6600 *C. albicans* gene-transcript levels, representing the entire genome, upon treatment of cells with 10 *μM* of itraconazole, revealed 296 genes to be responsive (see ref. *175*). A total of 116 gene transcript levels were at least 2.5-fold decreased, and 180 were similarly increased. A global upregulation of *ERG* genes in response to azole treatment was observed. *ERG11* and *ERG5* were found to be approx 12-fold upregulated. In addition, a significant upregulation was observed for *ERG6, ERG1, ERG3, ERG4, ERG10, ERG9, ERG26, ERG25, ERG2, ID11, HMGS, NCP1,* and *FEN2,* all genes known to be involved in ergosterol biosynthesis (Fig. 1). These two examples clearly demonstrate that the study of the transcriptome can help us to better understand the MOA of known drugs and to elucidate how potentially new drug candidates work. Results from the latter approach in the antifungal field have yet to be demonstrated or reported.

Transcriptional Fingerprints

The creation of large databases of expression profiles ("fingerprints") of many different genetically crippled strains and/or cells treated with compounds affecting a

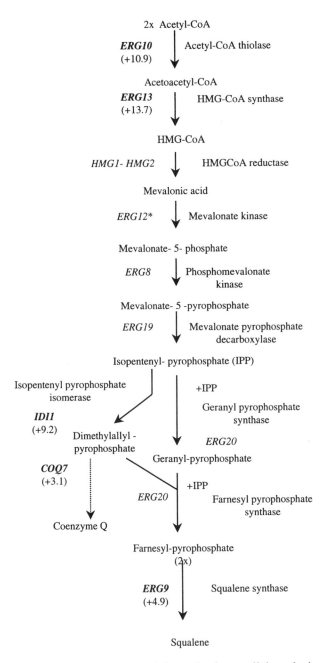

Fig. 1. The expression patterns generated from the in parallel analysis of all genes in a microorganism can provide information about how drugs achieve their therapeutic effect: transcript profiles revealed a global upregulation of *C. albicans ERG* genes in response to itraconazole treatment (ref. *175;* responsive genes are shown in bold, fold changes are shown in between brackets). This finding is in agreement with previous studies showing that this pathway is the target of azoles, and is responsive to modulations in ergosterol levels.

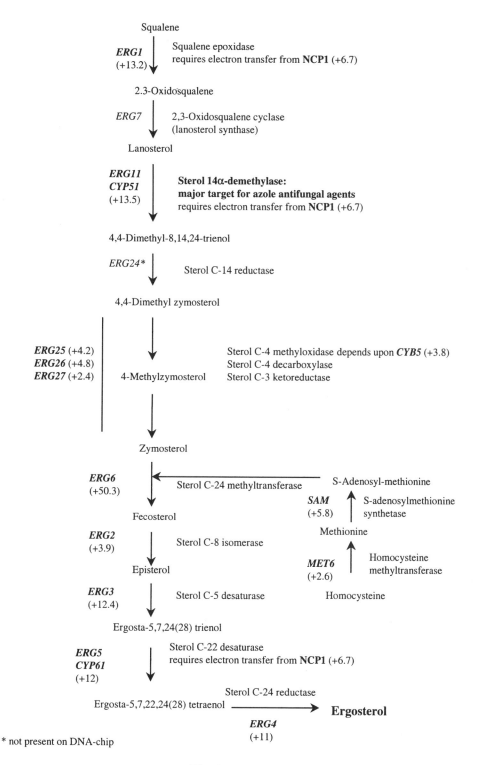

Fig. 1. *(Continued).*

broad variety of targets enables us to predict the function of a gene or the MoA of a compound simply by comparing its fingerprint to the ones available in the database. This approach is based on the assumption that the phenotype and resulting fingerprint of a drug-treated cell should be very similar to the phenotype of a cell in which the gene encoding the target protein has been genetically inactivated. Transcriptional fingerprints have already proven useful, for example, in revealing the target (his3) of the immunosuppressive drug 3-aminotriazole or tracolimus *(177)*. The same expression fingerprint was obtained in yeast cells treated with tracolimus and yeast cells carrying a null mutation in the tracolimus target, establishing that genetic and pharmacological ablation of a gene function results in similar changes in gene expression. Also in the classification of cancer types *(178,179)* and drugs (by mode of action and/or toxicity; *see* refs. *180–182*) this approach has proven valuable. Related to this is the observation in both bacteria and yeasts that underexpression of any component of a process (e.g., underexpression of a gene because of a genetic alteration) leads to increased sensitivity to an inhibitor of a relevant step in that process *(183–185)*.

Regulatory Networks

Changes in genome expression patterns generated by using genome microarrays can also provide valuable clues about regulatory mechanisms, cellular functions, and biochemical pathways. Jelinsky and Samson explored the response of *S. cerevisiae* to carcinogenic agents, and found groups of co-regulated genes exhibiting upstream regions with known and novel regulatory sequence motifs *(186)*. One group of co-regulated genes contained a number of DNA excision repair genes and a large selection of protein degradation genes whose transcription was apparently modulated by the proteasome-associated protein Rpn4. Regulatory networks between base excision repair and proteasomes were thus revealed by transcriptional profiling of damaged yeast cells. Many similar types of studies are now being conducted and reported, thereby continuously increasing our understanding of how gene expression is regulated and how pathways are connected.

Identification of Virulence Factors

As traditional genetic techniques to identify virulence determinants are time-consuming, these are now being quickly replaced by microarray methods. Gene-expression patterns in pathogens can be studied both in vitro and in an infection model in vivo. In addition, pathogens (cells) can now be elegantly separated from "contaminating" host tissue by laser-capture microdissection *(187)*. By using multiple rounds of linear amplification (based on cDNA synthesis from mRNA and subsequent in vitro transcription), it becomes feasible to monitor the expression of large numbers of genes, beginning with only a few cells.

CONCLUDING REMARKS

Thousands of genes are being discovered for the first time by sequencing the genomes of various organisms, reminding us that many processes remain to be explored at the molecular level. DNA microarrays provide a very useful tool for this exploration. The potential of DNA microarrays to elucidate MoA is supported by several findings such as ours, showing that the majority of genes in the ergosterol biosynthetic pathway are responsive to itraconazole, a drug known to target this pathway. As the genome sequences of several fungal pathogens gradually become available in both private and public databases, genome-wide transcript profiling will soon be an essential tool to understand the mode of action of novel antifungal compounds. However, as not all cellular processes are controlled at the level of gene expression (transcription), protein profiling will most certainly prove to be a very helpful complementary approach *(188).* The importance of protein-based methods is that they measure the final expression product rather than an intermediate. They also enable the detection of post-translational protein modifications. However, it remains a fact that protein-based approaches are generally more difficult and less sensitive, and have a lower throughput than RNA-based ones. The availability of the complete sequence of several microbial genomes, combined with the ongoing technological advances, is sure to change the face and the pace of antifungal drug discovery.

REFERENCES

1. Odds FC. Pathogenic fungi in the 21st century. Trends Microbiol 2000; 8:200–201.
2. Hartman PG, Sanglard D. Inhibitors of ergosterol biosynthesis as antifungal agents. Curr Pharmaceut Des 1997; 3:177–208.
3. Warnock DW. Introduction to the management of fungal infection in the compromised host. In: Warnock DW. Richardson MD (eds). Fungal Infection in the Compromised Patient, 2nd ed,/Chichester: John Wiley & Sons, 1990, pp. 23–53.
4. Kibbler CC. Epidemiology of fungal infections. In: Kibbler CC, Mackenzie DWR, Odds FC (eds). Principles and Practice of Clinical Mycology, Chichester: John Wiley & Sons, 1996, pp. 13–21.
5. Ampel NM. Emerging disease issues and fungal pathogens associated with HIV infection. Emerg Infect Dis 1996; 2:109–116.
6. Klepser ME, Ernst EJ, Pfaller MA. Update on antifungal resistance. Trends Microbiol 1997; 5:372–375.
7. Pfaller MA, Jones RN, Messer SA, Edmond MB, Wenzel RP. National surveillance of nocosomial blood stream infection due to Candida albicans: frequency of occurrence and antifungal susceptibility in the SCOPE program. Diagn Microbiol Infect Dis 1998; 31:327–332.
8. Viscoli C, Girmenia C, Marinus A, Collette L, Martino P, Vandercam B, et al. Candidemia in cancer patients: a prospective, multicenter surveillance study by the Invasive Fungal Infection Group (IFIG) of the European Organization for Research and Treatment of Cancer (EORTC). Clin Infect Dis 1999; 28:1071–1079.
9. Meis JFGM, Ruhnke M, de Pauw BE, Odds FC, Siegert W, Verwey PE. Candida dubliniensis candidemia in patients with chemotherapy-induced neutropenia and bone marrow transplantation. Emerg Infect Dis 1999; 5:150–153.
10. Brandt ME, Harrison LH, Pass M, Sofair AN, Huie S, Li R-K, et al. Candida dubliniensis fungemia: the first four cases in North America. Emerg Infect Dis 2000; 6:46–49.
11. Patterson TF, Kirkpatrick WR, White M, Hiemenz JW, Wingard JR, Dupont B, et al. Invasive aspergillosis. Disease spectrum, treatment practices, and outcomes. 13 Aspergillus Study Group. Medicine (Baltimore) 2000; 79:250–260.
12. Powderly WG. Cryptococcal meningitis in HIV-infected patients. Curr Infect Dis Rep 2000; 2:352–357.
13. Buchanan KL, Murphy JW. What makes Cryptococcus neoformans a pathogen? Emerg Infect Dis 1998; 4:71–83.
14. Dei-Casa E. Pneumocystis infections: the iceberg? Med Mycol 2000; 38 (Suppl 1):23–32.

15. Yale SH, Limper, AH. Pneumocystis carinii pneumonia in patients without acquired immunodeficiency syndrome: associated disorders and prior corticosteroid therapy. Mayo Clin Proc 1996; 71:5–13.

16. Hennequin C, Thierry A, Richard GF, Lecointre G, Nguyen HV, Gaillardin C, et al. Microsatellite typing as a new tool for identification of Saccharomyces cerevisiae strains. J Clin Microbiol 2001; 39:551–559.

17. Sheehan DJ, Hitchcock CA, Sibley CM. Current and emerging azole antifungal agents. Clin Microbiol Rev 1999; 12:40–79.

18. Wheat J. Endemic mycoses in AIDS: a clinical review. Clin Microbiol Rev 1995; 8:146–159.

19. Lortholarly O, Dupont B. Antifungal prophylaxis during neutropenia and immunodeficiency. Clin Microbiol Rev 1997; 10:477–504.

20. Marques SA, Robles AM, Tortorano AM, Tuculet MA, Negroni R, Mendes RP. Mycoses associated with AIDS in the Third World. Med Mycol 2000; 38 (Suppl 1):269–279.

21. Antinori AS, Ridolfo AL, Corbellino M, Galimberti L, Santambrogio S, Bonaccorso C, et al. Disseminated histoplasmosis in patients with AIDS. Recenti Prog Med 2000; 91:362–364.

22. Pier AC, Cabañes FJ, Chermette R, Ferreiro L, Guillot J, Jensen HE, Santurio, JM. Prominent animal mycoses from various regions of the world. Med Mycol 2000; 38 (Suppl 1):47–58.

23. Chaturvedi V, Ramani R, Gromadzki S, Rodeghier B, Chang H-G, Morse DL. Coccidioidomycosis in New York State. Emerg Infect Dis 2000; 6:25–29.

24. Viviani MA, Tortorano AM. Unusual mycoses in AIDS patients. In: Vanden Bossche H, Mackenzie DWR, Cauwenbergh G, Van Cutsem J, Drouhet E, Dupont, B. eds). Mycoses in AIDS Patients, New York: Plenum Press, 1990, pp. 147–153.

25. Dupont B, Crewe Brown HH, Westermann K, Martins MD, Rex JH, Lortholary O, et al. Mycoses in AIDS. Med Mycol 2000; 38(Suppl 1): 259–267.

26. Polak A, Mode of action studies. In: Ryley JF (ed). Chemotherapy of Fungal Diseases, Berlin: Springer Verlag, 1990: 153–182.

27. Vanden Bossche H, Marichal P, Odds FC. Molecular mechanisms of drug resistance in fungi. Trends Microbiol 1994; 2:393–400.

28. Bolard J. Mechanism of action of an anti-Candida drug: amphotericin B and its derivatives. In: Prasad R, (ed). Candida albicans. Cellular and Molecular Biology, Berlin: Springer Verlag, 1991, pp. 214–238.

29. Vanden Bossche H, Koymans L, Moereels H. P450 inhibitors of use in medical treatment: focus on mechanisms of action. Pharmacol Ther 1995; 67:79–100.

30. Vanden Bossche H, Koymans L. Cytochromes P450 in fungi. Mycoses 1998; 41 (Suppl 1): 32–38.

31. Petranyl G, Ryder NS, Stutz A. Allylamine derivatives: new class of synthetic antifungal agents inhibiting fungal squalene epoxidase. Science 1984; 224:1239–1241.

32. Ryder NS, Mieth H. Allylamine antifungal drugs. Curr Top Med Mycol 1992; 4:158–188.

33. Walsh TJ, Viviani M-A, Arathoon E, Chiou C, Ghannoum M, Groll AH, et al. New targets and delivery systems for antifungal therapy. Med Mycol 2000; 38 (Suppl 1): 335–347.

34. Groll AH, Walsh TJ. MK-0991 Merck & Co. Curr Opin Anti-infect Invest Drugs 1999; 1:334–345.

35. Vanden Bossche H. Chemotherapy of human fungal infections. In: Lyr H, (ed). Modern Selective Fungicides Jena: Gustav Fisher Verlag, 1995, pp. 431–484.

36. Verweij PE, de Pauw BE, Meis JF. Voriconazole Pfizer Ltd. Curr Opin Anti-infect Invest Drugs 1999; 1:361–372.

37. Perea S, Fothergill AW, Sutton DA, Rinaldi MG. Comparison of in vitro activities of voriconazole and five established antifungal agents against different species of dermatophytes using a broth macrodilution method. J Clin Microbiol 2001; 39:385–388.

38. Espinel-Ingroff AV. Sch-56592 Schering-Plough. Curr Opin Anti-infect Invest Drugs 1999; 1:377–384.

39. Georgopapadakou NH. BMS-207147 Eisai Co Ltd. Curr Opin Anti-infect Invest Drugs 1999; 1:373–376.

40. Watkins WJ, Renau TE. Progress with antifungal agents and approaches to combat fungal resistance. Ann Rep Med Chem 2000; 35:157–167.

41. Hawser S. LY-303366 Eli Lilly & Co. Curr Opin Anti-infect Invest Drugs 1999; 1:353–360.

42. Petraitis V, Petraitiene R, Groll AH, Sein T, Scaufele RL, Lyman CA, et al. Dosage-dependent antifungal efficacy of V-echinocandin (LY303366) against experimental fluconazole-resistant oropharyngeal and esophageal candidiasis. Antimicrob Agents Chemother 2001; 45:471–479.

43. Georgopapadakou NH. Sharman Pharmaceuticals. Curr Opin Anti-infect Invest Drugs 1999; 1:346–352.

44. Gargallo-Viola D. Sordarins as antifungal compounds. Curr Opin Anti-infect Invest Drugs 1999; 1:297–305.

45. Martinez A, Aviles P, Jimenez E, Caballero J, Gargallo-Viola D. Activities of sordarins in experimental models of candidiasis, aspergillosis, and pneumocystosis. Antimicrob Agents Chemother 2000; 44:3389–3394.

46. De Lucca AJ, Walsh T. Antifungal peptides: novel therapeutic compounds against emerging pathogens. Antimicrob Agents Chemother 1999; 43:1–11.

47. Heidler SA, Radding JA. Inositol phosphoryl transferases from human pathogenic fungi. Biochim Biophys Acta 2000; 1500:147–152.

48. Zhong W, Jeffries MW, Georgopapadakou NH. Inhibition of inositol phosphorylceramide synthase by aureobasidin A in Candida and Aspergillus species. Antimicrob Agents Chemother 2000; 44:651–653.

49. Fostel JM, Lartey PA. Emerging novel antifungal agents. Drug Discover Today 2000; 5:25–32.

50. Odds FC. Antifungal therapy. In: Kibbler CC, Mackenzie DWR, Odds FC (ed). Principles and Practice of Clinical Mycology, Chichester: Jhon Wiley & Sons, 1996, pp. 35–48.

51. Vermes A, Guchelaar HJ, Dankert J. Flucytosine: a review of its pharmacology, clinical indications, pharmacokinetics, toxicity and drug interactions. J Antimicrob Chemother 2000; 46:171–179.

52. Polak A, Scholer HJ. Mode of action of 5-fluorocytosine. Rev Institut Pasteur Lyon 1980; 13:233–244.

53. Fanos V, Cataldi L. Amphotericin B-induced nephrotoxicity: a review. J Chemother 2000; 12:463–470.

54. Sarosi GA. Amphotericin B still the 'gold standard' for antifungal therapy. Postgrad Med 1990; 88:151–166.

55. Graybill JR, Tollemar J, Torres-Rodriguez JM, Walsh TJ, Roilides E, Farmaki E. Antifungal compounds: controversies, queries and conclusions. Med Mycol 2000; 38 (Suppl 1): 323–333.

56. Williams DJ, Marten RM, Sarkany I. Oral treatment of ringworm with griseofulvin. Lancet 1958; 2:1212–1213.

57. Degreef H. Onychomycosis. Br J Clin Pract 1990; 44 (Suppl 71): 91–97.

58. Mohrenschlager M, Schnopp C, Fesq H, Strom K, Beham A, Mempel M, et al. Optimizing the therapeutic approach in tinea capitis of childhood with itraconazole. Br J Dermatol 2000; 143:1011–1015.

59. Vanden Bossche H, Willemsens G, Cools W, Lauwers WFJ, Le Jeune L. Biochemical effects of miconazole on fungi: inhibition of ergosterol biosynthesis in Candida albicans. Chem-Biol Interact 1978; 21:59–78.

60. Vanden Bossche H. Biochemical targets for antifungal azole derivatives: hypothesis on the mode of action. Curr Top Med Mycol 1985; 1:313–351.

61. Vanden Bossche H, Willemsens G, Cools W, Cornelissen F, Lauwers F, Van Cutsem J. In vitro and in vivo effects of ketoconazole on sterol synthesis. Antimicrob Ag Chemother 1980; 17:922–928.

62. Vanden Bossche H, Bellens D, Cools W, Gorrens J, Marichal P, Verhoeven H, et al. Cytochrome P-450: target for itaconazole. Drug Develop Res 1986; 8:287–298.

63. Hitchcock CA. Cytochrome P-450-dependent 14α-sterol demethylase of Candida albicans and its interaction with azole antifungals. Biochem Soc Trans 1991; 19:782–787.

64. Vanden Bossche H, Marichal P, Gorrens J, Bellens D, Coene M-C, Lauwers W, et al. Mode of action of antifungals of use in immunocompromised patients. Focus on Candida glabrata and Histoplasma capsulatum. In: Vanden Bossche H, Mackenzie DWR, Cauwenbergh G, Van Cutsem J, Drouhet E, Dupont, B, (eds). Mycoses in AIDS Patients. New York: Plenum Press, 1990, pp. 223–243.

65. Vanden Bossche H, Marichal P, Le Jeune L, Coene M-C, Gorrens J, Cools W. Effects of itraconazole on cytochrome P-450-dependent sterol 14α-demethylation and reduction of 3-ketosteroids in Cryptococcus neoformans. Antimicrob Agents Chemother 1993; 37:2101–2105.

66. Marichal P, Gorrens J, Laurijssens L, Vermuyten K, Van Hove C, Le Jeune L, et al. Accumulation of 3-ketosteroids induced by itraconazole in azole resistant clinical Candida albicans isolates. Antimicrob Agents Chemother 1999; 43:2663–2670.

67. Thienpont D, Van Cutsem J, Van Gerven F, Heeres J, Janssen PAJ. Ketoconazole—a new broad spectrum orally active antimycotic. Experientia 1979; 35:606–607.

68. Daneshmend TK, Warnock DW. Clinical pharmacokinetics of ketoconazole. Clin Pharmacokinet 1988; 14:13–34.

69. Graybill JR, Galgiani J, Stevens D, Dismukes W, Cloud G, and the NIAID Mycoses Study group. Progress in treatment of systemic mycoses: recent trials of the mycoses study group. In: Iwata K, Vanden Bossche H, (eds). In vitro and in vivo evaluation of antifungal agents, Amsterdam: Elsevier Science Publishers, 1986, pp.247–257.

70. Vanden Bossche H. Inhibitors of P450-dependent steroid biosynthesis: from research to medical treatment. J Steroid Biochem Mol Biol 1992; 43:1003–1021.

71. Venkatakrishnan K, von Moltke LL, Greenblatt DJ. Effects of the antifungal agents on oxidative drug metabolism: clinical relevance. Clin Pharmacokinet 2000; 38:111–180.

72. Heeres J, Backx LJJ, Van Cutsem J. Antimycotic azoles. Synthesis and antifungal properties of a series of novel triazole-3-ones. J Med Chem 1984; 27:894–900.

73. Richardson K, Cooper K, Marriott MS, Tarbit MH, Troke PF, Whittle PJ. Discovery of fluconazole, a novel antifungal agent. Rev Infect Dis 1990; 12:S267–S271.

74. Cauwenbergh G, De Doncker P. Itraconazole (R51211): a clinical review of its antimycotic activity in dermatology, gynecology, and internal medicine. Drug Dev Res 1986; 8:317–323.

75. Kauffman CA, Carver PL. Antifungal agents in the 1990s. Current status and future developments. Drugs 1997; 53:539–549.

76. Harousseau JL, Dekker AW, Stamatoullas-Bastard A, Fassas A, Linkesch W, Gouveia J, et al. Itraconazole oral solution for primary prophylaxis of fungal infections in patients with hematological malignancy and profound neutropenia: a randomized, double-blind, double-placebo, multicenter trial comparing itraconazole and amphotericin B. Antimicrob Agents Chemother 2000; 44:1887–1893.

77. Vanden Bossche H, Dromer F, Improvisi I, Lozano-Chiu M, Rex JH, Sanglard D. Antifungal drug resistance in pathogenic fungi. Medical Mycol 1998; 36 (Suppl 1):119–128.

78. Espinel-Ingroff A, Warnock DW, Vaquez JA, Arthington-Skaggs BA. In vitro antifungal susceptibilty methods and clinical implications of antifungal resistance. Medical Mycol 2000; 38 (Suppl 1):293–304.

79. Marichal P. Mechanisms of resistance to azole antifungal compounds. Curr Opin Anti-infect Invest Drugs 1999; 1:318–333.

80. Marr KA, Lyons CN, Ha K, Rustad TR, White TC. Inducible azole resistance associated with a heterogeneous phenotype in Candida albicans. Antimicrob Agents Chemother 2001; 45:52–59.

81. Goldman M, Cloud GA, Smedema M, LeMonte A, Connolly P, McKinsey DS, et al. Does long-term itraconazole prophylaxis result in in vitro azole resistance in mucosal Candida albicans isolates from persons with advanced human immunodeficiency virus infection? The National Institute of Allergy and Infectious Diseases Mycoses study group. Antimicrob Agents Chemother 2000; 44:1585–1587.

82. Weig M, Muller F-MC. Synergism of voriconazole and terbinafine against Candida albicans isolates from human immunodeficiency virus-infected patients with oropharyngeal candidiasis. Antimicrob Agents Chemother 2001; 45:966–968.

83. Perez A. Terbinafine: broad new spectrum of indications in several subcutaneous and systemic and parasitic diseases. Mycoses 1999; 42 Suppl 2:111–114.

84. De Backer MD, Nelissen B, Logghe M, Viaene J, Loonen I, Vandoninck S, et al. An antisense-based functional genomics approach for identification of genes critical for growth of Candida albicans. Nat Biotechnol 2001; 19:235–241.

85. Groll AH, De Lucca AJ, Walsh TJ. Emerging targets for the development of novel antifungal therapeutics. Trends Microbiol 1998; 6:117–124.

86. Heidler SA, Radding JA. The AURI gene in Saccharomyces cerevisiae encodes dominant resistance to the antifungal agent aureobasidin A (LY295337). Antimicrob Agents Chemother 1995; 39:2765–2769.

87. Nagiec MM, Nagiec EE, Baltisberger JA, Wells GB, Lester RL, Dickson RC. Sphingolipid synthesis as a target for antifungal drugs. Complementation of the inositolphosphorylceramide synthase defect in a mutant strain of Saccharomyces cerevisiae by the AUR1 gene. J Biol Chem 1997; 272:9809–9817.

88. Endo M, Takesako K, Kato I., Yamaguchi H. Fungicidal action of aureobasidin A, a cyclic depsipeptide antifungal antibiotic, against Saccharomyces cerevisiae. Antimicrob Agents Chemother 1997; 41:672–676.

89. Hashida-Okado T, Yasumoto R, Endo M, Takesako K, Kato I. Isolation and characterization of the aureobasidin A-resistant gene, aur1R, on Schizosacchromyces pombe: roles of Aur1p+ in cell morphogenesis. Curr Genet 1998; 33:38–45.

90. http://www-sequence.stanford.edu:8080/genbank/AF013799.

91. Kuroda M, Hashida-Okado T, Yasumoto R, Gomi K, Kato I, Takesako K. An aureobasidin A resistance gene isolated from Aspergillus is a homolog of yeast AUR1, a gene responsible for inositolphosphorylceramide (IPC) synthase activity. Mol Gen Genet 1999; 261:290–296.

92. Ogawa A, Hashida-Okado T, Endo M, Yoshioka H, Tsuruo T, Takesko K, et al. Role of ABC transporters in aureobasidin A resistance. Antimicrob Agents Chemother 1998; 42:755–761.

93. Tobin MB, Peery RB, Skatrud PL. Genes encoding multiple drug resistance like proteins in Aspergillus fumigatus and Aspergillus flavus. Gene 1997; 200:11–23.

94. Balkovec JM. Non-azole antifungal agents. Annu Rep Med Chem 1998; 33:173–182.

95. Mandala, SM, Harris GH. Isolation and characterization of novel inhibitors of sphingolipid synthesis: australifungin, viridiofungins, rustimicin, and khafrefungin. Methods Enzymol 1999; 311:335–348.

96. Vanden Bossche H, Marichal P. Gorrens J, Bellens D, Moereels H, Janssen PAJ. Mutation in cytochrome P450-dependent 14α-demethylase results in decreased affinity for azole antifungals. Biochem Soc Trans 1990; 18:56–59.

97. Kirsch DR, Lai MH, O'Sullivan J. Isolation of the gene for cytochrome P450 L1A1 (lanosterol 14α-demethylase) from Candida albicans. Gene 1988; 68:229–237.

98. Lai MH, Kirsch DR. Nucleotide sequence of cytochrome P450L1A1 (lanosterol 14α-demethylase) from *Candida albicans*. Nucleic Acids Res 1989; 17:804.

99. Marichal P, Koymans L, Willemsens S, Bellens D, Verhasselt P, Luyten W, et al. Contribution of mutations in the cytochrome P450 14α-demethylase (Erg11p, Cyp51p) to azole resistance in Candida albicans. Microbiology 1999; 145:2701–2713.

100. Sanglard D, Ischer F, Koymans L, Bille J. Amino acid substitutions in the cytochrome P450 lanosterol 14α-demethylase (CYP51A1) from azole-resistant Candida albicans clinical isolates contribute to resistance to azole antifungal agents. Antimicrob Agents Chemother 1998; 42:241–253.

101. Kelly SL, Lamb DC, Kelly DE. Y132H substitution in Candida albicans sterol 14α-demethylase confers fluconazole resistance by preventing binding to haem. FEMS Microbiol Lett 1999; Nov. 15, 180(2):171–175.

102. Asai K, Tsuchimori N, Okonogi K, Perfect JR, Gotoh O, Yoshida Y. Formation of azole-resistant Candida albicans by mutation of sterol 14-demethylase P450. Antimicrob Agents Chemother 1999; 43:1163–1169.

103. Lamb DC, Kelly D, Schunck WH, Shyadehi AZ, Akhtar M, Lowe DJ, et al. The mutation T315A in Candida albicans sterol 14α-demethylase causes reduced enzyme activity and fluconazole resistance through reduced affinity. J Biol Chem 1997; 272:5682–5688.

104. Kelly SL, Lamb DC, Loeffler J, Einsele H, Kelly DE. The G464S amino acid substitution in Candida albicans sterol 14α-demethylase causes fluconazole resistance in the clinic through reduced affinity. Biochem Biophys Res Commun 1999; 262:174–179.

105. White TC. The presence of an R467K amino acid substitution and loss of allelic variation correlate with an azole-resistant lanosterol 14α-demethylase in Candida albicans. Antimicrob Agents Chemother 1997; 41:1488–1494.

106. Lamb DC, Kelly DE, White TC, Kelly SL. The R464K amino acid substitution in Candida albicans sterol 14α-demethylase causes drug resistance through reduced affinity. Antimicrob Agents Chemother 2000; 44:63–67.

107. Skaggs BA, Alexander JF, Pierson CA, Scweitzer KS, Chun KT, Foegel C, et al. Cloning and characterization of the Saccharomyces cerevisiae C-22 sterol desturase gene, encoding a second cytochrome P-450 involved in ergosterol biosynthesis. Gene 1996; 169:105–109.

108. Kelly SL, Lamb DC, Baldwin BC, Corran AJ, Kelly DE Characterization of Saccharomyces cerevisiae CYP61, sterol delta 22-desaturase, and inhibition by azole antifungal agents. J Biol Chem 1997; 272:9986–9988.

109. Lamb DC, Maspahy S, Kelly DE, Manning NJ, Geber A, Bennett JE, et al. Purification, reconstitution, and inhibition of cytochrome P-450 sterol Δ^{22}-desaturase from the pathogenic fungus Candida glabrata. Antimicrob Agents Chemother 1999; 43:1725–1728.

110. Lamb DC, Kelly DE, Baldwin BC, Kelly SL. Differential inhibition of human CYP3A4 and Candida albicans CYP51 with azole antifungal agents. Chem Biol Interact 2000 125:165–175.

111. Vanden Bossche H, Marichal P, Odds FC, Le Jeune L, Coene MC. Characterization of an azole-resistant Candida glabrata isolate. Antimicrob Ag Chemother 1992; 36:2602–2610.

112. Vanden Bossche H, Warnock DW, Dupont B, Kerridge D, Sen GS, Improvisi L, et al. Mechanisms and clinical impact of antifungal drug resistance. J Med Vet Mycol 1994; 32:180–202.

113. Marichal P, Vanden Bossche H, Odds FC, Nobels G, Warnock DW, Timmermans V, et al. Molecular biological characterization of an azole-resistant Candida glabrata isolate. Antimicrob Ag Chemother 1997; 41:2229–2237.

114. Marichal P, Vanden Bossche H. Mechanisms of resistance to azole antifungals. Acta Biochim Pol 1995; 42:509–516.

115. Vanden Bossche H. Mechanisms of antifungal resistance. Rev Iberoam Micol 1997; 14:44–49.

116. White TC, Marr KA, Bowden RA. Clinical, cellular, and molecular factors that contribute to antifungal drug resistance. Clin Microbiol Rev 1998; 11:382–402.

117. Sanglard D, Isher F, Calabrese D, de Micheli M, Bille J. Multiple resistance mechanisms to azole antifungals in yeast clinical isolates. Drug Resistance Updates 1998; 1:255–265.

118. Ryley JF, Wilson RG, Barrett-Bee KJ. Azole resistance in Candida albicans. Sabouraudia 1984; 22:53–93.

119. Sanglard D, Kuchler K, Ischer F, Pagani L, Monod M, Bille J. Mechanisms of resistance to azole antifungal agents in Candida albicans isolates from AIDS patients involve specific multidrug transporters. Antimicrob Agents Chemother 1995; 39:2378–2386.

120. Venkateswarlu K, Denning DW, Manning NJ, Kelly SL. Resistance to fluconazole in Candida albicans from AIDS patients correlated with reduced intracellular accumulation of drug. FEMS Microbiol Lett 1995; 131:337–341.

121. Marichal P, Gorrens J, Coene M-C, Le Jeune L, Vanden Bossche H. Origin of differences in susceptibility of Candida krusei to azole antifungal agents. Mycoses 1995; 38:111–117.

122. Venkateswarlu K, Denning DW, Manning NJ, Kelly SL. Reduced accumulation of drug in Candida krusei accounts for itraconazole resistance. Antimicrob Agents Chemother 1996; 40:2443–2446.

123. Miyazaki H, Miyazaki Y, Geber A, Parkinson T, Hitchcock C, Falconer DJ, et al. Fluconazole resistance associated with drug efflux and increased transcription of a drug transporter gene, PDH1, in Candida glabrata. Antimicrob Agents Chemother 1998; 42:1695–1701.

124. Sanglard D, Ischer F, Calabrese D, Majcherczyk PA, Bille J. The ATP binding cassette transporter gene CgCDR1 from Candida glabrata is involved in the resistance of clinical isolates to azole antifungal agents. Antimicrob Agents Chemother 1999; 43:2753–2765.

125. Moran GP, Sanglard D, Donelly SM, Shanley DB, Sullivan DJ, Coleman DC. Identification and expression of multidrug transporters responsible for fluconazole resistance in Candida dubliniensis. Antimicrob Agents Chemother 1998; 42:1819–1830.

126. Venkateswarlu K, Taylor M, Manning NJ, Rinaldi MG, Kelly SL. Fluconazole tolerance in clinical isolates of Cryptococcus neoformans. Antimicrob Agents Chemother 1997; 41:748–751.

127. de Waard MA, Van Nistelrooy JGM. An energy-dependent efflux mechanism for fenarimol in a wild-type strain and fenarimol-resitant mutants of Aspergillus nidulans. Pestic Biochem Physiol 1980; 13:255–266.

128. Lees ND, Broughton MM, Sanglard D, Bard M. Azole susceptibility and hyphal formation in a cytochrome P450-deficient mutant of Candida albicans. Antimicrob Agents Chemother 1990; 34:831–836.

129. Jensen-Pergakes KL, Kennedy MA, Lees ND, Barbuch R, Koegel C, Bard M. Sequencing, disruption, and characterization of the Candida albicans sterol methyltransferase (ERG6) gene: drug susceptibilty studies in erg6 mutants. Antimicrob Agents Chemother 1998; 42:1160–1167.

130. de Waard MA, Van Nistelrooy JGM. Mechanism of resistance to fenarimol in Aspergillus nidulans. Pestic Biochem Physiol 1979; 10:219–229.

131. de Waard MA, Van Nistelrooy JGM. Antagonistic and synergistic activities of various chemicals on the toxicity of fenarimol to Aspergillus nidulans. Pestic Sci 1982; 13:279–286.

132. Goffeau A, Park J, Paulsen IT, Jonniaux JL, Dinh T, Mordant P, et al. Multidrug-resistant transport proteins in yeast: complete inventory and phylogenetic characterization of yeast open reading frames within the major facilitator superfamily. Yeast 1997; 13:43–54.

133. Decottignies A, Goffeau A. Complete inventory of the yeast ABC proteins. Nat Geneti 1997; 15:137–145.

134. Marr K, Lyons CN, Rustad T, Bowden RA, White T. Rapid, transient fluconazole resistance in Candida albicans is associated with increased mRNA levels of CDR. Antimicrob Agents Chemother 1998; 42:2584–2589.

135. Prasad R, De Wergifosse P, Goffeau A, Balzi E. Molecular cloning and characterization of a novel gene of Candida albicans, CDR1, conferring multiple resistance to drugs and antifungals. Curr Genet 1995; 27:320–329.

136. Sanglard D, Ischer F, Monod M, Bille J. Cloning of Candida albicans genes conferring resistance to azole antifungal agents: characterization of CDR2, a new multidrug ABC transporter gene. Microbiology 1997; 143:405–416.

137. Sanglard D, Ischer F, Monod M, Bille J. Susceptibilities of Candida albicans multidrug trans-porter mutants to various antifungal agents and other metabolic inhibitors. Antimicrob Agents Chemother 1996; 40:2300–2305.

138. Albertson GD, Niimi M, Cannon RD, Jenkinson HF. Multiple efflux mechanisms are involved in Candida albicans fluconazole resistance. Antimicrob Agents Chemother 1996; 40:2300–2305.

139. Balan I, Alarco AM, Raymond M. The Candida albicans CDR3 gene codes for an opaque-phase transporter. J Bacteriol 1997; 179:7210–7218.

140. Franz R, Michel S, Morschhauser J. A fourth gene from the Candida albicans CDR family of ABC transporters. Gene 1998; 220:91–98.

141. Fling M, Kopf J, Tamarkin A, Gorman JA, Smith HA, Koltin Y. Analysis of a Candida albicans gene that encodes a novel mechanism for resistance to benomyl and methotrexate. Mol Gen Genet 1991; 227:318–329.

142. Katiyar SK, Edlind TD. Identification and expression of multidrug resistance-related ABC transporter genes in Candida krusei Med Mycol 2001; 39:109–116.

143. Barchiesi F, Calabrese D, Sanglard D, Falconi di Francesco L, Caselli F, Giannini D, et al. Experimental induction of fluconazole resistance in Candida tropicalis ATCC750. Antimicrob Agents Chemother 2000; 44:1578–1584.

144. Thornewell SJ, Peery TJ, Skatrud PL. Cloning and characterization of CneMDR1: a Cryptococ-cus neoformans gene encoding a protein related to multidrug resistance proteins. Gene 1997; 201:21–29.

145. Spitzer SG, Spitzer ED. Identification of a Cryptococcus neoformans sequence belonging to the major facilitator superfamilty (MFS). In: Program and Abstracts of the 97th General meeting of ASM, 1997; Abstract F26.

146. Slaven JW, Anderson MJ, Sanglard D, Dixon GK, Bille J, Roberts IS, et al. Induced expression of a novel ABC transporter gene adr1 from Aspergillus fumigatus in response to itraconazole. In: Program and Abstracts of the 39th ICAAC. 1999; Abstract No. 447.

147. Del Sorbo G, Andrade AC, Van Nistelrooy JGM, Van Fan JAL, Balzi E, De Waard MA. Mul-tidrug resistance in Aspergillus nidulans involves novel ATP-binding cassette transporters. Mol Gen Genet 1997; 254:417–426.

148. Kolaczkowski M, Goffeau A. Active efflux by multidrug transporters as one of the strategies to evade chemotherapy and novel practical implications of yeast pleiotropic drug resistance. Phar-macol Ther 1997; 76:219–242.

149. Dogra S, Krishnamurthy S, Gupta V, Dixit BL, Gupta CM, Sanglard D, et al. Asymmetric dis-tribution of phosphatidylethanolamine in C.albicans: possible mediation by CDR1, a mul-tidrug transporter belonging to ATP binding cassette (ABC) superfamily. Yeast 1999; 15:111–121.

150. Smriti D, Prasad R. CDR1p, which confers multidrug resistance in Candida albicans, is a gen-eral phospholipid translocase. In: Program and Abstracts of the 39th ICAAC. 1999; Abstract No. 2078.

151. Sanglard D, Ischer F, Monod M, Dogra S, Prasad R, Bille J. Analysis of the ATP-binding cas-sette (ABC)-transporter gene CDR4 from Candida albicans. In: Abstract Book 5th ASM Can-dida Candidiasis Conference, 1999; Abstract C27, p.56.

152. Wu T, Wright K, Hurst SF, Morrison CJ. Enhanced extracellular production of aspartyl pro-teinase, a virulence factor, by Candida albicans isolates following growth in subinhibitory con-centrations of fluconazole. Antimicrob Agents Chemother 2000; 44:1200–1208.

153. Maesaki S, Marichal P, Hossain MA, Sanglard D, Vanden Bossche H, Kohno S. Synergistic effects of tracrolimus and azole antifungal agents against azole-resistant Candida albicans strains. J Antimicrob Chemother 1998; 42:747–753.

154. Egner K, Rosenthal FE, Kralli A, Sanglard D, Kuchler K. Genetic separation of FK506 susceptibility and drug transport in the yeast Pdr5 ATP binding cassette multidrug resistance transporter. Mol Biol Cell 1998; 9:523–543.

155. Egner R, Bauer BE, Kuchler K. The transmembrane domain 10 of the yeast Pdr5p ABC antifungal efflux pump determines both substrate specificity and inhibitor susceptibility. Mol Microbiol 2000; 35:1255–1263.

156. Goffeau A, Barrell BG, Bussey H, Davis RW, Dujon B, Feldmann H, et al. Life with 6000 genes. Science 1996; 274:563–574.

157. The C. elegans sequencing consortium. Genome sequence of the nematode C. elegans: a platform for investigating biology. Science 1998; 282:2012–2018.

158. Adams MD, Celniker SE, Holt RA, Evans CA, Gocayne JD, Amanatides PG, et al. The genome sequence of Drosophila melanogaster. Science 2000; 287:2185–2195.

159. Broder S, Venter JC. Whole genomes: the foundation of new biology and medicine. Curr Opin Biotechnol 2000; 11(6):581–585.

160. Moir DT, Shaw KJ, Hare RS, Vovis GF. Genomics and antimicrobial drug discovery. Antimicrob Agents Chemother 1999; 43(3):439–446.

161. Rosamond J, Allsop A. Harnessing the power of the genome in the search for new antibiotics. Science 2000; 287:1973–1976.

162. Venter JC, Adams MD, Myers EW, Li PW, Mural RJ, Sutton GG, et al. The sequence of the human genome. Science 2001; 291:1304–1351.

163. Casadevall A. Antibody-based therapies for emerging infectious diseases. Emerg Infect Dis 1996; 2(3):200–208.

164. Brown PO, Botstein D. Exploring the new world of the genome with DNA microarrays. Nat Genet 1999; 21:33–37.

165. Duggan DJ, Bittner M, Chen Y, Meltzer P, Trent JM. Expression profiling using cDNA microarrays. Nat Genet 1999; 21:10–14.

166. Graves DJ. Powerful tools for genetic analysis come of age. Trends Biotechnol 1999; 17(3):127–134.

167. van Hal NL, Vorst O, van Houwelingen AM, Kok EJ, Peijnenburg A, Aharoni A, et al. The application of DNA microarrays in gene expression analysis. J Biotechnol 2000; 78:271–280.

168. Lennon GG, Lehrach H. Hybridization analyses of arrayed cDNA libraries. Trends Genet 1991; 7:314–317.

169. Southern EM, Case-Green SC, Elder JK, Johnson M, Mir KU, Wang L, Williams, JC, et al. Arrays of complementary oligonucleotides for analysing the hybridisation behaviour of nucleic acids. Nucleic Acids Res 1994; 22:1368–1373.

170. Zhao N, Hashida H, Takahashi N, Misumi Y, Sakaki Y. High-density cDNA filter analysis: a novel approach for large-scale, quantitative analysis of gene expression. Gene 1995; 156:207–213.

171. De Risi JL, Yver VR, Brown PO. Exploring the metabolic and genetic control of gene expression on a genomic scale. Science 1997; 278:680–686.

172. Spellman PT, Sherlock G, Zhang MQ, Iyer VR, Anders K, Eisen MB, et al. Comprehensive identification of cell cycle-regulated genes of the yeast Saccharomyces cerevisiae by microarray hybridisation. Mol Biol Cell 1998; 9:3273–3297.

173. Eisen MB, Spellman PT, Brown PO, Botstein D. Cluster analysis and display of genome-wide expression patterns. Proc Natl Acad Sci USA 1998; 95(25):14,863–14,868.

174. Chu S, DeRisi J, Eisen M, Mulholland J, Botstein D, Brown PO, Herskowitz I. The transcriptional program of sporulation in budding yeast. Science 1998; 282:699–705.

175. De Backer MD, Ilyina T, Ma X-S, Vandoninck S, Luyten WHML, Vanden Bossche H. Genomic profiling of the response of Candida albicans to itraconazole treatment using a DNA microarray. Antimicrob Agents Chemother 2001; 45:1660–1670.

176. Bammert GF, Fostel JM. Genome-wide expression patterns in Saccharomyces cerevisiae: comparison of drug treatments and genetic alterations affecting biosynthesis of ergosterol. Antimicrob Agents Chemother 2000; 44:1255–1265.

177. Marton MJ, DeRisi JL, Bennett HA, Iyer VR, Meyer MR, Roberts CJ, et al. Drug target validation and identification of secondary drug target effects using DNA microarrays. Nat Med 1998; 4:1293–1301.

178. Golub TR, Slonim DK, Tamayo P, Huard C, Gaasenbeek M, Mesirov JP, et al. Molecular classification of cancer: class discovery and class prediction by gene expression monitoring. Science 1999; 286:531–537.

179. Alizadeh AA, Eisen MB, Davis RE, Ma C, Lossos IS, Rosenwald A, et al. Distinct types of diffuse large B-cell lymphoma identified by gene expression profiling. Nature 2000; 403:503–510.

180. Gray NS, Wodicka L, Thunnissen AM, Norman TC, Kwon S, Espinoza FH, et al. Exploiting chemical libraries, structure and genomics in the search for kinase inhibitors. Science 1998; 281:533–538.

181. Rosania GR, Chang YT, Perez O, Sutherlin D, Dong H, Lockhart DJ, et al. Myoseverin: a microtubule binding molecule with novel cellular effects. Nat Biotechnol 2000; 18:304–308.

182. Hu JS, Durst M, Kerb R, Truong V, Ma JT, Khurgin E, et al. Analysis of drug pharmacology towards predicting drug behaviour by expression profiling using high-density oligonucleotide arrays. Ann NY Acad Sci 2000; 919:9–15.

183. Moehle CM. Patent application RiboGene Inc., 1995; PCT WO 95/11969.

184. Numata K, Yamamoto H, Hatori M, Miyaki T, Kawaguchi H. Isolation of an aminoglycoside hypersensitive mutant and its application in screening. J Antibiot 1986; 39:994–1000.

185. Oliver S. Redundancy reveals drugs in action. Nat Genet 1999; 21:245–246.

186. Jelinsky SA, Estep P, Church GM, Samson LD. Regulatory networks revealed by transcriptional profiling of damaged Saccharomyces cerevisiae cells: Rpn4 links base excision repair with proteasomes. Mol Cell Biol 2000; 20(21):8157–8167.

187. Emmert-Buck MR, Bonner RF, Smith PD, Chuaqui RF, Zhuang Z, Goldstein SR, et al. Laser capture microdissection. Science 1996; 274:998–1001.

188. Blackstock WP, Weir MP. Proteomics: quantitative and physical mapping of cellular proteins. Trends Biotechnol 1999; 17(3):121–127.

Cryptococcus neoformans

A Molecular Model for the Study of Fungal Pathogenesis and Drug Discovery in the Genomic Era

Jennifer K. Lodge and John R. Perfect

INTRODUCTION

Cryptococcus neoformans is a worldwide opportunistic fungal pathogen that causes central nervous system (CNS) infections in both immunocompetent and immunosuppressed patients. During the AIDS pandemic, the increase in rates of infection and difficulties in management have been amplified. Current antifungal treatments have been extensively studied, but there are still reports of 10–25% acute mortality in medically advanced countries, and in countries with less resources more than 50% of patients will die within 2 wk of being diagnosed. Thus, new targets for antifungal therapies are being sought. Genomics will accelerate the search for new targets for antifungal drugs, and *C. neoformans* is an ideal model system for these studies.

Medical Importance of **Cryptococcus neoformans**

Clinical Aspects and Patient Populations

AIDS patients are extremely vulnerable to opportunistic fungal infections *(1–3)*. *Cryptococcus neoformans* (for review *see* refs. *4,5*) is an opportunistic pathogen that frequently causes pulmonary infections and meningoencephalitis *(6,7)*, particularly in patients with AIDS. It has been estimated that 7–10% of patients with AIDS will develop cryptococcosis, which is fatal if left untreated and is a leading cause of death in immunocompromised patients.

Current Antifungal Therapies

The recommended treatments for cryptococcosis *(8)* are the azoles—fluconazole or intraconazole—or amphotericin B. These can be used alone or in combination with 5-flucytosine. 5-flucytosine, which targets pyrimidine biosynthesis, is not used alone because of the high frequency of development of resistant strains *(9)*. Amphotericin B binds to ergosterol and has significant toxicity, but lipid formulations of amphotericin B can reduce some of this toxicity. The azoles inhibit ergosterol biosynthesis and are better tolerated than amphotericin B, but fluconazole is fungistatic, and may require lifelong therapy to prevent relapse in AIDS patients who do not respond to HAART *(7,10)*. Newer triazoles—such as voriconazole and posaconazole—hold promise, but

From: *Pathogen Genomics: Impact on Human Health*
Edited by: K. J. Shaw © Humana Press Inc., Totowa, NJ

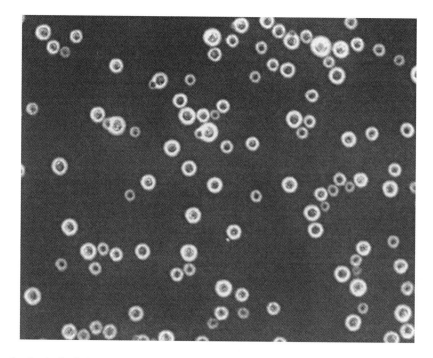

Fig. 1. An india ink stain of *Cryptococcus neoformans* grown under conditions that induce capsule formation.

still target ergosterol biosynthesis. New antifungals that inhibit cell wall formation are effective against several species of fungi, but not *Cryptococcus neoformans*. Fluconazole-resistant *C. neoformans* strains are emerging *(11),* and long-term treatment, including prophylactic therapy *(12)* with fluconazole and poor responses to HAART, are likely to accelerate this trend.

Biology of C. neoformans

Cryptococcus neoformans is a basidiomycetous fungus that is generally isolated as a haploid yeast (for review, *see* ref. *13*) (Fig. 1) although diploids have been identified in nature *(14).* There are two mating types (Matα and Mat a), which can undergo recognition, fusion, and formation of a mycelium. A structure called a basidium is formed from the mycelium, and spores are then produced from the surface of the basidium. Certain haploid strains (MATα) have also been shown to produce basidiospores under specific nutrient deprivations *(15).* Based on the size of the basidospore and its resistance to desiccation, it is possible that the basidospore is the infectious propagule, although it has not yet been identified in nature.

C. neoformans has a Worldwide Distribution

There are several serotypes based on capsular structural differences, and currently they are classified into three varieties, although the nomenclature changes as further genetic information is studied. Presently, serotypes A and D comprise *C. neoformans* var. *grubii* and var. neoformans, respectively. Serotypes B and C comprise *C. neofor-*

mans var. *gattii* Serotypes A and D, compared to B and C, have clinical and environmental differences. For instance, serotypes A and D are found in North America and Europe and are opportunistic pathogens, whereas serotypes B and C are predominantly found in subtropical regions associated with Eucalyptus trees, and generally infect normal hosts.

Genetics

C. neoformans usually grows as a haploid yeast. In *Cryptococcus neoformans* var. *neoformans,* there is a well-defined sexual cycle with two mating types, a and α Marked strains are available for crosses and genetic analysis. Congenic mating pairs are available, and one member of a pair, JEC21, is the type strain for the *C. neoformans* genome project. A thermally regulated, stable diploid has been created *(16),* which may be useful for assessing the phenotype of mutations in a diploid and determining if a gene is essential for vegetative growth. Recently, a *Cryptococcus neoformans* var. *grubii* strain that is *MATa* has been identified *(17,18).* This finding may help to make congenic pairs of this most common variety, since previously all strains of this variety that would mate were *MATα.*

Molecular Genetics

C. neoformans grows well in the laboratory in both rich and minimal media at temperatures ranging from 24°C to 37°C. It can easily be grown in liquid culture or on agar plates. The molecular genetics of *C. neoformans* has advanced significantly in the last decade. Methods for DNA and RNA preparation are well established. Analysis of chromosomes by CHEF gel is available, and shows variability in sizes and numbers between strains *(19,20).* Transformation systems using electroporation *(21)* or biolistic delivery *(22)* have been developed with many selectable markers, including *URA5 (21)* encoding orotidine-5′-phosphate decarboxylase, *ADE2 (22)* encoding phosphoribosylaminoimidazole carboxylase, *NMT1 (23)* encoding N-myristoyltransferase, hygromycin B resistance *(24),* G418 resistance *(25),* phleomycin resistance *(25),* and nourseothricin resistance *(26).* Targeted gene replacement by homologous recombination has also proved highly successful and is now commonplace *(27,28,29).* Homologous recombination rates for variety *grubii* serotype A range from 2% to 50% *(27,30–34)* depending on the allele. Detailed studies controlling for locus specificity and length of homology for recombination rates are just beginning, and preliminary data from the Lodge laboratory suggests that as little as 50 basepairs of homology can promote homologous recombination, although not efficiently. Earlier studies using electroporation as the DNA delivery method suggest that variety *neoformans* was less effective at homologous recombination, with rates ranging from 0.001–0.1% *(28,35,36).* However, recent findings suggest that the DNA delivery method is critical: variety *neoformans* transformed by biolistic techniques achieve a homologous recombination rates similar to serotype A *(29)* ranging from 1–4%. With low efficiency, variety *gattii* strains can be transformed, but homologous recombination remains elusive.

Pathogenesis

Animal Models

A major advantage of *Cryptococcus neoformans* in the study of fungal pathogenesis and drug targets is the outstanding animal models of disease. Since *Cryptococcus* can be both a primary and secondary pathogen, the animal models can mimic both disease states. Mice are the most useful, and models using intranasal, intravenous (iv), or intracerebral inoculation can help to address organ-specific immunity issues *(4)*. The infection is subacute, with easily used end points of quantitative cultures or survival. With both transgenic mice for specific immune defects or exogenous immune suppression (corticosteroids or cyclophosphamide), the impact of host factors can be controlled. A complementary model has been the corticosteroid-treated rabbit model of cryptococcal meningitis *(37)*. It requires severe immunosuppression to allow a reproducible infection in this species. In fact, it mimics the lack of a cerebrospinal fluid (CSF) inflammatory response typically seen in AIDS patients with cryptococcal meningitis. Many antifungal trials have been performed in this model, and it has correctly predicted human response to drugs in all cases studied. For instance, amphotericin B is very potent despite low CSF levels; itraconazole has CNS activity despite poor penetration into the subarachnoid space; and fluconazole does not kill yeasts as rapidly as amphotericin B in the CSF. The rabbit model also allows for the ability to serially remove yeast cells from a clinically relevant site and examine gene or protein expression patterns. Both these animal model systems have been used to examine the impact of single or double gene-specific null mutants and their complemented strain compared to the wild-type parent in classic virulence studies. In our studies, over two dozen specific null mutants have been studied, with about two-thirds exhibiting attenuation of virulence at several grades, one-third demonstrating no virulence phenotypes, and one null mutant with hypervirulence *(38,39)*. It is clear that attenuation of null mutants can range from statistical evidence that the null mutant does not reach wild-type fitness but still produces disease to strains that simply cannot survive in the host. Although the rabbit and mouse models vary in species, route of inoculation, and use of immunosuppression, most null mutants have been concordant in their outcomes. However, as expected, there are genes important in one model but not in another, such as the urease *(URE1)* gene. The *URE1* mutant has no impact on growth within the rabbit CSF, but is attenuated for virulence in both the iv and intranasal murine model *(34)*. The use of two robust animal models allows the investigators to more closely eliminate host-range determinants so that identified gene targets are more likely to be relevant in human disease rather than be rabbit- or murine-model specific. The clear end points, multiple models and species, and reproducibility of results make the animal models for cryptococcosis a major advantage in molecular studies of pathogenesis and drug targets.

Virulence Factors of C. neoformans

Fungal virulence factors have been the subject of intense study over the past decade (for review *see* refs. *40–43*). Generally, putative virulence factors are identified by observation of a correlation between the presence of the factor and virulence, by isolation and virulence testing of specific mutants which lack the factor, or by analogy to other systems combined with directed replacement of a gene responsible for the factor. Targeted gene disruption (gene knockout) and comparison to the wild-type parent in an animal model has become the standard for determination of the importance of particular genes or phenotypes to virulence *(44)*. An important additional control is a demonstration that supplying a complete functional copy of the deleted gene in the attenuated mutant will restore virulence. These approaches require that a phenotype or gene be suspected of being important for virulence and taken through these molecular Koch's postulates. Several virulence factors of *C. neoformans* and the signal transduction pathways required to express them have been identified. These include the alpha mating type and the production of the polysaccharide capsule, melanin, urease, and phospholipase, and growth at high temperatures 37–39°C.

SIGNAL TRANSDUCTION

C. neoformans has at least three signal transduction pathways (for review *see* ref. *45*), which differentially regulate mating, filamentation, growth, and haploid fruiting *(13,31,32,46–49)*. Two of these pathways are associated with heterotrimeric G proteins and kinase cascades, similar to those found in other fungi. At least one of the G protein-mediated pathways regulates the expression of the known virulence factors such as melanin and capsule biosynthesis. Two others—one through a *RAS* protein and another through calcineurin—regulate the ability to grow at high temperatures and thus the ability to produce disease.

ASSOCIATION WITH THE ALPHA-MATING TYPE

Analysis of clinical isolates of *C. neoformans* showed that there was a strong bias toward the alpha mating type in the majority of the isolates, suggesting the possibility that the cells with the alpha mating type were more virulent *(50)*. Testing of isogenic *MATα* and *MATα* cells revealed that the *MATα* cells were more virulent *(51)*. Another contributing factor to the high frequency of *MATα* strains found in clinical isolates is that the alpha mating type undergoes haploid fruiting under specific conditions and produces spores that may be the infectious propagules, thus allowing the *MATα* strains to produce more infectious particles than the strains carrying the *MATα* locus *(15)*. The importance of the alpha-mating type locus in morphogenesis and virulence is now being studied one gene at a time.

POLYSACCHARIDE CAPSULE

C. neoformans produces a large polysaccharide capsule during infection of a mammalian host and in vitro under specific growth conditions *(52,53)*. Acapsular mutants have been isolated and found to be significantly less virulent *(54)*. Four capsule synthesis genes—*CAP59, CAP60, CAP64,* and *CAP10*—were cloned by complementation to acapsular mutants. The contribution to capsule formation of the isolated genes was further established by targeted gene disruption of each of the four genes and testing of each disruptant in an animal model *(28,35,55,56)*. In addition, disruption of the *MAN1* gene encoding phosphomannose isomerase reduces capsule production and has profound effects on virulence in which the yeast is completely eliminated from the host *(57)*. There are many unique genes associated with the capsule structure, and more have recently been identified. It will be important to merge this genetic approach with an understanding of the biochemistry of this complex but extremely important structure.

MELANIN PRODUCTION

C. neoformans produces melanin under particular in vitro and in vivo conditions *(58)*. Because melanin is a potential antioxidant, mutants that were unable to synthesize melanin were identified and shown to be less virulent than wild-type *(59)*. A gene that encodes a laccase *(60)* was isolated, and a targeted disruption in the laccase gene was made. The resulting null mutant was shown to be less virulent than wild-type, and confirmed the central importance of this phenotype for virulence *(36)*.

UREASE PRODUCTION

Urease is an enzyme that catalyzes the hydrolysis of urea, and thus alters the pH of the surrounding environment. It is found in many bacterial and fungal species, and has been shown to be a virulence factor in several other systems. A urease gene was isolated from *C. neoformans* and subjected to targeted gene disruption. The disruptants had attenuated virulence in murine inhalation and iv inoculation models, but not in an immunocompromised rabbit cryptococcal meningitis *(34)*. Urease has also been shown to have an impact on the TH1/TH2 immune response to *C. neoformans (61)*.

PHOSPHOLIPASE B PRODUCTION

Phospholipase B hydrolyzes ester linkages in phospholipids and has been shown to be a virulence factor in other systems (reviewed in ref. *62*), including *Candida albicans (63)*. Analysis of many different clinical isolates of *C. neoformans* have exposed an association of high levels of secreted phospholipase with virulence *(64–66)*, and knockout of a gene encoding a phospholipase B showed an attenuation of virulence in rabbits and mice *(67)*. Both this gene and *IPC* gene have been shown to be important for the growth of *C. neoformans* on the intracellular level *(68)*.

Other Possible Virulence Factors

Based on other fungal systems and on our current understanding of *C. neoformans* biology, one might also expect that genes involved in mannitol production *(69)*, Fe assimilation *(70)*, Ca binding *(71)*, adhesion *(72,73)*, cell-wall production, and secreted proteases *(74,75)* are important for virulence. There are a myriad of potential targets to explore in *C. neoformans* pathobiology.

The Search for New Antifungal Targets

New targets for the treatment of cryptococcal meningitis must be identified—preferably targets that would be applicable to all pathogenic fungi, including *Candida albicans, Pneumocystis carinii, Aspergillus fumigatus, Histoplasma capsulatum*, and *Coccidioides immitis*. The ideal target would be an enzyme that is essential for viability of the pathogenic fungi, so that when inhibited, the fungi die quickly. A fungicidal inhibitor may be crucial for treating fungal infections in an immunocompromised patient because the patient's immune system is poorly equipped to clear all the organisms. The ideal target should also be unique to fungi, so that fungal-specific inhibitors with no toxicity to a human host could be designed. Genomics will provide a wealth of information to identify new targets through genes with a homologue in other fungal systems, but no direct homologue in mammalian systems either in structure or function.

Fungal Cell Wall

One newer target for antifungal therapy is the enzymes involved in synthesis of the cell wall *(76,77)*. A major advantage of targeting cell-wall synthesis is that these enzymes are unique to fungi, and some inhibitors of (1,3)-beta-D-glucan synthase have been successfully developed, including the pneumocandins, echinocandins, papulacandins, and acidic terpenoid inhibitors *(78–80)*. Unfortunately, these compounds are not effective against all fungi. *C. neoformans* in particular appears to be resistant to the pneumocandins and the echinocandins *(81,82)*. Recently, the glucan synthase homologue *(FSK1)* has been cloned and shown to be essential in *C. neoformans (83)*. Interestingly, the *C. neoformans FSK1* homologue is highly conserved with other fungal *FSK1* genes, and retains the residues believed to be important for echinocandin susceptibility. Further studies on understanding the reduced effectiveness of present candins against *C. neoformans* could lead to better compounds, since the target remains an attractive anticryptococcal area.

Essential Genes

Another approach to drug targets is to identify proteins that are essential for growth. In fact, few classic virulence targets have been drug activity sites, but targets for ability to grow remain most successful. Essential proteins are appealing targets because their inhibition has the potential to kill all of the infecting fungi quickly, allowing an immunocompromised patient to completely clear the organisms and prevent relapse. Unfortunately, essential proteins often have homologous human counterparts with similar substrate specificities, making the development of a species-specific inhibitor difficult.

Demonstration that a gene is essential for viability in *C. neoformans* has been problematic and has been done on a gene-by-gene basis. MyristoylCoA:protein *N*-myristoyl transferase *(NMT1)* was demonstrated to be essential by development of a temperature-sensitive mutant based on a similar mutation found in *S. cerevisiae NMT1 (27,84)*. If a gene cannot be disrupted, it is suspected of being essential. However, it is important to show that recombination can occur at that locus. One method used to demonstrate that topoisomerase I is essential for viability in *C. neoformans (33)* is to transform the yeast with a wild-type copy of the putative essential gene, and compare the rate of gene disruption at the endogenous locus between the wild-type strain and the strain with the extra copy of the gene. If no knockouts can be obtained in the wild-type strain, but can be obtained in the strain with the extra copy, then one can infer that the gene is likely to be essential, as was shown for topoisomerase I *(33)*. A similar approach was used to demonstrate that a B-1,3 glucan synthase gene *(FKS1)* was essential for *C. neoformans*. The strategy was to develop two gene-disruption vectors, only one of which would disrupt gene function. The other innocuous vector could homologously recombine at the *FKS1* locus, but the disruption vector could not *(83)*.

Some essential enzymes that have been studied as potential antifungal targets either have no human counterpart (phosphoribosylaminoimidazole carboxylase, 38; inositol-phosphoryl ceramide synthase, 68) or have distinct substrate specificities (*NMT1, 84–86;* elongation factor 3, 87; topoisomerase I, 33). Other studies with DNA topoisomerase I *(88)* suggest an alternative approach that does not require an enzyme to be essential—when topoisomerase I is inhibited while it is bound to DNA, the genomic DNA is sufficiently damaged to cause cell death.

Thus far, the use of inducible promoters has not successfully demonstrated that a gene is essential. An important consideration is the level of enzyme required compared to the level of enzyme present in steady state. If an enzyme is present in much larger concentrations than actually required for viability, reducing but not eliminating the enzyme may not show a growth defect. This has occurred with both *TOP1* and *IPC1*, in which under a *GAL7* inducible promoter the gene can be regulated, but there is still enough expression under noninducible conditions for the strains to survive. Quantitation of the steady-state level of the enzyme and knowing how much enzyme is actually needed for the yeast to survive also will help choose targets for antifungal therapies. An enzyme that requires 80% inhibition to cause cell death may make a better target than an enzyme that requires 99.9% inhibition *(85)*.

Recently, the use of anti-sense RNA and RNAi have been applied successfully to *C. neoformans (89)*. It has been used with both whole transcripts and oligonucleotides. This tool can help in analyzing essential genes, and could possibly be developed into a molecular drug-treatment strategy that has already been used in human cytomegalic virus infections.

C. neoformans AS A MODEL SYSTEM FOR GENOME-WIDE FUNCTIONAL GENOMICS AND PROTEOMIC ANALYSIS OF PATHOGENESIS AND DEVELOPMENT OF ANTIFUNGAL THERAPIES

C. neoformans is a pathogenic fungus that is ripe for functional genomic or proteomic approaches to analysis of pathogenesis and development of new antifungal targets. *C. neoformans* has several advantages over all other fungal pathogens for comparative genomics, microarrays, genome-wide targeted gene disruption, and proteome-wide studies. First, a successful genome-sequencing project is underway, and will be completed in 2003. Second, *C. neoformans* is easily grown and manipulated in the laboratory. Third, the tools for molecular genetic analysis, such as transformation and homologous recombination, are relatively straightforward and well-documented in *C. neoformans*. Fourth, it has a haploid genome that facilitates creating knockout mutants. Fifth, multiple, robust animal models for cryptococcal meningitis have been well-established.

Genomic Analysis of C. neoformans

A concerted effort to obtain the complete genomic sequence of *Cryptococcus neoformans* began in 1999 and has been highly successful (For review, *see* ref. *90*). The genome of *C. neoformans* has been estimated to be 21–24 Mb *(20)*, with an A+T content close to 50%, and multiple introns in most of the genes encoding proteins. The genome project began in February of 1999 at a meeting held in St. Louis, MO to establish a genome project. There was consensus that the first strain to be sequenced would be serotype D, JEC21, but that a serotype A strain known as H99 should also be the subject of comparative genomics projects because it is a better model for virulence and host-response studies. As a direct result of this meeting, two grants from NIH-NIAID were funded to sequence the JEC21 genome to four- to five fold coverage, and to sequence cDNAs and their genomic clone counterparts to establish intron/exon junctions. A third grant from NIH-NIAID has recently been awarded that will fund further random shotgun sequencing, assembly, and additional annotation. In June 2001, a second *C. neoformans* genome meeting was held. At this meeting, data from the sequencing projects was presented, and plans are being developed for the identification of genes and the annotation of the genome. Dr. James Kronstad presented a bacterial artificial chromosome (BAC) mapping project that forms the basis of a physical map, and Dr. Rytas Vigalas presented a genetic map of *C. neoformans*. The linking of these two maps to the sequencing efforts will speed assembly and completion of the genome sequence. Projects in comparative genomes, functional genomics, and proteomics were presented.

Stanford University

Dr. Ron Davis is the principal investigator and Dr. Richard Hyman is the scientist overseeing the project. In this project, M13 libraries with ~2-kb inserts were made from sheared DNA from JEC21. The clones are being sequenced and the data is available on the Stanford DNA Sequencing and Technology Center website: http://sequence-www.stanford.edu/group/C.neoformans/index.html

The project has proceeded rapidly. Data was entered beginning in March 1999. Funding for the project was begun in March 2000. The data can be downloaded and is searchable. More recently, data are being obtained with the ABI3700 automated sequencing machine, and offer higher quality and length. The first genome assembly was done on October 2000, and generated 3900 contigs averaging 3000 bp in length and covering 12.9 Mb of genome sequence. The second assembly took place in May 2001, and generated 3666 contigs covering 18.6 Mb. In September of 2001, Dr. Hyman announced that the random shotgun sequencing phase of the project ended with sevenfold coverage.

The Institute for Genome Research (TIGR)

In 2000, the NIH-NIAID policy on genome projects changed, limiting the organisms eligible for genome-sequencing projects. *C. neoformans* was one of the five eligible organisms. An application from Dr. Claire Fraser at TIGR received funding in March 2001. The scope of this project is to provide an additional fourfold coverage of the *C. neoformans* genome using random shotgun sequencing of plasmids with small, medium, and large genomic inserts. The use of plasmid vectors that can provide linked sequence information and inserts of various sizes will aid rapid and effective genome assembly. Genomic information obtained by TIGR will be combined with the data from the projects at Stanford University and the University of Oklahoma to assemble the complete genome. Open reading frames (ORFs) will be identified and annotated. The time frame for completion of entire genome of serotype D strain JEC21 is the end of 2002. In September 2001, Dr. Fraser and Dr. Brendan Loftus announced that the TIGR portion of the random-sequencing phase of the project was complete, with 150 million bp of quality sequence, for a nominal coverage of six fold. TIGR has placed data on its website: http://www.tigr.org/tdb/edb2/crypt/htmls/

University of Oklahoma

Dr. Juneann Murphy is the principal investigator for the second grant, which is focused on intron/exon boundary identification. *C. neoformans* has multiple introns in most of its genes. As a pilot project, a normalized cDNA library from the serotype A strain H99 was made, and 5′ and 3′ ends of 1400 cDNAs were sequenced and are available on the website: http://www.genome.ou.edu/cneo.html

The data on this website can be downloaded via ftp. The reads have been blasted against GENBANK and against themselves, and the homologies are available on the website. cDNAs with significant homology to known proteins have been assembled into 421 contigs, each comprised of data from 1 to 20 traces. The goal of this project is to identify enough intron/exon junctions that gene-finding programs can be optimized for *C. neoformans*. In the course of this project, a cDNA library from serotype D, JEC21 has been created and will be normalized. At least 4000 cDNAs from the normalized library will be sequenced. Primers will be designed, and the corresponding genomic clones from selected cDNAs will be cloned and sequenced. The cDNA and genomic-clone sequences will be compared to identify intron/exon boundaries. This information will be used to optimize parameters of the gene-finding software.

THE FUTURE OF DRUG DISCOVERY AND PATHOGENESIS STUDIES IN C. *neoformans*

Proteomics

Proteomics is the Study of the Entire Protein Complement of an Organism

Proteomics allows us to examine a comprehensive array of proteins in an organism and to identify the genes for proteins of interest (for review *see* refs. *91–93*). The quantity of each protein can be determined, so that changes in the quantity or modifications of a specific protein in response to changes in environment can be correlated. Proteomics examines the steady-state levels and modifications of a large percentage of the proteins in a population of cells. Changes in the environment cause changes in the relative abundance of some proteins, cause new proteins to be induced, and alter protein modifications. Proteomics allows us to observe these changes and to identify the protein that has changed. Several factors could cause the change in the intensity of a protein spot, including induction of its mRNA, stabilization of its mRNA, increase in its translation rate, reduction in its turnover rate, or a change in its post-translational modifications. Proteomics has the advantage over examination of mRNA levels, because it is a more accurate picture of gene expression and modification.

Proteomics examines the end point of any of these changes—the amount of protein and its state of modification. At this time, this provides the most accurate picture available of the state of the cell under specific conditions. Proteomics may be superior to functional genomic methods that measure mRNA abundance because there can be a poor correlation between the mRNA levels and protein levels.

Proteomics and identification of antifungal targets

Proteomics will be useful for drug development in several ways. First, treatment of an organism with sublethal doses of an antibiotic will often induce proteins that are in the same pathway as the mechanism of action (MOA) of that compound. Treatment of fungal cells with compounds with antifungal activity but unknown MOA and analysis of the proteins whose expression is affected can help pinpoint the mechanism of action of new antifungals that are discovered through routine screening for antifungal activity. Secondly, proteomics will be useful for identification of new targets within a known pathway. For example, ergosterol (or ergosterol biosynthesis) has been the major target of antifungal therapy for many years. Identification of proteins induced during amphotericin or fluconazole treatment may lead to the development of additional targets in this essential fungal pathway. Third, proteins that are highly induced during pathogenesis may be essential for growth in an animal. Identification of these proteins will further elucidate mechanisms of pathogenesis and potentially lead to novel antifungal targets.

Requirement for a C. neoformans *specific protein database*

Proteomics will require the development of a database for the identification of Cryptococcus proteins. The matching of a protein spot on a gel to a gene requires relatively accurate information about the potential proteins that are made by an organism. Most *C. neoformans* genes have many introns, and the current gene-finding programs are not likely to correctly identify all the exons and introns. Most of the current gene-finding research has focused on simple organisms with high gene density and few or no introns, or on organisms such as Drosophila or humans with low gene density and long introns. Some genes with homology to genes in other systems are being identified by basic linear alignment search tool (BLAST)-searches, but many genes do not have obvious homologs. Because the cDNA sequencing project will be sequencing entire cDNAs and not just the 3′ ends, and will sequence the genomic copy of the cDNA, it will be valuable for developing a protein database by providing information about splice junctions as well as identifying genes. Yet many genes will be missing from the cDNA database because of low levels of expression under the specific growth conditions in which the mRNA was harvested. Are now available protocols in both our laboratories in which proteins can be efficiently removed and isolated from *C. neoformans* for further sequence identifications.

Comparative Genomics

Cryptococcus neoformans represents an ideal microorganism for the study of evolutionary biology. With its three varieties, a comparative genomic study can be undertaken. It has been found through allele mapping that although *Cryptococcus neoformans* var. *grubii* and *Cryptococcus neoformans* var. *neoformans* are similar, they diverged from each other over 20 million years ago. When examining gene sequences, there is generally a 5–6% difference in nucleotide sequence between varieties and polymerase chain reaction (PCR) fingerprinting yields different patterns. Until recently, the MATa locus of *grubii* was not found to be functional, and sequence of the mitochondrial genome of the two varieties shows vast differences in size and structure (F. Dietrich, personal communication). Furthermore, even the genetic basis of the virulence composite has differed at one locus *(STE12)* and probably others *(47,49)*. The variety *gattii* has even more clinical and ecological differences compared to the other two varieties, and will be a third group to study in comparative genomics. As the variety *neoformans* genome sequence is completed, it will be important for the variety *grubii,* the most common variety of clinical disease, to also be sequenced and annotated for study. For this purpose, Fred Dietrich at Duke University has started the sequencing of the *grubii* genome, and these early sequences can be found at http://cneo.genetics.duke.edu. There are plans from an Australian group to begin sequencing the *gattii* genome. The power of these sequencing efforts will be to perform comparative genomics and to begin to understand the organization and evolution behind these important basidiomycetous human pathogens.

Analysis of the Transcriptome

Information gleaned by examination of the levels of mRNAs under specific conditions can be used in a similar manner as the analysis of protein levels described here. Pathways induced by antifungal agents with no known MOA can be identified and new targets in known pathways may be identified under certain in vitro conditions. Transcription profiling may also be used to understand *C. neoformans* gene regulations in the host.

Gene-Expression Analysis

Several methods have been used to detect differential gene expression of several specific environmental conditions in *C. neoformans,* such as elevated temperature, and specifically from cells taken directly from the host. These include cDNA library subtraction, differential display reverse-transcriptase-PCR (RT-PCR), and construction of an in vivo expression technology (IVET) system using green fluorescent protein (GFP) as a marker. Jim Kronstad has adopted serial analysis of gene expression (SAGE) to *C. neoformans* to detect differential gene expression. Three important findings have arisen from these studies. First, although labor-intensive, these methods can detect differential gene expression. Second, it is clear that even in the host there must be continuously changing signals during infection that can change gene expression. For example, it took almost 1 wk of infection in CSF before the pheromone gene of *C. neoformans* had its expression induced *(94)*. It emphasizes the dynamic and complexity of gene-expression profiles. Third, despite the detection of up- or downregulated genes, the importance of these genes to a particular phenotype still requires rigorous site-directed mutants and determination of phenotype that is not assured simply by understanding its regulation during these screening devices.

Microarrays

These types of studies are becoming more common in model organisms and in humans. They can both help and add to the complexity of transcriptional profiling. Presently, the studies are expensive and require careful quality control. However, as the cryptococcal genome sequence is completed, an obvious use of this data is to create microarray chips for the research community. Joe Heitman's laboratory has created a mini chip with a series of selected genes to perform limited but rapid transcriptional profiling in *C. neoformans. (90).*

Global Analysis of Gene Function

Genome-wide mutagenesis and subsequent analysis of mutants will be powerful tools for the identification of potential antifungal targets and pathogenesis genes. Techniques have been developed in other systems that will be useful for analysis of *C. neoformans* genes. Targeted gene-disruption studies in diploids followed by tetrad analysis have been exceptionally useful in *S. cerevisiae* to determine which genes are essential for vegetative growth *(95),* and thus potential antifungal targets. A stable diploid strain has been developed in *C. neoformans,* but a targeted gene disruption has not been demonstrated in a diploid to date. In addition, analysis of spores will be more difficult in the basidiomycetes than in the ascomycetes. Other promising techniques will use inducible expression of RNAs to will inhibit gene expression in *C. neoformans* in a conditional manner.

Inducible Repression of a Gene by RNA

Modulation of gene expression by anti-sense RNA or RNAi is a promising device to determine whether a gene is essential or not. Anti-sense RNA is the expression of an

RNA that is complementary to the normal mRNA of the gene, and RNAi is the expression of a double-stranded RNA from a portion of the gene. The mechanisms for both of these techniques are being explored in other systems. These expression techniques are being used in other systems that are less amenable to targeted gene deletion, such as *C. albicans,* a fungus that is an obligate diploid *(96),* and *C. elegans,* a worm *(97).* In *C. neoformans,* anti-sense RNA under the control of an inducible *GAL7* promoter has been shown to inhibit expression of a nonessential gene, *LACC,* and an essential gene, *CNB1 (89).* RNAi has been shown to work in *C. neoformans* using an actin promoter on nonessential genes including *CAP59* and *ADE2* (H. Liu and T. Doering, *personal communication).* Because gene disruptions in nonessential genes are relatively easy in *C. neoformans,* the utility of gene-expression inhibition by gene-specific RNA expression will be to analyze essential genes. Inducible promoters must be further identified for use in this technology so that large-scale experiments examining every coding sequence can be done to identify essential genes as potential antifungal targets.

"Bar Coding" and Mass Analysis of Virulence Determinants

To determine genes that are essential for pathogenesis, individual genes can be disrupted and their phenotype can be assessed in an animal model. This process can be relatively expensive in time considerations, numbers of animals used, and dollar costs. Mixtures of mutants can facilitate the identification of some (but perhaps not all) genes needed for pathogenesis. Inserting unique DNA tag identifiers (signature tags or bar codes) in mutants allows researchers to follow the mutant through the infection process, even if that mutant is mixed with many others. Bar coding in *S. cerevisiae* has facilitated the analysis of many mutants mixed together *(98,99).* Signature-tagged mutagenesis is a technique that was developed in *Salmonella typhimurium (100),* and has been applied to several other systems, including *C. neoformans (101).* It was demonstrated that using a tail-vein inoculation, at least 100 strains could be mixed together and each strain participated in the infection *(101).* Of 600 mutants generated by random insertions, four mutants had significant, reproducible phenotypes. Three were less virulent in the mouse model, and one was hypervirulent. Combining this signature-tag technique with targeted gene disruptions would allow the contribution of every gene in the *C. neoformans* genome to be tested using a relatively small number of animals. Assuming that there are likely to be 6000–8000 genes in the *C. neoformans* genome, mutants in every gene could be tested in mixtures of 45 mutants in less than 200 animals.

CONCLUSION

A genome sequence for *C. neoformans* is revolutionizing our methods in the study of this serious human pathogen. The last decade has witnessed the development of an infrastructure in molecular biology, genetics, immunology, and animal models for *C. neoformans* that will allow the research world to capitalize on this fungal pathogen in the study of functional genomics and pathogenesis. This model fungal pathogen can further be exploited to identify new broad-spectrum antifungal targets at the molecular and biochemical level.

REFERENCES

1. Dismukes WE. Cryptococcal Meningitis in patients with AIDS. J Infect Dis 1988; 157:859–860.

2. Dupont B, Graybill JR, Armstrong D, et al. Fungal infections in AIDS patients. J Med Vet Mycol 1992; 30:19–28.

3. Samonis G, Bafaloukos D. Fungal infections in cancer patients: an escalating problem. In Vivo 1992; 6:183–194.

4. Casadevall A, Perfect JR. "Cryptococcus neoformans." Washington, DC: ASM Press, 1998, pp. 1–53.

5. Mitchell TG, Perfect JR. Cryptococcosis in the era of AIDS—100 years after the discovery of Cryptococcus neoformans. Clin Microbiol Rev 1995; 8:515–548.

6. Levitz SM. The ecology of Cryptococcus neoformans and the epidemiology of cryptoccocosis. Rev Infect Dis 1991; 13:1163–1169.

7. White MH, Armstrong D. Cryptococcosis. Infect Dis Clin North Am 1994; 8:383–398.

8. Saag MS, Graybill RJ, Larsen RA, Pappas PG, Perfect JR, Powderly WG, et al. Practice guidelines for the management of cryptococcal disease. Infectious Diseases Society of America. Clin Infect Dis 2000; 30:710–718.

9. Whelan WL. The genetic basis of resistance to 5-fluorocytosine in Candida species and Cryptococcus neoformans. CRC Crit Rev Microbiol 1987; 15:45–46.

10. Powderly WG, Saag MS, Cloud GA, et al. A controlled trial of fluconazole or amphotericin B to prevent relapse of cryptococcal meningitis in patients with the acquired immunodeficiency syndrome. N Engl J Med 1992; 326:793–798.

11. Paugam A, Dupouy-Camet J, Blanche P, et al. Increased fluconazole resistance of Cryptococcus neoformans isolated from a patient with AIDS and recurrent meningitis. Clin Infect Dis 1994; 19:975–976.

12. Powderly WG, Finkelstein DM, Feinberg J, et al. A randomized trial comparing fluconazole with clotrimazole troches for the prevention of fungal infections in patients with advanced human immunodeficiency virus infection. N Engl J Med 1995; 332:700–705.

13. Alspaugh JA, Davidson RC, Heitman J. Morphogenesis of Cryptococcus neoformans In: Ernst JF, Schmidt A (eds). Dimorphism in Human Pathogenic and Apathogenic Yeasts. Basel, Switzerland, Karger 2000, pp. 217–238.

14. Kwon-Chung KJ A new genus, Filobasidiella, the perfect state of Cryptococcus neoformans. Mycologia 1975; 67:1197–1200.

15. Wickes BL, Mayorga ME, Edman U, and Edman JC. Dimorphism and haploid fruiting of Cryptococcus neoformans: association with the alpha-mating type. Proc Natl Acad Sci USA 1996; 93:7327–7331.

16. Sia RA, Lengeler KB, Heitman J. Diploid strains of the pathogenic basidiomycete Cryptococcus neoformans are thermally dimorphic. Fungal Genet Biol 2000; 29:153–163.

17. Lengeler KB, Wang P, Cox GM, Perfect JR, Heitman J. Identification of the MATa mating-type locus of Cryptococcus neoformans reveals a serotype A MATa strain thought to have been extinct. Proc Natl Acad Sci USA 2000; 97:14,455–14,460.

18. Keller SM, Cogliati M, Esposto MC, Wickes BL, Viviani MA. Characterization of a Cryptococcus neoformans serotype A MATa strain. Abstract. 2nd Cryptococcus neoformans Genomics Meeting, 2001.

19. Perfect JR, Ketabchi N, Cox GM, Ingram CI, Beiser C. Karyotyping of Cryptococcus neoformans as an epidemiological tool. J Clin Microbiol 1993; 31:3305–3309.

20. Wickes BL, Moore TDE, Kwon-Chung KJ. Comparison of the electrophoretic karyotypes and chromosomal location of ten genes in the two varieties of Cryptococcus neoformans. Microbiology 1994; 140:543–550.

21. Edman JC, Kwon-Chung KJ. Isolation of the URA5 gene from Cryptococcus neoformans var. neoformans and its use as a selective marker for transformation. Mol Cell Biol 1990; 10:4538–4544.

22. Toffaletti DL, Rude TH, Johnston SA, Durack DT, Perfect JR. Gene transfer in Cryptococcus neoformans by use of biolistic delivery of DNA. J Bacteriol 1993; 175:1405–1411.

23. Lodge JK, Jackson-Machelski E, Higgins M, Devadas B, McWherter CA, Gordon JI. Genetic and biochemical studies establish that the fungicidal effect of a fully depeptidized inhibitor of Cryptococcus neoformans myristoylCoA:protein N-myristoyltransferase is Nmt dependent. J Biol Chem 1998; 273:12,482–12,491.

24. Cox GM, Toffaletti DL, Perfect JR. A dominant selection system for use in Cryptococcus neoformans. J Med Vet Mycol 1996; 34:385–391.

25. Hua JH, Meyer JD, Lodge JK. Development of positive selectable markers for the fungal pathogen, Cryptococcus neoformans. Clin Diagn Lab Immunol 2000; 7:125–128.

26. McDade HC, Cox GM. A new dominant selectable marker for use in Cryptococcus neoformans. Medical Mycology 2001; 39:151–154.

27. Lodge JK, Jackson-Machelski E, Toffaletti DL, Perfect JR, Gordon JI. Targeted gene replacement demonstrates that myristoyl-CoA:protein N-myristoyltransferase is essential for viability of Cryptococcus neoformans. Proc Natl Acad Sci USA 1994b; 91:12,008–12,012.

28. Chang YC, Kwon-Chung KJ. Complementation of a capsule-deficient mutation of Cryptococcus neoformans restores its virulence. Mol Cell Biol 1994; 14:4912–4919.

29. Davidson RC, Cruz MC, Sia RA, Allen B, Alspaugh JA, Heitman J. Gene disruption by biolistic transformation in serotype D strains of Cryptococcus neoformans. Fungal Genet Biol 2000; 29:38–48.

30. Alspaugh JA, Cavallo LM, Perfect JR, Heitman J. RASl regulates filamentation, mating and growth at high temperature of Cryptococcus neoformans. Mol Microbiol 2000; 36:352–365.

31. Odom A, Muir S, Lim E, Toffaletti DL, Perfect J, Heitman J. Calcineurin is required for virulence of Cryptococcus neoformans. EMBO J 1997; 16:2576–2589.

32. Cruz MC, Sia RA, Olson M, Cox GM, Heitman J. Comparison of the roles of calcineurin in physiology and virulence in serotype D and serotype A strains of Cryptococcus neoformans. Infect Immun 2000; 68:982–985.

33. Del Poeta M, Toffaletti DL, Rude TH, Dykstra CC, Heitman J, Perfect JR. Topoisomerase I is essential in Cryptococcus neoformans: Role in pathobiology and as an antifungal target. Genetics 1999; 152:167–178.

34. Cox GM, Mukherjee J, Cole GT, Casadevall A, Perfect JR. Urease as a virulence factor in experimental cryptococcosis. Infect Immun 2000; 68:443–448.

35. Chang YC, Penoyer LA, Kwon-Chung KJ. The second capsule gene of Cryptococcus neoformans, CAP64, is essential for virulence. Infect Immun 1996; 64:1977–1983.

36. Salas SD, Bennett JE, Kwon-Chung KJ, Perfect JR, Williamson PR. Effect of the laccase gene CNLAC1, on virulence of Cryptococcus neoformans. J Exp Med 1996; 184:377–386.

37. Perfect JR, Lang SDR, Durack DT. Chronic cryptococcal meningitis. Am J Pathol 1980; 101:177–194.

38. Perfect JR, Toffaletti DL, Rude TH. The gene encoding phosphoriboxylaminoimidazole carboxylase (ADE2) is essential for growth of Cryptococcus neoformans in cerebrospinal fluid. Infect Immun 1993; 61:4446–4451.

39. Alspaugh JA, Pukkila-Worley R, Harashima T, Cavallo LM, Funnel D, Cox GM, et al. Adenylyl cyclase functions downstream of the Gα protein GPA1 and controls mating and pathogenicity. J Euk Cell 2002; in press.

40. Perfect JR, Wong B, Chang YC, Kwon-Chung KJ, Williamson PR. Cryptococcus neoformans: virulence and host defenses Medical Mycology 1998; 36 (Suppl 1):79–86.

41. Hamilton AJ, Goodley J. Virulence factors of Cryptococcus neoformans. Curr Top Med Mycol 1996; 7:19–42.

42. Buchanan KL, Murphy JW. What makes Cryptococcus neoformans a pathogen? Emerg Infect Dis. 1998; 4:71–83.

43. Kozel TR. Virulence factors of Cryptococcus neoformans. Trends Microbiol 1995; 3:295–299.

44. Kwon-Chung KJ. Gene disruption to evaluate the role of fungal candidate virulence genes. Curr Opin Microbiol 1998; 1:381–389.

45. Alspaugh JA, Perfect JR, Heitman J. Signal transduction pathways regulating differentiation and pathogenicity of Cryptococcus neoformans. Fungal Genetics and Biology 1998; 25:1–14.

46. Alspaugh JA, Perfect JR, Heitman J. Cryptococcus neoformans mating and virulence are regulated by the G-protein alpha subunit GPA1 and cAMP. Genes Dev 1997; 11:3206–3217.

47. Chang YC, Wickes BL, Miller GF, Penoyer LA, Kwon-Chung KJ. Cryptococcus neoformans STE12alpha regulates virulence but is not essential for mating. J Exp Med 2000; 191:871–882.

48. Gorlach J, Fox DS, Cutler NS, Cox GM, Perfect JR, Heitman J. Identification and characterization of a highly conserved calcineurin binding protein, CBP1/calcipressin, in Cryptococcus neoformans EMBO J 2000; 19:3618–3629.

49. Wang P, Perfect JR, Heitman J. The G-protein beta subunit GPB1 is required for mating and haploid fruiting in Cryptococcus neoformans. Mol Cell Biol 2000; 20:352–362.

50. Kwon-Chung KJ, Bennett JE. Distribution of a and alpha mating types of Cryptococcus neoformans among natural and clinical isolates. Am J Epidemiol 1978; 108:337–340.

51. Kwon-Chung K, Edman JC, Wickes BL. Genetic association of mating types and virulence in Cryptococcus neoformans. Infect Immun 1992; 60:602–605.

52. Cherniak R, Sundstrom JB. Polysaccharide antigens of the capsule of Cryptococcus neoformans. Infect Immun 1994; 62:1507–1512.

53. Granger DL, Perfect JR, Durack DT. Virulence of Cryptococcus neoformans. Regulation of capsule synthesis by carbon dioxide. J Clin Investing 1985; 76:508–516.

54. Kwon-Chung KJ, Rhodes JC. Encapsulation and melanin formation as indicators of virulence in Cryptococcus neoformans. Infect Immun 1986; 51:218–223.

55. Chang YC, Kwon-Chung KJ. Isolation of the third capsule-associated gene, CAP60, required for virulence in Cryptococcus neoformans. Infect Immun 1998; 66:2230–2236.

56. Chang YC, Kwon-Chung KJ. Isolation, characterization, and localization of a capsule-associated gene, CAP10, of Cryptococcus neoformans. J Bacteriol 1999; 181:5636–5643.

57. Wills EA, Roberts IS, Del Poeta M, Rivera J, Casadevall A, Cox GM, et al. Identification and characterization of the Cryptococcus neoformans phosphomannose isomerase-encoding gene, MAN1, and its impact on pathogenicity. Mol Microbiol 2001; 40:610–620.

58. Casadevall A, Rosas AL, Nosanchuk JD. Melanin and virulence in Cryptococcus neoformans. Curr Opin Microbiol 2000; 3:354–358.

59. Rhodes JC, Polacheck I, Kwon-Chung KJ. Phenoloxidase activity and virulence in isogenic strains of Cryptococcus neoformans. Infect Immun 1982; 36:1175–1184.

60. Williamson PR. Biochemical and molecular characterization of the diphenol oxidase of Cryptococcus neoformans: Identification as a laccase. J Bacteriol 1994; 176:656–664.

61. Deepe GS, Romani L, Calich ULG, Molinari-Madlum EEW, Arruda EWI, Arruda C, et al. Knock-out mice as experimental models of virulence. Med Mycology 2000; 38:(Suppl 1) 87–98.

62. Schmiel DH, Miller VL. Bacterial phospholipases and pathogenesis. Microbes and Infection 1999; 1:1103–1112.

63. Leidich SD, Ibrahim AS, Fu Y, Koul A, Jessup CJ, Vitullo J, et al. Cloning and disruption of caPLB1, a phospholipase B gene involved in the pathogenicity of Candida albicans. J Biol Chem 1998; 273:26,078–26,086.

64. Chen SC, Muller M, Zhou JZ, Wright LC, Sorrell TC Phospholipase activity in Cryptococcus neoformans: a new virulence factor? J Infect Dis 1997a; 175:414–420.

65. Chen SC, Wright LC, Santangelo RT, Muller M, Moran VR, Kuchel PW, et al. Identification of extracellular phospholipase B, lysophospholipase, and acyltransferase produced by Cryptococcus neoformans. Infect Immun 1997b; 65:405–411.

66. Chen SC, Wright LC, Golding JC, Sorrell TC. Purification and characterization of secretory phospholipase B, lysophospholipase and lysophospholipase/transacylase from a virulent strain of the pathogenic fungus Cryptococcus neoformans. Biochem J 2000; 347:431–439.

67. Cox GM, McDade HC, Chen SC, Tucker SC, Gottfredsson M, Wright LC, et al. Extracellular phospholipase activity is a virulence factor for Cryptococcus neoformans. Mol Microbiol 2001; 39:166–175.

68. Luberto C, Toffaletti DL, Wills EA, Tucker SC, Casadevall A, Perfect JR, et al. Roles for inositol-phosphoryl ceramide synthase 1 (IPC1) in pathogenesis of C. neoformans. Genes Dev 2001; 15:201–212.

69. Chaturvedi VP, Flynn T, Niehaus WG, Wong B. Stress tolerance and pathogenic potential of a mannitol-mutant of Cryptococcus neoformans. Microbiology 1996; 142:937–943.

70. Nyhus KJ, Jacobson ES. Genetic and physiologic characterization of ferric/cupric reductase constitutive mutants of Cryptococcus neoformans. Infect Immun 1999; 67:2357–2365.

71. Batanghari JW, Deepe GS, Jr DiCera E, Goldman WE. Histoplasma aquisition of calcium and expression of CBP1 during intracellular parasitism. Mol Microbiol 1998; 27:531–539.

72. Cormack BP, Ghori N, Falkow S. An adhesin of the yeast pathogen Candida globrata mediating adherence to human epithelial cells. Science 1999; 285:578–582.

73. Brandhorst T, Klein B. Cell wall biogenesis of Blastomyces dermatitdis. Evidence for a novel mechanism of cell surface localization of a virulence-associated adhesin via extracellular release and reassociation with cell wall chitin. J Biol Chem 2000; 275:7925–7934.

74. Brueske CH. Proteolytic activity of a clinical isolate of Cryptococcus neoformans. J Clin Microbiol 1986; 23:631–633.

75. Hube B. Extracellular proteinases of human pathogenic fungi. Contribution to Microbiology 2000; 5:126–137.

76. Bulawa CE. Genetics and molecular biology of chitin synthesis in fungi. Annu Rev Microbiol 1993; 47:505–534.

77. Marcilla A, Mormeneo S, Elorza MV, et al. Wall formation by Candida albicans yeast cells: synthesis, secretion and incorporation of two types of mannoproteins. J Gen Microbiol 1993; 139:2985–2993.

78. Bartizal K, Abruzzo G, Trainor C, Krupa D, Nollstadt K, Schmatz D, et al. In vitro antifungal activities and in vivo efficacies of 1,3-beta-D-glucan synthesis inhibitors L-671,329, L-646,991, tetrahydroechinocandin B, and L-687,781, a papulacandin. Antimicrob Agents Chemother 1992; 36:1648–1657.

79. Kurtz MB, Douglas C, Marrinan J, Nollstadt K, Onishi J, Dreikorn S, et al. Increased antifungal activity of L-733,560, a water-soluble, semisynthetic pneumocandin, is due to enhanced inhibition of cell wall synthesis. Antimicrob Agents Chemother 1994; 38:2750–2757.

80. Onishi J, Meinz M, Thompson J, Curotto J, Dreikorn S, Rosenbach M, et al. Discovery of novel antifungal (1,3)-beta-D-glucan synthase inhibitors. Antimicrob Agents Chemother 2000; 44:368–377.

81. Abruzzo GK, Flattery AM, Gill CJ, et al. Evaluation of water-soluble pneumocandin analogs L-733560, L-705589 and L-731373 with mouse models of disseminated aspergillosis, candidiasis, and cryptococcosis. Antimicrob Agents Chemother 1995; 39:1077–1081.

82. Krishnarao TV, Galgiani JN. Comparison of the in vitro activities of the echinocandin LY303366, the pneumocandin MK-0991, and fluconazole against Candida species and Cryptococcus neoformans. Antimicrob Agents Chemother 1997; 41:1957–1960.

83. Thompson JR, Douglas CM, Li W, Jue CK, Pramanik B, Yuan X, et al. A glucan synthase FKS1 homolog in Cryptococcus neoformans is single copy and encodes an essential function. J Bacteriol 1999; 181:444–453.

84. Lodge JK, Johnson RL, Weinberg RA, Gordon JI. Comparison of myristoylCoA:protein N-myristoyltransferases from three pathogenic fungi—Cryptococcus neoformans, Histoplasma capsulatum, and Candida albicans. J Biol Chem 1994a; 269:2996–3009.

85. Lodge JK, Jackson-Machelski E, Devadas B, Zupec M, Getman DP, Kishore N, et al. N-myristoylation of Arf proteins in Candida albicans: an in vivo assay for evaluating antifungal inhibitors of myristoylCoA:protein N-myrisotyltransferase. Microbiology 1997; 143:357–366.

86. Weinberg RA, McWherter CA, Freeman SK, et al. Genetic studies reveal that myristoylCoA:protein N-myristoyltransferase is an essential enzyme in Candida albicans. Mol Microbiol 1995; 16:241–250.

87. Belfield GP, Tuite MF. Translation elongation Factor 3:a fungus-specific translation factor? Mol Microbiol 1993; 9:411–418.

88. Fostel JM, Montgomery DA, Shen LL. Characterization of DNA topoisomerase I from Candida albicans as a target for drug discovery. Antimicrob Agents Chemother 1992; 36:2131–2138.

89. Gorlach JM, McDade HC, Perfect JR, Cox GM. Antisense repression in Cryptococcus neoformans as a laboratory tool and potential antifungal strategy. Microbiology 2002; 148:213–219.

90. Heitman J, Casadevall A, Lodge JK, Perfect JR. The Cryptococcus neoformans genome sequencing project. Mycopathalogia 2001; 148:1–7.

91. Gygi SP, Aebersold R. Mass spectrometry and proteomics. Curr Opin in Chem Biology 2000; 4:489–494.

92. Gygi SP, Rist B, Aebersold R. Measuring gene expression by quantitative proteome analysis. Curr Opin Biotechnol 2000; 11:396–401.

93. O'Donovan C, Apweiler R, Bairoch A. The human proteomics initiative (HPI). Trends Biotechnol 2001; 19:178–181.

94. Del Poeta M, Toffaletti DL, Rude TH, Sparks SD, Heitman J. Cryptococcus neoformans differential gene expression detected in vitro and in vivo with green fluorescent protein. Infect Immun 1999; 67:1812–1820.

95. Winzeler EA, Shoemaker DD, Astromoff A, Liang H, Anderson K, Andre B, et al. Functional characterization of the Saccharomyces cerevisiae genome by gene deletion and parallel analysis. Science 1999; 285:901–906.

96. De Backer MD, Nelissen B, Logghe M, Viaene J, Loonen I, Vandoninck S, et al. An antisense-based functional genomics approach for identification of genes critical for growth of Candida albicans. Nat Biotechnol 2001; 19:235–241.

97. Fraser AG, Kamath RS, Zipperlen P, Martinez-Campos M, Sohrmann M, Ahringer J. Functional genomic analysis of C. elegans chromosome I by systematic RNA interference. Nature 2000; 408:325–330.

98. Shoemaker DD, Laskari DA, Morris D, Mittmann M, Davis RW. Quantitation phenotypic analysis of yeast deletion mutants using a highly parallel molecular bar-coding strategy. Nat Genet 1996; 14:450–456.

99. Hughes TR, Marton MJ, Jones AR, Roberts CJ, Stoughton R, Armour CD, et al. Functional discovery via a compendium of expression profiles. Cell 2000; 102:109–126.

100. Hensel M, Shea JE, Gleeson C, Jones MD, Dalton E, Holden DW. Simultaneous identification of bacterial virulence genes by negative selection. Science 1995; 269:400–403.

101. Nelson RT, Hua J, Pryor B, Lodge JK. Identification of virulence mutants of the fungal pathogen Cryptococcus neoformans using signature-tagged mutagenesis. Genetics 2001; 157:935–947.

14

Antifungal Target Selection in *Aspergillus nidulans*

Using Bioinformatics to Make the Difference

Rosanna Pena-Muralla, Patricia Ayoubi, Marcia Graminha, Nilce M. Martinez-Rossi, Antonio Rossi, and Rolf A. Prade

INTRODUCTION

Microbes are both beneficial and detrimental to humans. They produce life-saving drugs, cause diseases, destroy crops, and contaminate feeds and foods. Although fungi do not cause outbreaks or pandemics, the incidence of fungal infections among the growing population of immunocompromised patients and the recurring establishment of drug resistance underscore the need for new drugs. A search strategy that may reveal novel targets suitable for drug development is the comparative analysis of fungal and human genomes. By comparing *Aspergillus nidulans* unigene ESTs to the nearly complete human genome, we found 387 nonhuman ESTs with predictable function, eight of which were essential in yeast. Moreover, phylogenetic reconstruction of a fatty-acid synthase demonstrates co-segregation of fungal alpha and beta subunits, which assemble into hetero-multimers, whereas the human polypeptide associates as a homodimer. Thus, the comparative approach identifies intrinsic differences between genomes and provides new genetic information for target selection, which may lead to drugs with reduced or no host interference.

The industrial sector employs filamentous fungi as the biotechnology-manufacturing units to produce everything from local, unique-tasting and flavored beer brews, chemically sophisticated pharmaceutical compounds, and life-saving human proteins. However, they are also pathogens that infect animals and plants—rotting and poisoning crops and causing economic loss to agribusinesses *(1)*. Human systemic and superficial mycoses are on the rise leading to increased health care costs *(2)*. In the United States alone, as much as $47 billion is spent annually to curb the increasing incidence of human microbial infections and antimicrobial resistance *(3)*. Finally, filamentous fungi are often used as tractable biochemical, genetic, and physiological models with extensive biological information restricted to a few model species, namely *Saccharomyces cerevisiae (4–10)*, *Neurospora crassa (11–13)*, and *Aspergillus nidulans* (14–17).

From: *Pathogen Genomics: Impact on Human Health*
Edited by: K. J. Shaw © Humana Press Inc., Totowa, NJ

ANTIFUNGAL TARGETS, DRUGS, AND RESISTANCE

By the end of the first half of the twentieth century, there were published reports on the therapeutic use of sulfonamides, benzimidazoles, hydroxystilbamidines, nystatin, amphotericin B, griseofulvin, and azoles. Although the number of antifungal agents was small compared to the abundance of antibiotics available for bacterial infections, fungal infections were usually easily treatable before the 1980s because they were often limited to superficial mycoses, athlete's foot, thrush caused by *Candida albicans*, cryptococcosis, ringworms (keratomycoses), and a few cases of deep-seated mycoses *(18–22)*.

Over the last two decades, however, the incidence of severe systemic fungal infections has increased significantly, mainly because of the explosive growth in the number of patients with compromised immune systems *(23)*. Opportunistic fungal infections are common among patients who have acquired immunodeficiency syndrome (AIDS), or have had medical procedures that artificially suppress the immune system, such as organ transplant, and chemotherapy *(24–26)*. *Aspergillus fumigatus, Candida albicans, Cryptococcus neoformans, Histoplasma capsulatum, Sporothrix schenckii,* and the dermatophytic fungi are the most prevalent pathogens among HIV-infected patients *(24)*, a population of over 36 million worldwide *(27)*.

Prior to the increase in the population of immunocompromised patients, treatments were directed primarily toward superficial mycoses, athlete's foot, and ringworms (keratomycoses). Antifungal formulations included typically mixtures of benzoic and salicylic acid (Whitfield's ointment), sulfur, gentian violet, potassium permanganate, aluminum chloride, or undecanoic acid *(28)*. Agents to treat systemic mycoses were rare until the advent of modern chemotherapy. Potassium iodide, hydroxystilbadine, and sulfonamides have been used to treat everything from sporotrichosis to paracoccidioidomycosis and histoplasmosis *(29)*.

Although the number of antifungals currently available on the pharmaceutical market (Table 1) has increased, the main antifungal target is ergosterol, the cholesterol analog found predominantly in fungal-cell membranes *(30)*. Membrane integrity is challenged in two ways: by interference caused by direct interaction of polyenes such as amphotericin B with ergosterol, and by inhibition of specific steps of sterol biosynthesis involving allylamines, thiocarbamates, azoles, and morpholines that limit the availability of ergosterol. Amphotericin B is a powerful antimycotic because it efficiently intercalates with ergosterol *(31,32)*, but is of limited use because of its poor solubility in water and toxicity to kidney and neural cells. Other antifungal drugs inhibit DNA synthesis as nucleoside analogs (flucytosine) *(33)*, or as inhibitors of mitosis (griseofulvin) *(26,34–38)*.

Despite the extensive selection of antifungals currently available on the pharmaceutical market, their mode of action involves a surprisingly small number of cellular targets, indicating that there should be additional differences significant enough to enable the design of compounds that preferentially interfere with essential fungal functions.

Overcoming the strong negative selective action of antifungals is difficult. However, once it is genetically acquired, resistance quickly spreads throughout the population because it confers a significant advantage for survival *(39–41)*. The problem of emerging resistance to existing drugs severely limits the efficacy and impact of all known

Table 1
Common antifungal drugs in the market and their cellular targets

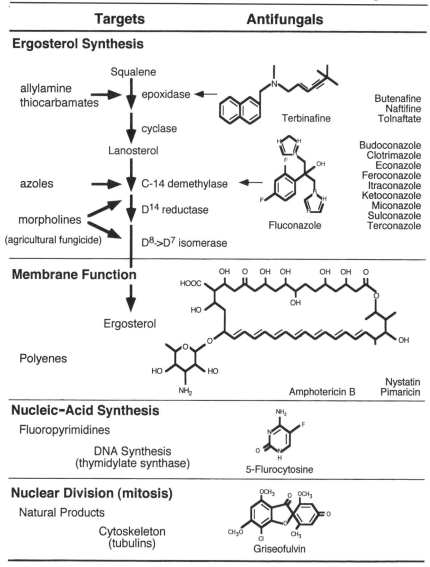

antifungals *(42–44)*. Documented resistance mechanisms are associated with active drug efflux *(45)*, membrane permeability reduction *(46)*, and overproduction *(47)* or compensatory mutations *(48)* of the target enzyme.

The initial step toward development of new antifungal drugs is the identification of cellular targets. Antifungal effectiveness directly correlates with the specificity by which drugs interact with the target pathogen without affecting the host. Thus, comparative genomics, which reveals intrinsic differences between fungal and human genomes, could be used to identify targets selective to fungi and harmless to man. A case in point is topoisomerase I in which critical differences in protein sequence of the enzyme in fungi and humans can be exploited to selectively target only the fungal topoisomerases *(49,50).*

THE GENOMICS APPROACH

Although fungi have not been the protagonists of major outbreaks, the significant incidence of fungal infections on the growing population of immune-compromised patients, coupled with the recurrent detection of drug resistance, drives the need to discover the novel targets and new drugs, and find other medical applications for existing drugs.

Extensive genome sequencing in both humans and fungi has enabled a more directed approach toward target discovery. Systematic comparative analysis of fungal (pathogen) genes with the human (host) gene complement generates genetic information that is essential to recognize potential drug targets and useful to the design of drugs and treatments.

Gene-complement estimates situate filamentous fungi within eight and ten thousand genes *(51),* with over 26,025 unique expressed sequence tags (ESTs) available from public resources (Ayoubi P., July 2001, *unpublished results*). Fungal ESTs represent a set of genetic information useful to identify potential targets via comparison against nearly all human (host) genes. Comparisons employing similarity-matching algorithms against human ESTs and unique polypeptide data sets *(52)* could generate a nonhuman gene list of potential targets for drug-screening experiments.

Fungal ESTs available in the public domain are primarily from model systems such as *Aspergillus (Emericella) nidulans* (12,457 from one condition), *Neurospora crassa* (10,850 and 9,075 from two conditions), and *Schizosaccharomyces pombe (8,118).* A limited number of publicly available ESTs from pathogens belong to a few species such as *Fusarium sporotrichoides* (7,498), *Blumeria graminis* (4,908), *Pneumocystis carinii* (3,896), *Pyricularia grisea* (2,556), *Metarhizium anisopliae* (1,693) and *Mycosphaerella graminicola* (1,158). For a complete and updated overview of fungal ESTs and their functional classification visit http://aspergillus-genomics.org.

The bioinformatics-based comparative method employed here relies on the prediction of function through similarity matching between DNA fragments of known function and anonymous fragments *(53,54).* Thus, functional equivalency relationships established through similarity matching are independent of chemical verification and based solely on sequence conservation between DNA fragments. Two homologous DNA sequences separated by speciation accumulate mutations over time *(55).* Only mutations that preserve function persist, and thus define regions of higher and lower conservation critical for the structure and function of a particular group of similar variants *(55).* To estimate the validity of such comparisons, an analysis of functional assignment based on similarity matching was made, which showed that errors stem mainly from multidomain proteins, convergent evolution, and variation in enzyme specificity, strongly suggesting that automated functional (enzyme) annotation should make use of fragments smaller than the full-length coding polypeptide *(56,57).* Moreover, other studies show that transfer of functional annotation between protein-sequence alignments is precise down to 40% amino-acid sequence identity, and grouping into enzymatic classification schemes at 25% identity levels *(58).*

Genes that fall within this group of shared conserved domains are orthologous if biochemical function is identical, regardless of whether a given protein is composed of two or more domains appearing in different configurations in multiple genes. To refer to the similarities between partial amino-acid sequences, as with the information derived from ESTs (sub-genomic fragments), we employ the term "analog" *(59)*.

Although a comparative approach with incomplete genome information may not be ideal and may not deliver all possible targets that are biologically feasible because of the difficulty to ascertain functional equivalency across evolutionary boundaries, it offers the possibility of unambiguously evaluating all the targets that are not detectable in the human genome. Thus, the comparative approach is ideal to determine the difference between genomes, even if the full genome-sequence information of one organism is incomplete. Comparisons between whole bacterial genomes and human genes have been reported, and were made by using minimal high-scoring pairs of 90 and 150 employing BLASTP and BLASTX variants, respectively *(20,33)*.

Here we have employed the *A. nidulans* EST unigene collection, compared it to the nearly complete gene complement in humans, and further analyzed the ESTs lacking a significant hit with any human amino acid sequence (Fig. 1). Initially, 4,595 unique ESTs were compared to all available human ESTs (3.3 million) and the resulting TBLASTX results were grouped into significant and insignificant hits with a cutoff value of $e = 10^{-4}$ (high-scoring pair ~100). The *A. nidulans* ESTs that failed to align to any human EST were further investigated by BLASTX comparison against the human polypeptide set (26,612 peptides). ESTs with no significant hits to human ESTs or polypeptides were further analyzed by BLASTX comparison against all other nonhuman organisms to predict the function of these nonhuman genes. We found 387 genes with no homology to humans, yet they were analogous to functions known in other taxonomic groups (Table 2).

Functional assignments through annotation transfer were based on expectation values less than $e = 10^{-16}$ (hsp $\geq$ 200), with an average percent (predicted) amino-acid sequence identity of 67%. The distribution of ESTs into functional categories was based on the Metabolic Pathways Database from Selkov and collaborators *(60)*.

Fig. 2 shows nonhuman *A. nidulans* EST distribution patterns of major cellular or metabolic categories, according to various analogous taxonomic groups. The majority of nonhuman genes fall within metabolism (87%), with only a limited number grouping with other cellular functions. Similar distribution patterns were obtained when the entire EST collection was sorted *(61)*, suggesting that significant differences were not detected at the higher classification levels.

Aromatic metabolism increased from 2.0% in the human-like ESTs to 6.5% in the nonhuman ESTs (Fig. 2) (Table 3). This marked dissimilarity validates the comparative approach used in this study by corroborating the remarkable absence of aromatic functions in mammals *(62)*. Carbohydrate metabolism (50%), electron transport (2.2%) and signal transduction (2.2%) are functional categories more related to animals than any other organismal group. In contrast, aromatic (6.5%) and essential (13.2%) compound metabolism, protein (12.4%), lipid (5.9%) synthesis, information pathways (4.6%), cell structure (1%), and transmembrane transport (3.1%) are categories more similar to plants than animals (Fig. 2).

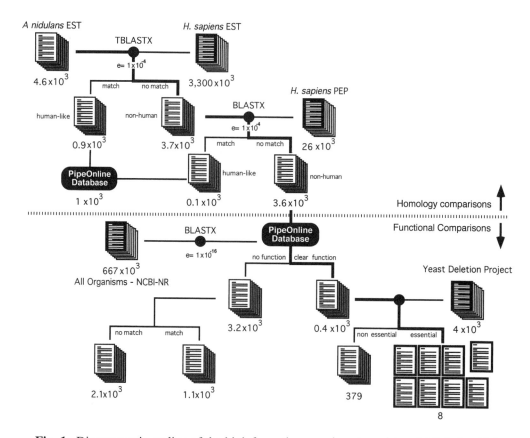

Fig. 1. Diagrammatic outline of the bioinformatics experiment used to establish *A. nidulans* human and nonhuman analogs. The *A. nidulans* 4,595 record-containing unigene data set was partitioned into human and nonhuman-like subsets via a two-step process with the BLAST cutoff value set at e=10⁻⁴. The first comparison was against human ESTs (3.3 million) using TBLASTX, and the second against all human proteins (26,612 unique ORFs) with BLASTX. The resulting nonhuman subset (3,557 records) was further subdivided into records with unclear (3,170) and clear function (387), employing the PipeOnline functional sorting algorithm with a BLASTX cutoff value set at e=10⁻¹⁶. The 387 nonhuman ESTs, which had a clear functional assignment, were further categorized by comparing them to the yeast deletion project and grouping them into essential (8 records) and nonessential (379 records). White-faced record stacks indicate *A. nidulans* ESTs; dark-faced records indicate comparison databases. Numbers under each database or database subset show an approximation of the data set sizes at each step of the comparative process. PipeOnline databases are accessible through http://aspergillus-genomics.org.

Table 3 compares the functional distribution between nonhuman, *A. nidulans* ESTs (subtracted collection) and all *A. nidulans* ESTs (the entire collection). In most categories, distribution of nonhuman ESTs coincides with the control. In a few cases, remarkable differences were observed. For example, the synthesis of aromatic compounds and sugar alcohols was increased by threefold and twofold respectively in the nonhuman subtracted ESTs. Alternatively, amino sugars, lipid, nucleotide and nucleic-acid synthesis categories were clearly underrepresented, with 0.3-, 0.6-, and 0.5-fold reductions, respectively.

Table 2
Homology-based partition of *A. nidulans* ESTs against gene-specific human DNA sequence and those of other organisms

| | | Partition[a] | | |
| | | | % | |
Homologous category	Unique ESTs	Genes	Analogy	Function
Total *A nidulans* ESTs	4,595	–	–	–
Nonhuman	3,557	77	–	–
Analogous to other organisms	387	–	11	–
Functionally classified	203	–	–	52
Functionally unclassified	184	–	–	48
Non-analogous	3,170	–	89	–
Human-like	1,039	23	–	–

[a] BLASTP cutoff value used for data set partition.

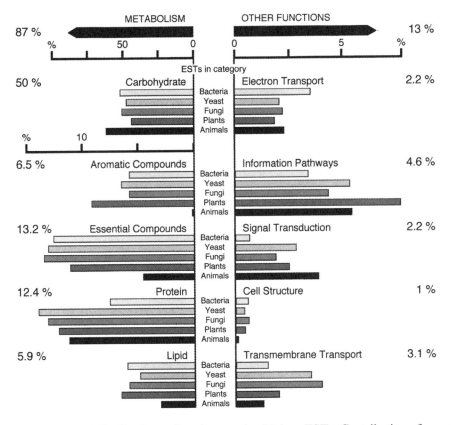

Fig. 2. Functional distributions of nonhuman *A. nidulans* ESTs. Contribution of a particular category expressed as the number of ESTs with clear functional assignment that fall within the depicted metabolic or cellular groups (WIT-MPW). ESTs within a particular group are also classified, whether they are more similar to bacteria, yeast, filamentous fungi, and plants or animals homologues.

Table 3
Functional distribution of *A. nidulans* ESTs non-homologous to human gene-specific DNA sequences

	Unique *A. nidulans* ESTs					
	Nonhuman ESTs				All ESTs (4,595)	
	Average		With function (380)[a]			
Functional category	HSP	Length (bp)	#	% (A)	% (B)	fold (A/B)
Electron transport	407	485	19	2.2	3.0	0.7
Information pathways	420	409	40	4.6	6.0	0.8
DNA modification and repair			11			
Translation and posttranslational modification			25			
Transcription and stress response			4			
Intermediate metabolism	395	438	751	87.0	87.0	1.0
Aromatic compounds			49	6.5	2.0	3.3
Anabolism			18	36.7		
Catabolism			31	63.3		
Carbohydrate			380	50.6	47.0	1.1
Main carbohydrate pathways			62	16.3	21.0	0.8
Monosaccharides			73	19.2	17.0	1.1
Dissaccharides			22	5.8	4.0	1.4
Polysaccharides			48	12.6	9.0	1.4
Sugar alcohols			36	9.5	5.0	1.9
Alcohols			47	12.4	11.0	1.1
Amino sugars			3	0.8	3.0	0.3
Organic acids			68	17.9	21.0	0.9
Other carbohydrates			21	5.5	7.0	0.8
Coenzymes and prosthetic groups			39	5.2	5.0	1.0
Essential elements			99	13.2	11.0	1.2
Lipid			44	5.9	10.0	0.6
Monocarbon compounds			17	2.3	2.0	1.1
Nucleotides and nucleic acids			28	3.7	7.0	0.5
Porphyrin			2	0.3		
Proteins, peptides and amino acids			93	12.4	16.0	0.8
Signal transduction	419	459	19	2.2	3.0	0.7
Cell structure	361	589	7	0.8		
Transmembrane transport	410	432	27	3.1	3.0	1.0

[a] = BLASTX cutoff value, e=10^{-16}

ESSENTIAL GENES AS POTENTIAL TARGETS

We found 387 nonhuman analogs with predictable functional assignments based on significant alignments with nonhuman organisms—e.g., plants, bacteria, yeast, and other fungi (Fig. 3A). These ESTs were further subgrouped as essential and nonessential genes, based on comparisons with the information available in *Saccha-*

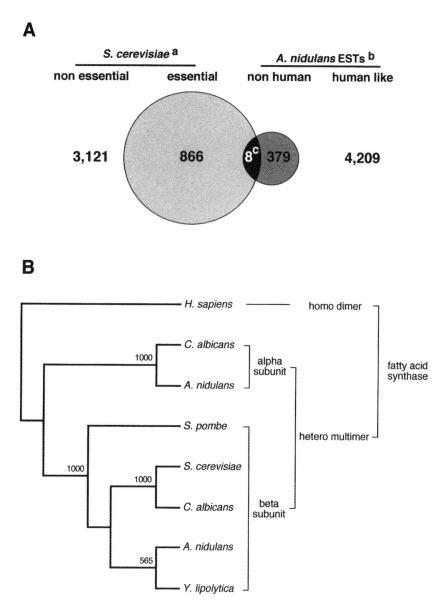

Fig. 3. Identification of essential, nonhuman *A. nidulans* EST analogs. (**A**) 387 nonhuman *A. nidulans* EST analogs were compared to 874 reported essential yeast genes, and eight matches were identified. (**B**) Rooted and bootstrapped phenogram of fatty-acid synthase. Full-length fatty-acid synthase amino-acid sequences were used to construct the tree. Fatty-acid synthase group is divided into three major classes: human, alpha, and beta subunits. The human enzyme functions as a homodimer and all other fatty-acid synthase function as hetero tetramers or hexamer.

[a] MIPS database (http://mips.gsf.de) of known essential (874) and nonessential (3,121) genes.

[b] 4,595 unique *A. nidulans* ESTs, may not represent real genes.

[c] Possible essential genes in both *S. cerevisiae* and *A. nidulans.*

Table 4
Nonhuman *A. nidulans* ESTs homologous to essential genes in yeast

Functional definition (yeast)	Yeast ORF			*A. nidulans* EST			Human ORF	
	Name	aa	e-value	Name	bp	e-value	Name	aa
Fatty acid synthase—fungi have two subunits (α) and (β), humans only one	*FAS1*	2051	4.00E-10	g9b02a1.f1	421	N/A	N/A	N/A
	FAS2	1887	7.00E-45	r7b10a1.r1	314	0.940	*SRD5B1*	326
Phosphoglycero mutase—*A. nidulans* gene heterologous to yeast	*GPM1*	247	(2.00E-74)[a]	z3b09a1.r1	454	0.005	*PYK2*	1006
Fructose bisphosphate aldolase—fungal FBA different from human	*FBA1*	359	4.00E-50	x5h11a1.r1	452	0.003	*KIAA1683*	1180
UTPG-1-phosphate uridylyltransferase—mammalian domain absent in fungi	*UGP1*	499	2.00E-18	x1e10a1.r1	489	0.050	*UGPP2*	508
Trehalose phosphate synthase—no human trehalose phosphate synthase to date (*A. nidulans* EST sequence heterologous to yeast)	*TPS1*	495	(4.00E-42)[b]	f0f11a1.r1	445	N/A	N/A	N/A
Histidine kinase—osmosensor in yeast	*SLN1*	1220	8.00E-09	c5e08a1.r1	517	0.001	*RAB2*	777
Unknown—component of yeast SAGA complex	*TRA1*	3744	4.00E-15	p0e05a1.r1	463	0.098	*KIAA0473*	913
Unknown—possibly involved in cell-cycle control in *S. pombe*	*ROT1*	256	8.00E-25	q0d09a1.r1	329	0.110	*IP3R3*	2671

[a] Score reported from alignment with *Aspergillus oryzae*

[b] Score reported from alignment with *Neurospora crassa*

romyces cerevisiae (63). Table 4 describes the comparative information of eight non-human *A. nidulans* ESTs that are essential and homologous to yeast genes: fatty acid synthase (yeast *FAS1*), phosphoglyceromutase (yeast *GPM1*), fructose bisphosphate aldolase (yeast *FBA1*), UTP glucose-1-phosphate uridylyltransferase (yeast *UGP1*), trehalose phosphate synthase (yeast *TPS1*), histidine kinase (yeast *SLN1*), and two homologues of unknown function (*TRA1* and *ROT1*).

One gene identified by this approach was a fatty acid synthase (FAS; EC.2.3.1.85), an essential gene in both *S. cerevisiae* and *A. nidulans* for the synthesis of long-chain fatty acids (>C12) from acetyl-CoA, malonyl-CoA and NADPH *(64,65)*.

Fig. 3B shows a rooted, bootstrapped phenogram calculated from multiple protein-sequence alignments, indicating evolutionary similarities and differences among FAS polypeptides. Fungal FAS (fFAS) have the same functional organization and the arrangement of catalytic domains in *A. nidulans, P. griseofulvum, C. carbonum, S. pombe,* and *C. albicans* are similar to *S. cerevisiae (66,68)* domains.

One structural distinction between human (hFAS) and fungal (fFAS) fatty acid synthase is that hFAS occurs in a homodimeric form, arranged in a "head-to-tail" manner to form two palmitate-synthesizing sites *(69)*. fFAS also operate as hetero-multimeric protein aggregates containing alpha (FAS1) and beta (FAS2) subunits *(70–73)*.

Catalytic activities and functional domain organization among human and fungal FAS polypeptides differ significantly. The thioesterase activity that determines fatty-acid-chain length in hFAS *(74)* is absent in fFAS, suggesting differentiated chain-length control—perhaps via the ketosynthase domain *(65)*. hFAS contains seven catalytic activities in one polypeptide: beta-ketoacyl synthase, acyl and malonyl trans-ferases, enoyl reductase, beta-ketoacyl reductase, acyl carrier, beta hydroxyacyl dehy-dratase, and thioesterase. The pentafunctional activities of fFAS are distributed along two polypeptides: the α polypeptide (with beta-ketoacyl synthase, beta-ketoacyl reduc-tase, and acyl-carrier domains), and the fFAS β subunit that carries acetyl transferase and malonyl-palmityl transferase activities.

In this study, in addition to the differences determined for fatty acid synthase, two genes involved in glycolysis, fructose bisphosphate aldolase (EC 4.1.2.13) and phos-phoglyceromutase (EC 5.4.2.1) were identified as potential candidates for antifungal drug development. Using a comparative genomics approach, we have determined that the predicted protein sequences of these genes differ from their human glycolytic pro-tein counterparts. For example, fungal aldolases are all class II—zinc binding, and pro-tein sequences differ from human class I Schiff-acid-type aldolases *(75,76)*. Furthermore, the observation that specific inhibition of glycolysis using 3-bromopyru-vic acid efficiently kills liver-tumor tissues and cancer cells in culture *(77)* gives promise to the effectiveness of glycolytic targets.

Traditionally, genes involved in central metabolism have not been examined as tar-gets for the development of antimicrobial compounds because of the implicit likeli-hood of inhibiting functionally similar host proteins involved in the same metabolic pathway. Although the mode of action for some bacterial antibiotic targets involves unique metabolic steps such as peptidoglycan synthesis, many bacterial antibiotics associate with ribosomal RNAs. Ribosome components are present in all living organisms, and thus are not unique to pathogenic bacteria, yet they are effective targets because the mode of action takes sequence heterology into consideration. Similarly, differences between fungal and human amino-acid sequences should reveal new cellular targets for antifungal drugs, even with overlapping biological function.

Comparisons based on orthologous or analogous relationships are therefore useful to reveal differences between two or more genomes. Target selection, via genome-wide comparisons and compiling functional information of the genetic dissimilarities, reveal genetic information helpful in designing drugs and identifying drug targets.

The amino acid sequence-based functional sorting of gene libraries is useful in the selection of target genes. For example, carbohydrate metabolism genes are slightly more likely to be similar to human genes than are genes involved in the synthesis of aromatic compounds (Fig. 2). Genes associated with synthesis of essential elements, such as protein or lipid synthesis, are more likely to be similar to plant genes. These differences, although subtle, could play an important role in determining the effectiveness of a particular target. Suppose that there is no limitations in testing randomly generated drugs that inhibit the activity of a particular gene classified under aromatic metabolism or essential compounds. Such drugs are more likely to be fungal-specific than a drug that acts on genes coding for functions associated with essential compound metabolism.

Although these computational approaches are effective in determining genetic variation between host and pathogen genomes as they contribute to the identification of potential targets, the effectiveness of such targets must also pass a chemical and biological validation process. Thus, screening based on genomic comparison represents the first in a series of steps leading to the discovery of novel drug therapies.

Based on predicted protein-sequence heterology to human proteins, a comparative genomics approach is likely to accelerate drug-target identification, as well as the development of antifungals and antimicrobials. These comparisons are made possible through extensive sequencing efforts in humans, fungi, and other organisms.

ACKNOWLEDGMENTS

Research in the laboratories of authors has been supported by the National Science Foundation (NSF 98-13360, RAP) and Fundação de Amparo á Pesquisa do Estado de São Paulo (FAPESP 98/13261-5, NMMR and MG and 99/09877-3, AR). RPM received support from Ateneo de Manila University, Philippines.

REFERENCES

1. Prade RA, Zhan D, Ayoubi P, Mort AJ. Pectins, pectinases and plant-microbe interactions. Biotechnol Genet Eng Rev 1999; 16:361–391.
2. Garber G. An overview of fungal infections. Drugs 2001; 61 (Suppl 1):1–12.
3. Paladino JA. Economic justification of antimicrobial management programs: implications of antimicrobial resistance. Am J Health Syst Pharm 2000; 57 (Suppl 2):S10–S12.
4. Johnston M. The yeast genome: on the road to the Golden Age. Curr Opin Genet Dev 2000; 10:617–623.
5. Dixon B. Yeast as factory and factotum. Biologist (London) 2000; 47:15–18.
6. Van Belle D, Andre B. A genomic view of yeast membrane transporters. Curr Opin Cell Biol 2001; 13:389–398.

7. Devaux F, Marc P, Jacq C. Transcriptomes, transcription activators and microarrays. FEBS Lett 2001; 498:140–144.

8. Rolland F, Winderickx J, Thevelein JM. Glucose-sensing mechanisms in eukaryotic cells. Trends Biochem Sci 2001; 26:310–317.

9. Kohlwein SD. The beauty of the yeast: live cell microscopy at the limits of optical resolution. Microsc Res Tech 2000; 51:511–529.

10. Bielinsky AK, Gerbi SA. Where it all starts: eukaryotic origins of DNA replication. J Cell Sci 2001; 114:643–651.

11. Bell-Pedersen D. Understanding circadian rhythmicity in *Neurospora crassa:* from behavior to genes and back again. Fungal Genet Biol 2000; 29:1–18.

12. Osherov N, May GS. The molecular mechanisms of conidial germination. FEMS Microbiol Lett 2001; 199:153–160.

13. Ebbole DJ. Carbon catabolite repression of gene expression and conidiation in Neurospora crassa. Fungal Genet Biol 1998; 25:15–21.

14. Sweeney MJ, Dobson AD. Molecular biology of mycotoxin biosynthesis. FEMS Microbiol Lett 1999; 175:149–163.

15. Adams TH, Wieser JK, Yu JH. Asexual sporulation in *Aspergillus nidulans.* Microbiol Mol Biol Rev 1998; 62:35–54.

16. Denison SH. pH regulation of gene expression in fungi. Fungal Genet Biol 2000; 29:61–71.

17. Hamer L, Pan H, Adachi K, et al. Regions of microsynteny in *Magnaporthe grisea* and *Neurospora crassa.* Fungal Genet Biol 2001; 33:137–143.

18. Elewski BE. Large-scale epidemiological study of the causal agents of onychomycosis: mycological findings from the Multicenter Onychomycosis Study of Terbinafine. Arch Dermatol 1997; 133:1317–1318.

19. Fridkin SK, Jarvis WR. Epidemiology of nosocomial fungal infections. Clin Microbiol Rev 1996; 9:499–511.

20. Mushegian AR, Koonin EV. A minimal gene set for cellular life derived by comparison of complete bacterial genomes. Proc Natl Acad Sci USA 1996; 93:10,268–10,273.

21. Petri MG, Konig J, Moecke HP, et al. Epidemiology of invasive mycosis in ICU patients: a prospective multicenter study in 435 non-neutropenic patients. Paul-Ehrlich Society for Chemotherapy, Divisions of Mycology and Pneumonia Research. Intensive Care Med 1997; 23:317–325.

22. White TC, Marr KA, Bowden RA. Clinical, cellular, and molecular factors that contribute to antifungal drug resistance. Clin Microbiol Rev 1998; 11:382–402.

23. Marques SA, Robles AM, Tortorano AM, Tuculet MA, Negroni R, Mendes RP. Mycoses associated with AIDS in the Third World. Med Mycol 2000; 38(Suppl 1):269–279.

24. Durden FM, Elewski B. Fungal infections in HIV-infected patients. Semin Cutan Med Surg 1997; 16:200–212.

25. Kaplan JE, Hanson D, Dworkin MS, et al. Epidemiology of human immunodeficiency virus-associated opportunistic infections in the United States in the era of highly active antiretroviral therapy. Clin Infect Dis 2000; 30(Suppl 1:)S5–S14.

26. Ghannoum MA, Rice LB. Antifungal agents: mode of action, mechanisms of resistance, and correlation of these mechanisms with bacterial resistance. Clin Microbiol Rev 1999; 12:501–517.

27. Schwartlander B, Stover J, Walker N, et al. AIDS. Resource needs for HIV/AIDS. Science 2001; 292:2434–2436.

28. Rippon JW. Medical Mycology. The Pathogenic Fungi and the Pathogenic Actinomycetes. Philadelphia: WB. Saunders Company, 1988, pp. 1–9.

29. Speller DCE. Other Antifungal Agents. In: DCE Speller (ed.). Antifungal Chemotherapy, London: John Wiley & Sons, 1980, pp. 183–210.

30. Weete JD, Gandhi SR. Sterols of the phylum zygomycota: phylogenetic implications. Lipids 1997; 32:1309–1316.

31. Charbonneau C, Fournier I, Dufresne S, Barwicz J, Tancrede P. The interactions of amphotericin B with various sterols in relation to its possible use in anticancer therapy. Biophys Chem 2001; 91:125–133.

32. Fournier I, Barwicz J, Tancrede P. The structuring effects of amphotericin B on pure and ergosterol- or cholesterol-containing dipalmitoylphosphatidylcholine bilayers: a differential scanning calorimetry study. Biochim Biophys Acta 1998; 1373:76–86.

33. Moir DT, Shaw KJ, Hare RS, Vovis GF. Genomics and antimicrobial drug discovery. Antimicrob Agents Chemother 1999; 43:439–446.

34. Georgopapadakou NH. Antifungals targeted to sphingolipid synthesis: focus on inositol phosphorylceramide synthase. Expert Opin Investig Drugs 2000; 9:1787–1796.

35. Chiou CC, Groll AH, Walsh TJ. New drugs and novel targets for treatment of invasive fungal infections in patients with cancer. Oncologist 2000; 5:120–135.

36. DiDomenico B. Novel antifungal drugs. Curr Opin Microbiol 1999; 2:509–515.

37. Klein LL, Li L. Design and preparation of cyclopeptamine antifungal agents. Curr Pharm Des 1999; 5:57–72.

38. Soteropoulos P, Vaz T, Santangelo R, et al. Molecular characterization of the plasma membrane H(+)-ATPase, an antifungal target in *Cryptococcus neoformans*. Antimicrob Agents Chemother 2000; 44:2349–2355.

39. Cowen LE, Sanglard D, Calabrese D, Sirjusingh C, Anderson JB, Kohn LM. Evolution of drug resistance in experimental populations of *Candida albicans*. J Bacteriol 2000; 182:1515–1522.

40. Vanden Bossche H, Dromer F, Improvisi I, Lozano-Chiu M, Rex JH, Sanglard D. Antifungal drug resistance in pathogenic fungi. Med Mycol 1998; 36(Suppl 1):119–128.

41. Moore CB, Sayers N, Mosquera J, Slaven J, Denning DW. Antifungal drug resistance in *Aspergillus*. J Infect 2000; 41:203–220.

42. Dick JD, Merz WG, Saral R. Incidence of polyene-resistant yeasts recovered from clinical specimens. Antimicrob Agents Chemother 1980; 18:158–163.

43. Bouchara JP, Zouhair R, Le Boudouil S, et al. In-vivo selection of an azole-resistant petite mutant of *Candida glabrata*. J Med Microbiol 2000; 49:977–984.

44. Defontaine A, Bouchara JP, Declerk P, Planchenault C, Chabasse D, Hallet JN. In-vitro resistance to azoles associated with mitochondrial DNA deficiency in *Candida glabrata*. J Med Microbiol 1999; 48:663–670.

45. Calabrese D, Bille J, Sanglard D. A novel multidrug efflux transporter gene of the major facilitator superfamily from *Candida albicans* (FLU1) conferring resistance to fluconazole. Microbiology 2000; 146:2743–2754.

46. Hitchcock CA, Barrett-Bee KJ, Russell NJ. The lipid composition and permeability to azole of an azole- and polyene-resistant mutant of Candida albicans. J Med Vet Mycol 1987; 25:29–37.

47. vanden Bossche H, Marichal P, Odds FC, Le Jeune L, Coene MC. Characterization of an azole-resistant *Candida glabrata* isolate. Antimicrob Agents Chemother 1992; 36:2602–2610.

48. Watson PF, Rose ME, Ellis SW, England H, Kelly SL. Defective sterol C5-6 desaturation and azole resistance: a new hypothesis for the mode of action of azole antifungals. Biochem Biophys Res Commun 1989; 164:1170–1175.

49. Cardenas ME, Cruz MC, Del Poeta M, Chung N, Perfect JR, Heitman J. Antifungal activities of antineoplastic agents: *Saccharomyces cerevisiae* as a model system to study drug action. Clin Microbiol Rev 1999; 12:583–611.

50. Fostel J, Montgomery D, Lartey P. Comparison of responses of DNA topoisomerase I from *Candida albicans* and human cells to four new agents which stimulate topoisomerase- dependent DNA nicking. FEMS Microbiol Lett 1996; 138:105–111.

51. Kupfer DM, Reece CA, Clifton SW, Roe BA, Prade RA. Multicellular ascomycetous fungal genomes contain more than 8000 genes. Fungal Genet Biol 1997; 21:364–372.

52. Zhuo D, Zhao WD, Wright FA, et al. Assembly, annotation, and integration of UNIGENE clusters into the human genome draft. Genome Res 2001; 11:904–918.

53. Schuler GD. Sequence alignment and database searching. Methods Biochem Anal 1998; 39:145–171.

54. Smith TF. The art of matchmaking: sequence alignment methods and their structural implications. Structure Fold Des 1999; 7:R7–R12.

55. Ophir R, Itoh T, Graur D, Gojobori T. A simple method for estimating the intensity of purifying selection in protein-coding genes. Mol Biol Evol 1999; 16:49–53.

56. Shah I, Hunter L. Predicting enzyme function from sequence: a systematic appraisal. Proc Int Conf Intell Syst Mol Biol 1997; 5:276–283.

57. Rost B. Twilight zone of protein sequence alignments. Protein Eng 1999; 12:85–94.

58. Wilson CA, Kreychman J, Gerstein M. Assessing annotation transfer for genomics: quantifying the relations between protein sequence, structure and function through traditional and probabilistic scores. J Mol Biol 2000; 297:233–249.

59. Benner SA, Gaucher EA. Evolution, language and analogy in functional genomics. Trends Genet 2001; 17:414–418.

60. Selkov EJ, Grechkin Y, Mikhailova N, Salkov E. MPW: the Metabolic Pathways Database. Nucleic Acids Res 1998; 26:43–45.

61. Prade RA, Ayoubi P, Krishnan S, Macwana S, Russel H. Accumulation of stress and inducer-dependent plant cell wall degrading enzymes during asexual development in *Aspergillus nidulans*. Genetics 2001; 157:957–967.

62. Reeds PJ. Dispensable and indispensable amino acids for humans. J Nutr 2000; 130:1835S–1840S.

63. Mewes HW, Heumann K, Kaps A, et al. MIPS: a database for genomes and protein sequences. Nucleic Acids Res 1999; 27:44–48.

64. Schuller HJ, Fortsch B, Rautenstrauss B, Wolf DH, Schweizer E. Differential proteolytic sensitivity of yeast fatty acid synthetase subunits alpha and beta contributing to a balanced ratio of both fatty acid synthetase components. Eur J Biochem 1992; 203:607–614.

65. Brown DW, Adams TH, Keller NP. *Aspergillus* has distinct fatty acid synthases for primary and secondary metabolism. Proc Natl Acad Sci USA 1996; 93:14,873–14,877.

66. Ahn JH, Walton JD. A fatty acid synthase gene in *Cochliobolus carbonum* required for production of HC-toxin, cyclo(D-prolyl-L-alanyl-D-alanyl-L-2-amino-9, 10-epoxi-8-oxodecanoyl). Mol Plant-Microbe Interact 1997; 10:207–214.

67. Wiesner P, Beck J, Beck KF, et al. Isolation and sequence analysis of the fatty acid synthetase FAS2 gene from *Penicillium patulum*. Eur J Biochem 1988; 177:69–79.

68. Zhao XJ, Cihlar RL. Isolation and sequence of the *Candida albicans* FAS1 gene. Gene 1994; 147:119–124.

69. Wakil SJ. Fatty acid synthase, a proficient multifunctional enzyme. Biochemistry 1989; 28:4523–4530.

70. Chirala SS, Kuziora MA, Spector DM, Wakil SJ. Complementation of mutations and nucleotide sequence of FAS1 gene encoding beta subunit of yeast fatty acid synthase. J Biol Chem 1987; 262:4231–4240.

71. Kottig H, Rottner G, Beck KF, Schweizer M, Schweizer E. The pentafunctional FAS1 genes of *Saccharomyces cerevisiae* and *Yarrowia lipolytica* are co-linear and considerably longer than previously estimated. Mol Gen Genet 1991; 226:310–314.

72. Mohamed AH, Chirala SS, Mody NH, Huang WY, Wakil SJ. Primary structure of the multifunctional alpha subunit protein of yeast fatty acid synthase derived from FAS2 gene sequence. J Biol Chem 1988; 263:12,315–12,325.

73. Schweizer E, Kottig H, Regler R, Rottner G. Genetic control of *Yarrowia lipolytica* fatty acid synthetase biosynthesis and function. J Basic Microbiol 1988; 28:283–292.

74. Tai MH, Chirala SS, Wakil SJ. Roles of Ser101, Asp236, and His237 in catalysis of thioesterase II and of the C-terminal region of the enzyme in its interaction with fatty acid synthase. Proc Natl Acad Sci USA 1993; 90:1852–1856.

75. Alefounder PR, Baldwin SA, Perham RN, Short NJ. Cloning, sequence analysis and over-expression of the gene for the class II fructose 1,6-bisphosphate aldolase of *Escherichia coli*. Biochem J 1989; 257:529–534.

76. Gamblin SJ, Davies GJ, Grimes JM, Jackson RM, Littlechild JA, Watson HC. Activity and specificity of human aldolases. J Mol Biol 1991; 219:573–576.

77. Ko YH, Pedersen PL, Geschwind JF. Glucose catabolism in the rabbit VX2 tumor model for liver cancer: characterization and targeting hexokinase. Cancer Lett 2001; in press.

15

Functional Genomics of *Histoplasma capsulatum*

Dimorphism and Virulence

Glenmore Shearer, Jr.

INTRODUCTION

Histoplasma capsulatum (*Hc*; teleomorph, *Ajellomyces capsulatus*) is the etiologic agent of histoplasmosis, one of the most common systemic fungal infections of humans. Estimates of the incidence of histoplasmosis in the United States alone are approx 500,000 per year *(1)*. The worldwide incidence is unknown but is almost certainly in the millions. The mold form grows in the soil and converts to the pathogenic yeast form in the lungs of the host after inhalation of mold fragments or spores. Typically, in individuals with healthy immune systems, the disease is a self-limiting respiratory infection with influenza-like symptoms. However, in some otherwise healthy people and especially in individuals with weakened immune systems, histoplasmosis is a systemic and life-threatening disease. In particular, *Histoplasma* is a common and serious opportunistic pathogen in cancer patients, organ transplant patients, and AIDS patients *(2,3)*.

Significant advances have been made in elucidating the molecular basis of dimorphism and virulence in *Hc*. Theoretically, any gene product that is critical for yeast formation/maintenance or necessary for survival within the host could serve as a therapeutic target. Several laboratories, including ours, are working to identify genes that are critical for mold-yeast dimorphism in *Hc*. Although no genes critical for the morphotype switch have been reported, several gene products required for survival within the host phagocyte have been identified *(4,5)*. Much has been learned by using existing low-throughput methods such as subtractive screening and differential display, and we are now poised to utilize new genomic tools which will allow *Hc* researchers to make more rapid progress in our efforts to understand dimorphism and virulence in this important human pathogen.

PHYSIOLOGY OF DIMORPHISM

The *Hc* organism exhibits the intriguing biological phenomenon of dimorphism, which is integral to its pathogenesis (reviewed in ref. *6*). In the soil, *Hc* grows as a saprophytic differentiated multicellular mold, but in the infected host *Histoplasma* grows in an undifferentiated form as a unicellular budding yeast. When spores or

From: *Pathogen Genomics: Impact on Human Health*
Edited by: K. J. Shaw © Humana Press Inc., Totowa, NJ

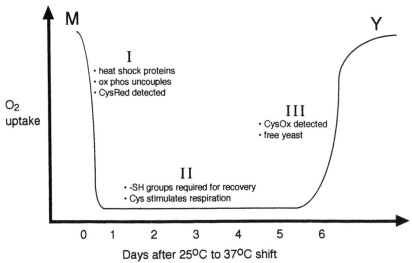

Fig. 1. Landmarks of the mold-to-yeast dimorphic shift.

mycelial fragments are inhaled, the organism converts to the yeast form. This mold-to-yeast (M–Y) conversion is critical for the disease process because cells treated to block this dimorphic shift cannot cause disease *(7)*. The M–Y or Y–M shift is easily seen in vitro by simply changing the incubation temperature to favor Y (e.g., 37°C) or M (e.g., 25°C). Because of interest in the biology of the multicellular/unicellular shift as well as its role in pathogenesis, several laboratories have done extensive studies on the cell biology, physiology, biochemistry, and more recently, the molecular biology, of dimorphism in *Hc*.

Maresca et al. *(8).* described three stages in the mold-to-yeast conversion in vitro as summarized in Fig. 1. In stage 1, the cells appear to undergo a shock response followed by a sharp drop in metabolic rate uncoupling of oxidative phosphorylation and loss of cytochromes. Early in stage 1, the cells begin expressing a yeast-specific enzyme, cystine reductase. In stage 2, which lasts about 2–4 days depending on the *Hc* strain, the metabolic rate as measured by oxygen consumption remains very low. At this stage, sulfhydryl-containing compounds (preferably cysteine) are required to progress to stage 3. Stage 3 is characterized by a rapid increase in metabolic rate, expression of a second yeast-specific enzyme (cysteine oxidase), and formation of yeast.

Clearly, -SH compounds, particularly cyst(e)ine, are important in the M–Y shift. Most strains of *Hc* are cysteine prototrophs in the mold form but cysteine auxotrophs in the yeast form because of the absence of sulfite reductase in the Y form *(9)*. The yeast form expresses cystine reductase and cysteine oxidase, and the mold form does not. Also, the sulfhydryl blocker PCMS (p-chloromercury- phenylsulfonic acid) inhibits the M–Y shift. A likely possibility is that cyst(e)ine and/or other -SH compounds are needed to modulate intracellular redox for the formation and/or maintenance of the yeast form. Further support is given to this idea by the results of Rippon, who showed that Y would grow at the nonpermissive temperature of 25°C if the redox potential was lowered (i.e., made more reducing) by passing a weak direct electrical current through the growth medium *(10)*.

THE GENOME OF HISTOPLASMA

Until recently, very little was known about the genome of *Hc*. The nuclear guanine plus cytosine (GC) content was reported to range from 45.4% to 49.8%, with an observed mean of 47.3% *(11)*. Analysis of the mitochondrial DNA of 23 isolates from human and animal sources by restriction-fragment-length polymorphism (RFLP) indicates that *Hc* can be grouped into three classes *(12)*. The only member in class 1 was the Downs strain. Class 2 isolates (e.g., G217B) were mostly from North America and the African *H. capsulatum var. duboisii*. Class 3 was composed mostly of isolates from Central America (e.g., G186B) and South America. More recent RFLP analysis with the yeast-specific clone *yps-3 (13)*, arbitrary primer polymerase chain reaction (PCR) *(14)*, and rDNA polymorphism analysis *(15)* have demonstrated that *Hc* is actually much more diverse than first believed.

Chromosome Number

Steele et al. *(16)* attempted to determine the chromosome number of *Hc* by analysis with contour-clamped homogenous electric field (CHEF) and field-inversion gel electrophoresis (FIGE). After solving the difficult problem of how to lyse *Hc* cells within agarose sample blocks, CHEF analysis and ethidium bromide staining revealed six bands in the Downs strain, three bands in the G217B strain, and four bands in the G186B strain. These putative chromosomal bands ranged from approx 2 Mb to more than 5.7 Mb in size. One interesting exception to this observation was the presence of a 0.5-Mb band seen only in G186B. FIGE analysis showed five bands in the Downs strain, two bands in G217B, and three bands in G186B. Because chromosomes can comigrate in these electrophoretic analyses, the investigators probed blots of the gels with several *Hc* genes and randomly selected fragments of *Hc* DNA to identify chromosome-specific probes. Comparison of the results from CHEF and FIGE blots showed that one CHEF band represented two chromosomes in the Downs strain. Without genetic linkage data, the chromosome number cannot be precisely determined, but we can estimate a minimum number from this electrophoretic analysis. The minimum chromosome number for these three strains is seven for Downs, three for G217B, and four for G186B. Clearly, there is significant variability in the electrophoretic mobility and putative chromosome number in these strains. The Downs strain in particular may not be representative of *Hc* strains, as discussed in the following section.

Ploidy, Genome Size, and Complexity

Recently my laboratory has conducted studies to determine the ploidy as well as the genome size and complexity of *Hc (17)*. Because the Downs strain has been used in many published experiments, but may be atypical based on the chromosome analysis described here, we included the Downs strain as well as a derivative of strain G186B (G186AS) in our studies. Nuclear DNA was isolated and analyzed by renaturation kinetics. Computer modeling of these results compared to control experiments with *E. coli* DNA showed that the Downs genome is approx 35 Mb, with 8% moderately repetitive sequences. In contrast, the G186AS genome is only 22 Mb, with less than 0.5% repetitive sequences. This difference is particularly striking in a "mini-Cot" reassociation experiment, which displays only the fastest reassociating components as shown in

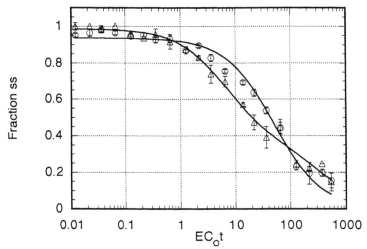

Fig. 2. Renaturation analysis of repetitive DNA from Downs (triangles) and G186AS (circles). Reprinted from ref. *17* by permission of the publisher.

Fig. 2. Clearly, the Downs strain has a larger and more complex repetitive component than G186AS.

As an independent method of genome size estimation, we used "genomic reconstruction" analysis—i.e., quantitative hybridization analysis with single-copy genes. This analysis also indicates that the Downs genome is atypical. Quantitative hybridization with *CAM1,* alpha tubulin, and beta tubulin probes indicated that these genes are in fact single copy in G186AS and yield an estimated haploid genome size of 24 Mb. In the Downs strain, however, only *CAM1* appears to be single copy; the tubulin probes hybridize to more than one locus at high stringency, which we believe is the result of duplication of some regions of the chromosome(s).

Analysis of DNA content per cell by fluorescent staining with propidium iodide followed by flow cytometry also indicates that the Downs strain has a larger genome than G186AS (Fig. 3). Comparison of peak channel numbers with similarly stained haploid, diploid, and tetraploid *Saccharomyces cerevisiae* reference strains was used to determine the quantity of DNA per cell. Each G186AS cell has approx 24 fg DNA (equivalent to 22 Mb of DNA), and Downs has approx 32 fg (equivalent to 30 Mb of DNA). Comparison of the DNA content per cell with the estimates of genome size indicates that *Hc* is haploid. Based on the analysis of G186AS, and our unpublished data from strains G217B and G186B, we believe the typical *Hc* genome to be approx 23 Mb in size with less than 1% repetitive sequences. The Downs strain, however, has a genome nearly 40% larger, and may be a partial diploid or aneuploid strain.

MOLECULAR BIOLOGY OF DIMORPHISM

Perhaps the most striking feature of *Hc* pathogenesis is the intimate link to mold/yeast dimorphism. The mold form is well-adapted for growth in the soil, particularly in areas enriched by animal excreta. In contrast, the yeast morphotype is well-suited for survival within the host phagocyte. The fact that *Hc* mycelia are not found in infected tissue gave rise to the hypothesis that only the yeast can cause disease. This

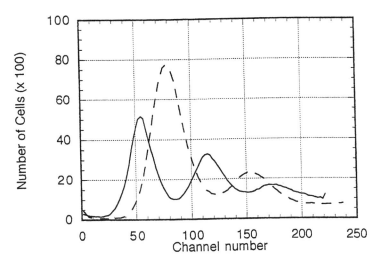

Fig. 3. Analysis of DNA content in propidium iodide stained cells by flow cytometry. Downs strain, dotted line; G186AS, solid line. Reprinted from ref. *17* by permission of the publisher.

concept that only the yeast is capable of productive infection is supported by experiments with the sulfhydryl blocker PCMS. *Hc* cells treated with 100 µ*M* PCMS for approx 24 h and then extensively washed can grow as mold, but cannot convert to yeast *(7)*. The PCMS effect is unidirectional: treated mold grow at 25°C but cannot convert to yeast at 37°C; treated yeast grow as yeast at 37°C and convert to mold at 25°C, but cannot shift back to yeast again at 37°C, as seen in untreated cultures. More interesting still is the finding that this block in the M–Y shift is still in effect after extensive washing and repeated transfers to fresh PCMS-free medium. Medoff et al. *(18)* discovered that the mold form of virulent strains of *Hc* treated with PCMS can grow at 37°C, but do so in the mold form. In contrast to untreated mycelia, the PCMS-treated mold cannot cause infection when injected into mice. This lack of pathogenicity is apparently not because the treated mold dies at the 37°C host temperature, because the mycelia can survive in vitro at this temperature. The fact that the treated mold survives at 37°C but cannot convert to yeast supports the necessity of yeast formation for pathogenicity. Although yeast formation is required for pathogenesis, it cannot be sufficient for disease, since there are several essentially avirulent *Hc* strains that appear to undergo a normal dimorphic shift in vitro.

Because the M–Y shift is a necessity for disease, an understanding of the molecular biology of dimorphism is valuable for biological as well as clinical reasons. Numerous studies have examined the intriguing cell biology and physiology of *Hc* dimorphism (see refs. *6,19*). Recently, several laboratories, including ours, have initiated studies of the molecular genetics of dimorphism. This process has been somewhat slow because of the absence of basic knowledge regarding the genome of *Hc* and the lack of several fundamental molecular tools.

Although *Hc* is a heterothallic ascomycete and sexual crosses can be done *(20)*, the spores have a low germination efficiency, and represent a significant aerosol biohazard. Thus, classical genetic experiments are generally not feasible with *Hc*. However, recent advances in methodology have allowed researchers to overcome this critical limitation by using molecular genetic tools that were previously unavailable for *Histoplasma.*

Transformation System

In the past, molecular genetic experiments have been quite difficult to conduct, because the powerful tools for transformation and gene disruption that are widely used in other systems were unavailable for *Hc.* Additional problems of poor plating efficiency and clumping of cells were solved by the development of HMM, a rich synthetic medium, and the isolation of nonclumping strains *(21).* Several laboratories have worked to develop a genetic transformation system for *Hc* by using these new tools. Preliminary experiments in my laboratory (unpublished) showed that it was possible to transform *Hc* strain G186AS with a circular plasmid carrying the bacterial hygromycin resistance marker, driven by promoters from filamentous ascomycetes such as *Aspergillus* sp., with a modified lithium acetate procedure. However, this method was quite inefficient, and typically resulted in ectopic integration or modification of the plasmid vector. The groundbreaking work in this area began in the Goldman laboratory in St. Louis. Worsham and Goldman isolated a mutant strain of *Hc* auxotrophic for uracil *(21),* and developed a genetic transformation system based on complementation of this mutant with the *Ura5* gene *(22).* Woods and Goldman *(23)* discovered that linear vectors with *Hc* telomeric repeats (GGGTTA) are far more efficient than circular plasmids, and are typically maintained by the transformed cells as episomes. The utility of telomere vectors carrying a uracil nutritional marker *(Ura5)* or the dominant hygromycin marker *(hph)* is now well-proven in *Hc.* The development of these tools and a high efficiency electroporation protocol (with nearly 10^5 transformants/μg) has made experiments previously unavailable to *Hc* researchers now quite feasible *(24).*

Gene Disruption

Early attempts to conduct targeted gene disruption were unsuccessful because *Hc* appears to have highly inefficient homologous recombination. The transformation of cells with large amounts of DNA results mostly in ectopic integration rather than targeted insertion. In 1998, Woods et al. *(25)* successfully disrupted the *Hc Ura5* gene by transforming Ura$^+$ cells with a Δ*Ura5::hph* construct to yield cells resistant to hygromycin (via the *hph* marker) and resistant to 5-FOA (5-fluoro orotic acid, which is toxic to Ura$^+$ cells). The relative efficiency was approx 1 allelic replacement per 1000 transformants. Recently, a positive/negative selection method has been developed by Sebghati et al. *(5),* which yields a much higher frequency of knockout mutants. A uracil auxotroph is transformed with a linear telomere plasmid containing a *Ura5* marker, and the target gene disrupted with the hygromycin marker. Growth for several weeks under uracil selection allows time for the double-crossover event to occur. Plating on agar medium containing hygromycin, uracil, and 5-FOA selects for the hygromycin marker and against the *Ura5* marker, thus favoring cells which have integrated the disrupted gene. Approximately 30% of the colonies appearing on the positive/negative selection plates are knockout mutants. Experiments in my laboratory with a slightly modified version of their protocol have yielded excellent results. We have recently constructed several knockout mutants of the mold-specific *MS8* gene (GenBank AF292398, isolated from our subtracted libraries as described here) in less than 3 wk. The disruption plasmid contained the *MS8* gene disrupted with the *hph* marker and approx 1.5 kb of 5′ flanking sequence and 1.5 kb of 3′ flanking sequence. Approximately one-third of the colonies on the positive/negative selection plates were *MS8* knockouts. Experiments are in progress to examine the effect(s) of this knockout on dimorphism.

Dimorphism-Regulated Genes

Because the M–Y transformation is critical for pathogenesis, several laboratories have attempted to identify the genes required for dimorphism. Since the tools for high-throughput genomics for *Hc* are only now becoming available, existing data has been derived from very laborious low-throughput methods such as differential hybridization methods, subtracted libraries, and differential display PCR.

Hsp82, cdc2, Ole1

Several gene transcripts upregulated in the yeast morphotype have been reported in the literature. Some are yeast-specific only in certain strains but not others, indicating that they cannot be required for dimorphism. As expected, heat-shock proteins are expressed quickly after the 25°C to 37°C shift used to induce the M–Y transformation in vitro. The *hsp82* gene, for example, is transiently upregulated after the temperature upshift *(26)*. The low-virulence Downs strain is apparently more sensitive to heat shock, since maximal expression of *hsp82* requires only 34°C rather than 37°C, as in the virulent G222B strain. Di Lallo et al. *(27)* reported that the *cdc2* transcript is expressed in both the mold and yeast, but is 3.4-fold more abundant in yeast. The *Ole1* gene, encoding a desaturase involved in regulating membrane fluidity, is expressed only in the yeast form of the virulent strain G217B, but is expressed in both M and Y in the Downs strain, and thus cannot be critical for dimorphism in general *(28)*. Two particularly interesting yeast-specific genes required for survival within host phagocytes *(CBP1)* or correlated with virulent strains *(yps-3)* have been reported.

Yps-3

Keath et al. *(29)* identified the yeast-specific clone *yps-3* by differential hybridization. Expression of *yps-3* was greatest in the high-virulence strain G217B, intermediate in the moderately virulent G186B strain, and not expressed in the low-virulence Downs strain. Because the Downs strain is dimorphic, *yps-3* cannot be essential to dimorphism, but does seem to correlate with virulence. The *yps-3* coding sequence is present in Downs genomic DNA, but has a 287-bp insertion sequence that disrupts the long open reading frame (ORF) as defined by the *yps-3* G217B cDNA *(30)*. The inserted sequence has some similarity to mobile genetic elements, but does not appear to be randomly distributed in the Downs genome. Both G217B and Downs have similar *yps-3* promoter regions; thus, Downs may be deficient in a trans-acting factor(s) needed for expression. A search of the GenBank database revealed that *yps-3* has little similarity to any known gene. Western blot analysis with polyclonal anti-yps-3 sera showed that the protein is present in the culture supernatant and cell-wall fraction of G217B *(31)*. No reactive bands were observed in any fraction of the Downs strain. Further analysis of *yps-3* and a second yeast-specific gene, *yps-21:E9,* showed that a 30-Kd nuclear protein, p30, recognized a decanucleotide motif, TCCTTTTTTT, in the putative promoter regions of both yps genes and the alpha-tubulin gene *(32)*. Surprisingly, since *yps-3* and *yps-21:E9* expression are yeast-specific, p30 was only detected in the mold form of G217B and not the yeast form. It is possible that the protein, denoted as p30M, may function as a repressor by itself or in combination with other trans-acting factors. The functions of *yps-3* and *yps-21:E9* are unknown.

CBP1

Patel et al. *(33)* isolated a calcium binding protein gene *(CBP1)* expressed only in the yeast form of *Hc*. Yeast cultures, but not mold cultures, release large quantities of the *CBP1* protein into the culture medium. The upregulation of *CBP1* in yeast may play a role in calcium acquisition within the macrophage phagolysosomes, and thus assist in intracellular parasitism. Analysis of *lacZ-CBP* fusion expression in *Hc* cells identified a 102-bp region required for expression. Basepair substitution experiments indicate that the sequences between 839 and 877 nt upstream of the start codon are the most critical for positive regulation in the yeast form. Recent studies have shown that *CBP1* is required for survival within the host phagocyte. A *cbp1*-knockout strain could not proliferate in mouse macrophage-like P388D1.D2 cells, yet complementation in trans with *CBP1* restored virulence *(5)*. *CBP1* is apparently not required for dimorphism, since *cbp1*-knockout mutants are still able to grow as yeast in calcium-supplemented media.

Although a number of yeast-specific and yeast-upregulated genes have been isolated, no genes required for *Hc* dimorphism have been reported in the literature as of April 2001. It is possible that some gene(s) critical for dimorphism are being overlooked by our general assumption that yeast-specific or yeast-upregulated genes are the most important regulators. Perhaps genes that are transcriptionally silent in the yeast morphotype play a vital role in dimorphism. For example, it may be necessary, to shut off certain mold-specific genes in order to form and maintain the yeast morphotype.

Default Model of Dimorphism

To illustrate this hypothesis, we may consider the following oversimplified but useful model of a "default" morphotype of *Hc*: mold default, yeast default, or neutral default (Fig. 4). If the mold form is the default form, expression of certain Y-specific genes would be required to shift the morphology away from the mold default (i.e., the M–Y shift requires activation of certain Y-specific genes). In contrast, if the yeast form is the default form, expression of certain M-specific genes are needed to shift the morphology away from the yeast default (i.e., mold formation requires upregulation of certain mold-specific genes, and thus the M–Y shift requires shutdown of these M-specific genes). In the neutral default model, the M–Y shift would require some combination of shutdown of M-specific genes and upregulation of Y-specific genes. In the latter two scenarios, an understanding of the role of these M-specific genes would be critical to elucidate the molecular biology of dimorphism. We have no compelling data to favor any of these scenarios *a priori*. The major difficulty is to distinguish genes that are up- or downregulated as the cause of the mophogenetic shift rather than simply as a result of the morphotype switch.

Recently, workers in my laboratory have begun to isolate mold-specific as well as yeast-specific genes from non-normalized subtracted libraries (those which favor abun-

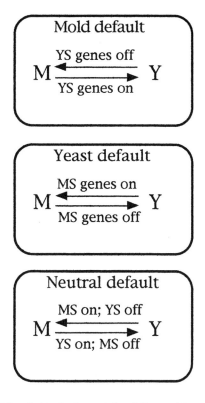

Fig. 4. Default models of dimorphism.

dant, differentially expressed transcripts) and normalized PCR-suppression subtracted libraries (which favor low-abundance, differentially expressed transcripts). Non-normalized subtracted libraries were prepared with a highly efficient modification of the enzyme-degrading subtraction method *(34)* by using rapid phenol emulsion hybridization *(35)*. Normalized subtracted libraries were prepared with a modification of the PCR suppression method *(36,37)*. From these libraries, we have isolated approx 8 unique M-specific genes and 6 unique Y-specific genes, representing both high-abundance and low-abundance transcripts. Studies are in progress to study their expression and construct knockout mutants to determine their possible roles in dimorphism.

VIRULENCE DETERMINANTS

In addition to searching for dimorphism genes, several laboratories have attempted to isolate genes that are critical for survival within the host. *Hc* is readily engulfed by phagocytic cells, and must survive in the hostile environment of the phagolysosome. Survival of *Hc* within this compartment has been shown to require yeast-protein synthesis *(38)*, suggesting that the yeast engage in an active defense. This is not surprising, since *Hc* yeast within the host phagocyte must survive a particularly harsh environment of nutrient limitation and attack by hydrolytic enzymes and reactive oxygen. Low-virulence strains are quickly killed in this environment, yet virulent strains are able to survive and proliferate. Several genes required for survival within the host phagocyte or correlated with virulence have been reported, as described here.

URA5

The first gene reported to be required for survival within phagocytes was the *Ura5* gene, which encodes orotidine-5′-monophosphate pyrophosphorylase. Retallack et al. *(4)* demonstrated that *ura5* mutant strains of *Hc* were incapable of causing infection in mice or in cultured mouse (RAW264.7) or human (U937) cells. Addition of uracil to the cell-culture medium, or supplying a *URA5* gene in trans, restored virulence to approximately the same level as seen with wild-type cells. Apparently, little free uracil is avialable within the phagolysosome during the infectious process.

Siderophores

Iron limitation by the infected host is a defense mechanism in bacterial as well as fungal infections *(39,40)*. Human serum, which is rich in unsaturated transferrin, inhibits *Hc* growth up to 50-fold, in part because of the ability of transferrin to sequester free iron *(41)*. Addition of iron to saturation or near saturation of total iron-binding capacity neutralizes the inhibitory effect. Iron limitation within phagocytic cells has also been shown to inhibit *Hc* growth. Treatment of mouse peritoneal macrophages with the intracellular iron-chelator deferoxamine inhibits the growth of *Hc* within the phagocyte. Exposure of the phagocytes to holotransferrin antagonizes the deferoxamine effect *(42)*.

A common method used by numerous microbes to grow in iron-poor environments is by secretion of siderophores that chelate iron. *Hc* has also been shown to secrete hydroxamate siderophores in culture *(43)*. Cells grown in media with less than 10 μ*M* iron produce detectable amounts of siderophores after 4 d of incubation at 37°C. Five hydroxamate siderophores have been identified: dimerum acid, acetyl dimerum acid, coprogen B, methyl coprogen B, and fusarinine (monomeric). Presumably, upregulation of one or more of the genes encoding these iron chelators promotes the survival of *Hc* yeast within the phagolysosome.

Calcium-Binding Protein

Batanghari et al. *(44)* isolated a gene encoding a calcium-binding protein *(CBP1)* that is not expressed in mold and upregulated in yeast in vitro and in vivo. Splenocytes from mice previously exposed to *Hc* yeast gave a positive proliferation response to purified *CBP1* protein, indicating that *CBP1* is expressed within the host. Knockout mutants of *CBP1* are incapable of destroying the macrophage-like cell line P388D1.D2, and do not cause disease in mice that are infected intranasally. Because the *cbp1*-knockout strains have the same generation time as wild-type yeast in broth culture, the lack of virulence is not caused by a general growth defect. Complementation in trans of *cbp1*-null strains with *CBP1* restored virulence to wild-type levels, confirming the requirement for *CBP1* in pathogenicity *(5)*.

PMA1

A possible mechanism for survival of *Hc* yeast within the host phagocyte is modulation of the acidic pH within the phagolysosome, which enhances activity of host hydrolytic enzymes. Eissenberg et al. *(45)* allowed P388D1 macrophages to engulf viable or methanol-killed *Hc* yeast and monitored vesicle pH. Phagolysosomes with viable *Hc* yeast had a pH of up to 2 U higher than vesicles with zymosan or nonviable *Hc*. Nearly neutral pH was maintained for up to 30 h in vesicles with live *Hc*. This effect was confined to vesicles with *Hc,* since vesicles containing zymosan within the same phagocyte showed normal acidification. The mechanism of this pH modulation is still unknown. One possibility is that the fungus may accomplish this by proton translocation via a plasma membrane H^+-ATPase such as the *PMA1* gene product *(46).*

Catalase

Hc yeast must also survive assault by reactive oxygen within the phagocyte. The fungistatic/fungicidal activity of murine alveolar and peritoneal macrophages is inhibited by catalase, indicating that H_2O_2 is involved. A likely possibility is that catalase produced by *Hc* cells in vivo help the yeast avoid damage from reactive compounds produced by the oxidative burst. *Histoplasma* cells produce significant amounts of catalase in vitro. Hamilton et al. *(47)* demonstrated that monoclonal antibodies (MAbs) against the M antigen, one of the major diagnostic antigens of histoplasmosis, were crossreactive against *Aspergillus niger* catalase. Zancope-Oliveira et al. have recently cloned the gene encoding the M antigen, and demonstrated that it shares significant amino-acid sequence similarity to catalases from several *Aspergillus* sp. *(48).*

Cell-Wall Composition

Cell-wall composition in *Hc* is also implicated in virulence. Most strains of *Hc* yeast give rise to somewhat rough colonies on agar plates, and tend to clump in liquid media. After extensive passage in culture, several smooth-colony, nonclumping variants have been isolated (so-called "smooth" strains). The smooth strains appear to undergo the normal M–Y dimorphism, but are far less virulent than the parental strains *(49).* Studies have shown that the smooth strains lack the α-(1,3)-glucan found in the walls of the virulent parental strains *(50).* The possible correlation of α-(1,3)-glucan levels with virulence is also observed in other pathogenic fungi. For example, strains of *Paracoccidioides brasiliensis (51)* and *Blastomyces dermatitidis (52)* with high levels of α-(1,3)-glucan are significantly more virulent than strains with reduced levels. An interesting hypothesis is that smooth variants may play a role in persistent infections that may later reactivate into clinical histoplasmosis *(53).*

A particularly intriguing feature of *Hc* growth is the apparent "quorum sensing" modulation of α-(1,3)-glucan content *(54). Hc* yeast growing within macrophages synthesize α-(1,3)-glucan constitutively. In contrast to this in vivo regulation, however, yeast growing in liquid culture medium modulate the α-(1,3)-glucan content, depending on culture density. When yeast cells synthesizing α-(1,3)-glucan are inoculated into growth medium at low cell densities, only about 30% of the cells have detectable α-(1,3)-glucan within their cell walls after 24 h. When the culture enters stationary phase, however, essentially every cell synthesizes α-(1,3)-glucan. Studies indicate that a soluble factor is released by the cells in α-(1,3)-glucan regulation. Cells inoculated into fresh medium that contained as little as 4% v/v of a filtrate from a dense culture remained positive for α-(1,3)-glucan.

Quorum sensing in bacteria involves the continuous release of a small mol-wt autoinducer. When the level of the autoinducer in the environment reaches a certain level (i.e., when the cell culture has reached a critical density), the cells respond by activating transcription of a subset of genes *(55,56)*. It is possible that *Hc* may have a similar signal to maintain α-(1,3)-glucan expression when the cells are within the host phagocyte. In contrast to the small mol wt of bacterial autoinducers, dialysis experiments indicate that the putative *Hc* autoinducer is larger than 6,000 daltons *(54)*.

THE FUTURE

The current state of knowledge regarding genomics in *Hc* is the result of the labors of many researchers who have used the low-throughput methodologies available to date. The field is now poised to utilize high-throughput methods, as recently highlighted by the human genome project. Recently, Anita Sil at the University of California at San Francisco and Lena Hwang at the University of California at Berkeley have begun development of DNA microarrays for *Hc* (A. Sil, *personal communication*). Approximately one-third of the *Hc* genome is represented in the array as 9600 random fragments ranging from 0.5 kb to 2 kb in size. Work is currently underway to construct a fully representative microarray. By screening the array with differentially labeled cDNAs, genes up- or down regulated in response to a particular stimulus can be identified. For example, the entire genome of *Hc* could be screened for dimorphism-regulated genes by probing the array with fluorescently labeled yeast and mold cDNA (e.g., green (Cy3) for yeast cDNA and red (Cy5) for mold cDNA). A few such experiments with a complete array would yield more data than all of the existing reports of subtractive screening, differential display, and other comparative methodologies.

In 1999, a Blue Ribbon Panel on Genomics was convened by the National Institutes of Health (NIAID) to identify priority organisms for future funding support for whole-genome sequencing projects. *Histoplasma capsulatum* was recently identified by the Panel as a priority organism. At least two groups are now considering sequencing the complete genome of at least one strain of *Hc*. Given the recent advances in automated sequencing, the 23-Mb *Hc* genome should be easily completed in just a few months. Perhaps by 2002 a complete *Hc* genome database will be available, which will be invaluable for comparative genomic studies, development of diagnostic probes, rapid identification of complete genes from sequence data derived from small expressed sequence tags, and other experimental approaches that are presently not feasible.

The availability of a *Hc*-genome-sequence database and DNA microarrays will give researchers the tools to quickly identify genes that may play roles in morphotype switching and pathogenesis. With this substantial improvement in our research armamentarium, it will be possible to accelerate studies to understand the molecular basis for dimorphism and the virulence of this important pathogen.

ACKNOWLEDGMENTS

I would like to thank G. Santangelo and P. Shearer for critical reading of this manuscript. The work from our laboratory was supported in part by grant AI49357 from the National Institutes of Health.

REFERENCES

1. Hammerman KJ, Powell KE, Tosh FE. The incidence of hospitalized cases of systemic mycotic infections. Sabouraudia 1974; 12:33–45.
2. Dixon DM, McNeil MM, Cohen ML, Gellin BG, La Montagne JR. Fungal infections: a growing threat. Public Health Rep 1996; 111:226–235.
3. Wheat LJ. Histoplasmosis in the acquired immunodeficiency syndrome. Curr Top Med Mycol 1996; 7:7–18.
4. Retallack DM, Heinecke EL, Gibbons R, Deepe GS, Woods JP. The URA5 gene is necessary for *Histoplasma capsulatum* growth during infection of mouse and human cells. Infect Immun 1999; 67:624–629.
5. Sebghati TS, Engle JT, Goldman WE. Intracellular parasitism by *Histoplasma capsulatum:* fungal virulence and calcium dependence. Science 2000; 290:1368–1372.
6. Maresca B, Kobayashi GS. Dimorphism in *Histoplasma capsulatum:* a model for the study of cell differentiation in pathogenic fungi. Microbiol Rev 1989; 53:186–209.
7. Medoff G, Sacco M, Maresca B, et al. Irreversible block of the mycelial-to-yeast phase transition of *Histoplasma capsulatum.* Science 1986; 231:476–479.
8. Maresca B, Lambowitz AM, Kumar VB, Grant GA, Kobayashi GS, Medoff G. Role of cysteine in regulating morphogenesis and mitochondrial activity in the dimorphic fungus *Histoplasma capsulatum.* Proc Natl Acad Sci USA 1981; 78:4596–4600.
9. Stetler DA, Boguslawski G. Cysteine biosynthesis in a fungus, *Histoplasma capsulatum.* Sabouraudia 1979; 17:23–34.
10. Rippon JW. Monitored environment system to control cell growth, morphology, and metabolic rate in fungi by oxidation-reduction potentials. Appl Microbiol 1968; 16:114–121.
11. Bawdon RE, Garrison RG, Fina LR. Deoxyribonucleic acid base composition of the yeastlike and mycelial phases of *Histoplasma capsulatum* and *Blastomyces dermatitidis.* J Bacteriol 1972; 111:593–596.
12. Vincent RD, Goewert R, Goldman WE, Kobayashi GS, Lambowitz AM, Medoff G. Classification of *Histoplasma capsulatum* isolates by restriction fragment polymorphisms. J Bacteriol 1986; 165:813–818.
13. Keath EJ, Kobayashi GS, Medoff G. Typing of *Histoplasma capsulatum* by restriction fragment length polymorphisms in a nuclear gene. J Clin Microbiol 1992; 30:2104–2107.
14. Kersulyte D, Woods JP, Keath EJ, Goldman WE, Berg DE. Diversity among clinical isolates of *Histoplasma capsulatum* detected by polymerase chain reaction with arbitrary primers. J Bacteriol 1992; 174:7075–7079.
15. Spitzer ED, Lasker BA, Travis SJ, Kobayashi GS, Medoff G. Use of mitochondrial and ribosomal DNA polymorphisms to classify clinical and soil isolates of *Histoplasma capsulatum.* Infect Immun 1989; 57:1409–1412.
16. Steele PE, Carle GF, Kobayashi GS, Medoff G. Electrophoretic analysis of *Histoplasma capsulatum* chromosomal DNA. Mol Cell Biol 1989; 9:983–987.
17. Carr J, Shearer G. Genome size, complexity, and ploidy of the pathogenic fungus *Histoplasma capsulatum.* J Bacteriol 1998; 180:6697–6703.
18. Medoff G, Kobayashi GS, Painter A, Travis S. Morphogenesis and pathogenicity of *Histoplasma capsulatum.* Infect Immun 1987; 55:1355–1358.
19. Maresca B, Kobayashi GS. Dimorphism in *Histoplasma capsulatum* and *Blastomyces dermatitidis* In: Dimorphism in Human Pathogenic and Apathogenic Yeasts. Ernst JF, Schmidt A (eds). Basel: Karger; 2000, pp. 201–216.
20. Kwon-Chung KJ. Emmonsiella capsulata: perfect state of *Histoplasma capsulatum.* Science 1972; 177:368–369.
21. Worsham PL, Goldman WE. Selection and characterization of ura5 mutants of *Histoplasma capsulatum.* Mol Gen Genet 1988; 214:348–352.

22. Worsham PL, Goldman WE. Development of a genetic transformation system for *Histoplasma capsulatum:* complementation of uracil auxotrophy. Mol Gen Genet 1990; 221:358–362.
23. Woods JP, Goldman WE. Autonomous replication of foreign DNA in *Histoplasma capsulatum:* role of native telomeric sequences. J Bacteriol 1993; 175:636–641.
24. Woods JP, Heinecke EL, Goldman WE. Electrotransformation and expression of bacterial genes encoding hygromycin phosphotransferase and beta-galactosidase in the pathogenic fungus *Histoplasma capsulatum.* Infect Immun 1998; 66:1697–1707.
25. Woods JP, Retallack DM, Heinecke EL, Goldman WE. Rare homologous gene targeting in *Histoplasma capsulatum:* disruption of the URA5Hc gene by allelic replacement. J Bacteriol 1998; 180:5135–5143.
26. Minchiotti G, Gargano S, Maresca B. Molecular cloning and expression of hsp82 gene of the dimorphic pathogenic fungus *Histoplasma capsulatum.* Biochim Biophys Acta 1992; 1131:103–107.
27. Di Lallo G, Gargano S, Maresca B. The *Histoplasma capsulatum* cdc2 gene is transcriptionally regulated during the morphologic transition. Gene 1994; 140:51–57.
28. Gargano S, Di Lallo G, Kobayashi GS, Maresca B. A temperature-sensitive strain of *Histoplasma capsulatum* has an altered delta 9-fatty acid desaturase gene. Lipids 1995; 30:899–906.
29. Keath EJ, Painter AA, Kobayashi GS, Medoff G. Variable expression of a yeast-phase-specific gene in *Histoplasma capsulatum* strains differing in thermotolerance and virulence. Infect Immun 1989; 57:1384–1390.
30. Keath EJ, Abidi FE. Molecular cloning and sequence analysis of yps-3, a yeast-phase-specific gene in the dimorphic fungal pathogen *Histoplasma capsulatum.* Microbiology 1994; 140:759–767.
31. Weaver CH, Sheehan KC, Keath EJ. Localization of a yeast-phase-specific gene product to the cell wall in *Histoplasma capsulatum.* Infect Immun 1996; 64:3048–3054.
32. Abidi FE, Roh H, Keath EJ. Identification and characterization of a phase-specific, nuclear DNA binding protein from the dimorphic pathogenic fungus *Histoplasma capsulatum.* Infect Immun 1998; 66:3867–3873.
33. Patel JB, Batanghari JW, Goldman WE. Probing the yeast phase-specific expression of the CBP1 gene in *Histoplasma capsulatum.* J Bacteriol 1998; 180:1786–1792.
34. Zeng J, Gorski RA, Hamer D. Differential cDNA cloning by enzymatic degrading subtraction (EDS). Nucleic Acids Res 1994; 22:4381–4385.
35. Miller RD, Riblet R. Improved phenol emulsion DNA reassociation technique (PERT) using thermal cycling. Nucleic Acids Res 1995; 23:2339–2340.
36. Diatchenko L, Lau YF, Campbell AP, et al. Suppression subtractive hybridization: a method for generating differentially regulated or tissue specific cDNA probes and libraries. Proc Natl Acad Sci USA 1996; 93:6025–6030.
37. Gurskaya NG, Diatchenko L, Chenchik A, et al. Equalizing cDNA subtraction based on selective suppression of polymerase chain reaction: cloning of Jurkat cell transcripts induced by phyto-hemaglutinin and phorbol 12-myristate 13-acetate. Anal Biochem 1996; 240:90–97.
38. Newman SL, Gootee L, Morris R, Bullock WE. Digestion of *Histoplasma capsulatum* yeasts by human macrophages. J Immunol 1992; 149:574–580.
39. Ratledge C, Dover LG. Iron metabolism in pathogenic bacteria. Annu Rev Microbiol 2000; 54:881–941.
40. Howard DH. Acquisition, transport, and storage of iron by pathogenic fungi. Clin Microbiol Rev 1999; 12:394–404.
41. Sutcliffe MC, Savage AM, Alford RH. Transferrin dependent growth inhibition of yeast-phase *Histoplasma capsulatum* by human serum and lymph. J Infect Dis 1980; 142:209–219.
42. Lane TE, Wu-Hsieh BA, Howard DH. Iron limitation and the gamma interferon-mediated anti-histoplasma state of murine macrophages. Infect Immun 1991; 59:2274–2278.

43. Howard DH, Rafie R, Tiwari A, Faull KF. Hydroxamate siderophores of *Histoplasma capsulatum.* Infect Immun 2000; 68:2338–2343.

44. Batanghari JW, Deepe GS, Di Cera E, Goldman WE. *Histoplasma acquisition* of calcium and expression of CBP1 during intracellular parasitism. Mol Microbiol 1998; 27:531–539.

45. Eissenberg LG, Goldman WE, Schlesinger PH. *Histoplasma capsulatum* modulates the acidification of phagolysosomes. J Exp Med 1993; 177:1605–1611.

46. Schafer MP, Dean GE. Cloning and sequence analysis of an H(+)-ATPase-encoding gene from the human dimorphic pathogen *Histoplasma capsulatum.* Gene 1993; 136:295–300.

47. Hamilton AJ, Bartholomew MA, Figueroa J, Fenelon LE, Hay RJ. Evidence that the M antigen of *Histoplasma capsulatum* var. *capsulatum* is a catalase which exhibits cross-reactivity with other dimorphic fungi. J Med Vet Mycol 1990; 28:479–485.

48. Zancope-Oliveira RM, Reiss E, Lott TJ, Mayer LW, Deepe GS. Molecular cloning, characterization, and expression of the M antigen of *Histoplasma capsulatum.* Infect Immun 1999; 67:1947–1953.

49. Klimpel KR, Goldman WE. Isolation and characterization of spontaneous avirulent variants of *Histoplasma capsulatum.* Infect Immun 1987; 55:528–533.

50. Klimpel KR, Goldman WE. Cell walls from avirulent variants of *Histoplasma capsulatum* lack alpha- (1,3)-glucan. Infect Immun 1988; 56:2997–3000.

51. San-Blas G, San-Blas F, Serrano LE. Host-parasite relationships in the yeastlike form of *Paracoccidioides brasiliensis* strain IVIC Pb9. Infect Immun 1977; 15:343–346.

52. Hogan LH, Klein BS. Altered expression of surface alpha- 1,3-glucan in genetically related strains of *Blastomyces dermatitidis* that differ in virulence. Infect Immun 1994; 62:3543–3546.

53. Eissenberg LG, Poirier S, Goldman WE. Phenotypic variation and persistence of *Histoplasma capsulatum* yeasts in host cells. Infect Immun 1996; 64:5310–5314.

54. Kugler S, Schurtz ST, Groppe EL, Goldman WE. Phenotypic variation and intracellular parasitism by *Histoplasma capsulatum.* Proc Natl Acad Sci USA 2000; 97:8794–8798.

55. Rumbaugh KP, Griswold JA, Hamood AN. The role of quorum sensing in the in vivo virulence of *Pseudomonas aeruginosa.* Microbes Infect 2000; 2:1721–1731.

56. de Kievit TR, Iglewski BH. Bacterial quorum sensing in pathogenic relationships. Infect Immun 2000; 68:4839–4849.

16

Gene-Finding in *Coccidioides immitis*

Searching for Immunogenic Proteins

Theo N. Kirkland and Garry T. Cole

INTRODUCTION

Coccidioides immitis is a primary fungal pathogen that lives in the soil of the desert Southwest. Like most medically important fungi that cause systemic disease, *C. immitis* exhibits different morphologies in its saprobic and parasitic phases, but is distinguished from other fungal pathogens by the unique morphogenetic features of its growth in host tissue (Fig. 1). Coccidioidomycosis, the disease caused by this pathogenic fungus, is also known as Valley Fever because the organism is prevalent in the San Joaquin Valley of Central California. *C. immitis* infections are caused by inhalation of the organism. The clinical spectrum of disease is broad, ranging from an asymptomatic infection to a rapidly fatal mycosis *(1)*. The most common clinical presentation is self-limited pneumonia, but in some cases the fungus can cause chronic cavitary pulmonary disease or disseminate beyond the lungs to the skin, bones, meninges, and other body organs. It has been estimated, primarily on the basis of skin tests, that there are between 25,000 and 100,000 new cases of human *C. immitis* infections each year in the United States. Approximately 5% of these new cases progress to disseminated disease.

Disseminated disease, especially meningitis, can be fatal. All forms of dissemination require prolonged treatment with antifungal drugs *(2)*. *C. immitis* meningitis must be treated for life *(3)*. The direct cost of medical supplies and sick leave for patients with Valley Fever has also escalated. In Kern County, California, located at the epicenter of the endemic region in that state, the accrued cost of the disease from 1991 to 1995 was estimated at more than $66 million. Although disseminated coccidioidomycosis is rare, and symptomatic coccidioidal pneumonia usually resolves without therapy, many of these patients are very ill for long periods of weeks to months. Dr. John Galgiani reported that a group of college students in Tucson who had coccidioidomycosis required an average of six clinic visits before the disease resolved *(4)*. Therefore, this can be an expensive illness in terms of medical costs and time lost from work or school, even when the infection resolves spontaneously. The vaccination of persons at risk of contacting coccidioidomycosis is a feasible approach to the control of this insidious fungal disease.

From: *Pathogen Genomics: Impact on Human Health*
Edited by: K. J. Shaw © Humana Press Inc., Totowa, NJ

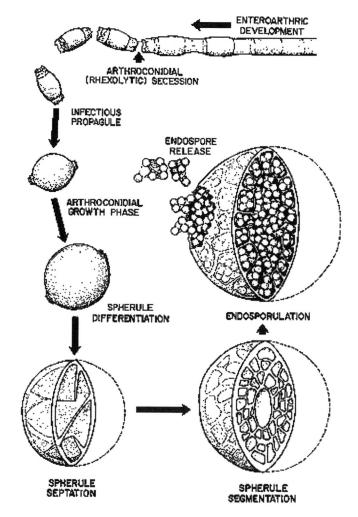

Fig. 1. The life cycle of *C. immitis* in human beings.

Recovery from coccidioidomycosis requires cell-mediated immunity. Patients who develop a positive skin test to *C. immitis* antigens tend to recover from their illness *(5)*. Those who have high titers of antibody to *C. immitis* are at higher risk for development of disseminated infection *(6)*. Since people who recover from *C. immitis* infection are almost never re-infected, natural immunity must be robust. In mice, T-lymphocytes are absolutely required for resistance to infection *(7)*. Mice can be successfully vaccinated by immunization with killed organisms or recombinant proteins *(8–10)*. For these reasons, there is great interest in the development of a vaccine against *C. immitis*.

GEOGRAPHIC DISTRIBUTION

Coccidioidomycosis is primarily found in the desert regions of Southern California, Arizona, Nevada, New Mexico, and West Texas. This large area is home to approximately 20% of the population of the United States. It also includes some of the most rapidly expanding cities in the nation, and attracts large numbers of visitors each year. The urban perimeters extend further into the desert each year, as exemplified by the Bakersfield region of California and the Phoenix-Tucson area of Arizona.

Many cases of coccidioidomycosis have also been reported in regions that are not hyperendemic, such as San Diego and Los Angeles *(1)*. Outbreaks of coccidioidomy-cosis have occurred among archaeology students digging in prehistoric Indian sites in Northern California. In 1977, a major dust storm blew soil from the San Joaquin Valley up into regions of Northern California, including San Francisco, Marin County, Santa Clara, and Monterey County. Immediately following the storm, numerous cases of coc-cidioidomycosis were reported in nonendemic regions of middle and Northern California. At the time, there was some concern that *C. immitis* may be able to seed and persist in the soil in these areas, but this has not occurred. The range of *C. immitis* includes West Texas and a large part of the desert regions of Northern Mexico. A few cases of coccidioidomycosis have also been reported in Central and South America. The largest South American endemic region is in Argentina, where the climate is dry and the soil conditions are similar to those in the desert Southwest of the United States. Despite these geographic limitations, physicians outside the endemic regions should consider coccidioidomycosis as a possible diagnosis of a respiratory infection if the patient has ever traveled through the desert Southwest or lived in an endemic area. Reactivation of a prior asymptomatic *C. immitis* infection is potential concern for an immunocompro-mised individual *(11)*.

MYCOLOGY

Arthroconidium Formation

The soil-inhabiting mycelial phase of *C. immitis* gives rise to infectious, airborne arthroconidia through what appears to be a simple process of fragmentation of hyphal elements. Single, cylindrical arthroconidia (approx $3–6 \times 2–4$ μm) are small enough to pass down the respiratory tree and reach the alveoli of the host. Most conidia, however, probably impact the mucosal lining of the upper respiratory tract. The ciliated epithe-lial cells lining the upper airways are capable of sweeping the mucus and entrapped fungal cells proximally toward the pharynx, where they are removed through the diges-tive tract. *C. immitis* conidia do not adhere to or germinate in the gastrointestinal tract.

Those arthroconidia that reach the terminal air sacs encounter alveolar macrophages. Evidence from experimental animal studies of coccidioidomycosis has indicated that host phagocytes are ineffective in the clearance of the infectious propag-ules *(12)*. Arthroconidia of *C. immitis* appear to be well-equipped with barriers to host defenses. The outer conidial-wall layer, which is derived from the original hyphal wall, is a hydrophobic sleeve that may have evolved as an adaptation for air dispersal of the soil saprobe. It may also serve as a passive barrier to destructive enzymes and oxidative products released by the host defense cells, and thereby contribute to survival of the pathogen in vivo.

Successful colonization of the host respiratory mucosa by *C. immitis* depends on conversion of arthroconidia to "round cells" or spherules. Little is known of the mor-phogenetic features of the initial stages of this saprobic to parasitic phase transition, and limited information is available on growth factors, which influence this process. A common requirement for such transitions among dimorphic fungal pathogens is an abrupt rise in temperature, typically from 25°C to 37°C. Thermal dimorphism in *Histoplasma capsulatum,* a related fungal respiratory pathogen, has been examined intensively. Morphogenetic events associated with transition from the hyphal to yeast phase in *H. capsulatum* are part of a complexity of physiological changes referred to as the heat-shock response. Studies of dimorphism in *H. capsulatum* have focused on identification of the "primary sensor" capable of monitoring temperature shifts, and the mechanisms by which molecular signals are transmitted from the sensor to the nucleus, where they ultimately influence expression of specific genes. These studies provide a model for the examination of thermal dimorphism in other fungal pathogens.

SPHERULE GROWTH AND SEGMENTATION

Growth

The isotropic growth phase of the spherule initially results in a spherule that may be 60 μm or more in diameter. A large central vacuole is usually observed in sectioned preparations of parasitic cells at this stage of development *(13)*. The vacuole has been suggested to be a source of internal turgor pressure, and is most likely an important reservoir for ions and macromolecules. Diametric growth of spherules, such as hyphal-tip elongation, probably relies on coordinated processes of turgor-driven expansion, plasticization of the pre-existing wall, and biosynthesis and intussusception of new-wall polymers. Isotropic growth of spherules is complete or nears completion when the process of segmentation begins *(13)*. Spherule segmentation is a process initiated by centripetal growth of the innermost-wall layer of the cell envelope. Ingrowth from various sites on the inner circumference of the spherule appears to be synchronous at the initiation of segmentation wall differentiation. Invaginated regions of newly synthesized wall fuse and give rise to isolated cytoplasmic compartments. The latter are further subdivided by cross-walls, to generate a multitude of small cytoplasmic units within the parental spherule. The central vacuole is still prominent at this stage.

Segmentation

Segmentation is apparently arrested when uninucleate, cytoplasmic compartments are formed. The segmentation wall then begins to undergo autolysis, and the central vacuole disappears as the uninucleate cells initiate differentiation into endospores. This event gives rise to approx 200–300 endospores per spherule. The endospores at this stage are typically 2–4 μm in diameter. Prior to endospore release from the maternal spherule, only fragments of the original segmentation wall remain. Breakdown of the segmentation apparatus may be partially caused by mechanical fractures in the rigid wall polymers as isotropic growth of the endospores is initiated. However, it is more likely that wall hydrolases secreted by the endospores are responsible for autolysis of the segmentation wall. Results of preliminary electron-microscopic studies of endosporulating spherules have revealed that chitin largely disappears within the spherule as endospores begin to form. At least two chitinases are expressed by *C. immitis (14)*. An understanding of their function(s) awaits molecular analyses of morphogenetic events in *C. immitis.* The endospores, although still contained within the maternal spherule, begin to undergo isotropic growth that results in rupture of the spherule wall. Under appropriate growth conditions, the endospores that are released give rise to a second generation of spherules, thus completing the parasitic cycle of *C. immitis.*

TAXONOMIC AFFINITY OF *C. immitis*

Sigler and Carmichael reintroduced the genus *Malbranchea* for soil saprobes with arthroconidia, which form by a process identical to that of *C. immitis (15).* Many of the true fungal pathogens of humans are placed in separate families of the order Onyge-nales, including agents of cutaneous infection in the Arthrodermataceae (*Trichophyton* and *Microsporum*), and respiratory pathogens in the Onygenaceae (*Coccidioides, Histoplasma,* and *Blastomyces*). Currah has argued that these two families include nat-ural groups of related ascomycetous fungi characterized by ascospore-cell walls that are smooth (Arthrodermataceae), or punctuate-reticulate (Onygenaceae), conidia, which form by lytic dehiscence mechanisms, and mycelia that have the ability to degrade keratin *(16).* Although strong morphologic evidence points to a close relation-ship between *C. immitis* and certain members of the Onygenaceae, results have not yet been confirmed.

Malbranchea also produces a sexual phase, and the teleomorph is known as *Uncinocarpus reesii.* This nonpathogenic, filamentous fungus, together with tele-morphs of other morphologically similar *Malbranchea* species, is classified in the Onygenales. Molecular evidence suggests that a close phylogenetic connection exists between *C. immitis* and *U. reesii (17).* Alignments of 18S rDNA sequences of *C. immitis, U. reesii,* and seven additional members of the Onygenaceae were compared, including *H. capsulatum, B. dermatitidis,* and five arthroconidium-producing soil saprobes accommodated in the genus *Malbranchea.* The 1,713-bp sequences of *U. reesii* rDNA differ from that of *C. immitis* by only 5 bp substitutions. Wagener parsi-mony analysis of these nine 18S rDNA sequences was performed together with com-parisons of sequences from seven additional pathogenic and nonpathogenic fungi obtained from the GenBank database. The maximum parsimony tree strongly sup-ports a close relationship between *C. immitis* and *U. reesii,* and argues that these taxa represent a monophyletic pair within the Onygenaceae. Despite this close evolution-ary relationship, *U. reesii* is not an animal pathogen.

GENOME STRUCTURE OF *C. immitis*

The *C. immitis* genome is 28 million bp in length, and is divided into four chromo-somes *(18).* No plasmids have been identified. *C. immitis* appears to be haploid in both the mycelial and spherule forms. The gene density is not known, but estimates from other filamentous fungi suggest that the genome codes for approx 12,000 proteins. *C. immitis* genes frequently contain introns, which makes gene identification more diffi-cult. The genes that have been characterized thus far have as many as eight introns, but most have 1–3 introns. The introns tend to be less than 100 bp long.

C. immitis has never been observed in a sexual state. However, recombination occurs at a rate that is higher than that expected by random mutation *(19).* Studies with anonymous molecular markers have shown that *C. immitis* isolates fall into two groups. Recombination occurs within each group, but the two groups do not recombine with each other. The mechanism of recombination is unclear *(19)*. The two groups of organisms are also geographically isolated from each other *(20)*. It has been proposed that these two groups of isolates represent two different species, but this proposal is controversial. Isolates from both groups cause human disease.

GENE-FINDING IN *C. immitis*

Preliminary sequencing of the *C. immitis* genome has been done in collaboration with Dr. Malcolm Gardner at the Institute for Genome Research. We have taken a two-pronged approach, using sequencing of expressed sequence tags (ESTs) and genomic sequencing. The ESTs were derived from a cDNA library made from spherule mRNA. Clones were randomly picked for DNA sequencing. The clones were sequenced from both ends with an average read length of 500 bp. The sequences were assembled by computer, and annotated by BLASTX analysis. The annotated EST database for *C. immitis,* which currently consists of 1,626 unique EST sequences, is available on the TIGR website at www.tigr.org.

Several genomic libraries with inserts from 2–10 Kb have been made and sequenced from each end. Because of an improvement in sequencing technology, the average read length increased to 650 bp. These sequences have also been assembled into contigs. Of the 6000 unique contigs analyzed to date, 25% have significant BLASTX matches to the nonredundant genomic NCBI database with an E value of $<10^{-4}$. As expected, the genes code for a wide variety of proteins. There is a bias toward highly conserved proteins, which tend to be "housekeeping" genes. However, a number of sequences present in the EST and genomic data are potential vaccine candidates.

The genomic sequence of *Neiserria meningitis* has been successfully used to predict protein-vaccine candidates for that organism. Potential candidates were defined as surface proteins or excreted proteins. We have defined potential vaccine candidates as proteins that are either expressed on the cell wall or excreted, and are not highly homologous to mammalian proteins. One vaccine candidate that has shown promise is the *C. immitis* cell-wall protein known as antigen 2, or the proline-rich antigen (Ag2/PRA) *(8)*. The function of this protein is unknown, but it is anchored to the cell wall by a glycophosphatidylinositol (GPI) linkage. Experiments in mice have shown that immunization with this protein significantly protects animals from *C. immitis* infection *(8,9)*. We have looked for other proteins that are predicted to be GPI-linked, based on homology with proteins that are GPI-linked in other fungi and have some promising preliminary data with one of these. Enzymes involved in modification of carbohydrate polymers during growth of the spherule are also promising candidates, since they should be exposed to the host immune system. There are several families of glucanases, glucoside transferases, and chitinases that are potential vaccine candidates. Secreted enzymes are also attractive possibilities as vaccines. We have identified a number of peptidases, as well as an alkaline phosphatase (Table 1). Homology to proteins that have been found to be immunogenic in other organisms, such as the heat-shock proteins, also suggests potential vaccine candidates. Using these guidelines, about 1% of the 6000 contigs tentatively identified thus far are potential candidates.

Of course, we cannot be sure that the proteins we have identified as potential vaccine candidates are immunogenic. We also know that not all cell-wall-associated proteins are effective vaccines in mice. In addition, we have found that some proteins that are

Table 1
Potential vaccine candidates

Category	Number
Peptidases	17
Glucan transferases	10
Glucanases	12
Heat-shock proteins	5
Misc. cell-wall-associated proteins	20

effective vaccines for other fungi are not an effective for *C. immitis (21)*. The hsp60 protein of *Histoplasma capsulatum* is an effective vaccine for experimental histoplasmosis in mice, but the *C. immitis* homologue, which is highly homologous to the *H. capsulatum* gene, is not an effective vaccine for *C. immitis* infection *(21)*. In addition, some cytoplasmic proteins are able to provide a modest amount of immunoprotection *(22)*. This may be the result of the release of cytoplasmic proteins as the organism ruptures when endospores are released. Nevertheless, these criteria seem to be reasonable ones for choosing vaccine candidates.

There are several options for testing vaccine candidates. We have found that surrogate markers such as T-cell proliferation in response to a given antigen are poor predictors of a successful vaccine *(8)*. In fact, Ag2/PRA elicits a very small proliferative response in T cells from *C. immitis*-immune mice. Therefore, we have chosen to conduct immunization and infectious challenge experiments. The immunization could be done with plasmids coding for the gene of interest, or with synthetic peptides conjugated to a carrier protein. Of these options, we currently favor synthetic peptides as the most efficient method for screening vaccine candidates.

We believe that genomic sequencing holds promise as a method for suggesting potential vaccine candidates. In addition, the sequence of genes involved in cell-wall synthesis, metabolism, cell division, and other essential functions will provide targets for drug development. Given the relatively low cost of DNA sequencing, we believe that determining the genomic sequence of *C. immitis* is a cost-effective way to better understand this fungus.

REFERENCES

1. Kirkland TN, Fierer J. Coccidioidomycosis: a reemerging infectious disease. Emerg Infect Dis 1996; 2:192–199.
2. Galgiani JN. Coccidioidomycosis. West J Med 1993; 159:153–171.
3. Dewsnup DH, Galgiani JN, Leviner BE, Sharkey-Mathis PK, Fierer J, Stevens DA. Is it ever safe to stop azole therapy for Coccidioides immitis meningitis? Ann Intern Med 1996; 124:305–310.
4. Kerrick SS, Lundergan LL, Galgiani JN. Coccidioidomycosis at a university health service. Am Rev Respir Dis 1985; 131:100–102.
5. Smith CE, Whiting EG, Baker EE, Rosenberger HG, Beard RR, Saito MT. The use of coccidioidin. Am Rev Tuberculosis 1948; 57:330–351.
6. Smith CE, Saito MT, Simons SA. Pattern of 39,500 serologic tests in coccidioidomycosis. JAMA 1956; 160:546–552.
7. Beaman L, Pappagianis D, Benjamini E. Mechanisms of resistance to infection with Coccidioides immitis in mice. Infect Immun 1979; 23:681–685.

8. Kirkland TN, Finley F, Orsborn KI, Galgiani JN. Evaluation of the proline-rich antigen of Coccidioides immitis as a vaccine candidate in mice. Infect Immun 1998; 66:3519–3522.

9. Abuodeh RO, Shubitz LF, Siegel E, Snyder S, Peng T, Osborn KI et al. Resistance to Coccidioides immitis in mice after immunization with recombinant protein or a DNA vaccine of a proline-rich antigen. Infect Immun 1999; 67:2935–2940.

10. Li K, Yu J, Hung C, Lehmann PF, Cole GT. Recombinant urease and urease DNA of Coccidioides immitis elicit an immunoprotective response against coccidioidomycosis in mice. Infect Immun 2001; 69:2878–2887.

11. Deresinski SC, Stevens DA. Coccidioidomycosis in compromised hosts—experience at Stanford University hospital. Medicine (Balt) 1974; 54:377–395.

12. Ampel NM, Galgiani JN. Interaction of human peripheral blood mononuclear cells with Coccidioides immitis arthroconidia. Cell Immunol 1991; 133:253–262.

13. Sun SH, Cole GT, Drutz DJ, Harrison JL. Electron-microscopic observations of the Coccidioides immitis parasitic cycle in vivo. J Med Vet Mycol 1986; 24:183–192.

14. Pishko EJ, Kirkland T, Cole GT. Isolation and characterization of two chitinase-encoding genes (cts1 and cts2) from the fungus Coccidioides immitis. Gene 1995; 167:173–177.

15. Sigler L, Carmichael JW. Taxonomy of malbranchea and some other hyphomycetes with arthroconidia. Mycotaxon 1976; 4:349–488.

16. Currah RS. Taxonomy of the onygenales: arthrodermataceae, gymnoascacease, myxotrichaceae and onygenaceae. Mycotaxon 1985; 24:1–216.

17. Pan S, Sigler L, Cole GT. Evidence for a phylogenetic connection between Coccidioides immitis and Uncinocarpus reesii (onygenaceae). Microbiology 1994; 140:1481–1494.

18. Pan S, Cole GT. Electrophoretic karyotypes of clinical isolates of Coccidioides immitis. Infect Immun 1992; 60:4872–4880.

19. Burt A, Carter D, Koenig G, Whute T, Taylor JW. Molecular markers reveal cryptic sex in the human pathogen Coccidioides immitis. Proc Natl Acad Sci USA 1996; 93:700–773.

20. Koufopanou V, Burt A, Taylor JW. Concordance of gene genealogies reveals reproductive isolation in the pathogenic fungus Coccidioides immitis. Proc Natl Acad Sci USA 1997; 94:5478–5482.

21. Deepe GS, Gibbons R, Brunner GD, Gomez FJ. A protective domain of heat-shock protein 60 from Histoplasma capsulatum. J Infect Dis 1996; 174:828–834.

22. Kirkland TN, Thomas PW, Finley F, Cole GT. Immunogenicity of a 48-kilodalton recombinant T-cell reactive protein of Coccidioides immitis. Infect Immun 1998; 66:424–431.

IV PROTOZOA

17

Toxoplasma gondii
A Model for Evolutionary Genomics and Chemotherapy

Jessica C. Kissinger, Michael J. Crawford, David S. Roos, and James W. Ajioka

INTRODUCTION: EVOLUTIONARY GENOMICS
OF *Toxoplasma gondii*

Effective chemotherapy requires the inhibition of critical molecular processes in the target pathogen without significantly impinging on those of the host. This simple principle requires that the host and pathogen must be different in some aspect, usually in a metabolic or structural pathway. However, apicomplexan parasites such as *Toxoplasma gondii* and the hosts that they infect are both eukaryotic organisms. Thus, finding unique drug targets in essential pathways is difficult, and requires extensive searches for unique processes that can serve as effective targets for drug design. The current treatment of toxoplasmosis reflects our former and very limited understanding of these parasites, as the drugs are confined to broad-spectrum antibiotics or variations on antibacterial compounds. Moreover, their specific mode of action in the parasite remained largely undefined until the advent of genetic, genomic and cellular methods of investigation (for reviews, *see* refs. *1–3*).

Three recent events have changed the drug-discovery landscape for *T. gondii* and other apicomplexan parasites: (1) The generation of *T. gondii* expressed sequence tags (ESTs) *(4,5)*, (2) The discovery of a plastid-like organelle, the "apicoplast," in apicomplexan parasites including *T. gondii (6–9)*, and (3) The complete genome sequence of an Apicomplexan parasite *(Plasmodium falciparum) (10,11)*. These investigations revealed a unique evolutionary history for *T. gondii* and the Apicomplexa. The evidence suggests that primary and secondary endosymbiotic events produced a "chimeric" cell with two organelles/organellar genomes and a "mosaic" nuclear genome composed of genetic material from various sources, including a photosynthetic algae. Collectively, these advances provide large-sequence data sets and a new evolutionary framework for the search for novel drug targets. We are now challenged with the development of biological and computational tools to exploit these resources for the identification and verification of new chemotherapeutic targets.

From: *Pathogen Genomics: Impact on Human Health*
Edited by: K. J. Shaw © Humana Press Inc., Totowa, NJ

Evolution of **T. gondii** *(Apicomplexans):* **Primary and Secondary Endosymbioses**

Eukaryotic cells are chimeric by their very nature, but the compositional complexity of a particular lineage depends upon their evolutionary history. Through a series of evolutionary events (endosymbioses), the organelle-containing eukaryotic cell was formed. Mitochondria and chloroplasts evolved through primary endosymbiotic events with alpha-proteobacteria and cyanobacteria, respectively. Each of these organelles contains remnants of its original genome, but in many cases, genes originally encoded in the organellar genome have been transferred to the host nuclear genome (Fig. 1A). The protein products of these nuclear-encoded organellar genes are then targeted back to the organelle, where they continue to function. A secondary endosymbiotic event between two eukaryotic cells may occur when one cell engulfs another cell, notably between a non-photosynthetic cell and a photosynthetic cell. Apicomplexan parasites (if not all alveolata *(12)* appear to have been derived by such a secondary endosymbiotic event (see Fig. 1B). The apicoplast organelle, surrounded by its four membranes, appears to be the major remnant of an alga engulfed in a secondary endosymbiosis *(8,13)*. The apicoplast organelle of *Toxoplasma gondii* and many other apicomplexan parasites has been sequenced in whole or in part, and is a bona fide highly reduced chloroplast genome with a gene content that provides little insight into the function of this essential organelle. However, from the perspective of chemotherapy, the discovery of this organelle and its evolutionary origin represented a critical breakthrough in the search for novel chemotherapeutic targets. The products encoded in the organellar genome or those encoded by organellar genes that have been transferred to the host nuclear genome (*see* Fig. 1) are of cyanobacterial or algal origin, and thus may serve as effective drug targets. In this way, *T. gondii* and other apicomplexan parasites can be viewed as evolutionary chimeras at the genetic and biochemical levels. The discussion that follows examines the variety of potential chemotherapeutic targets that exist (mitochondrial, plastid, algal, and nuclear), and the techniques and tools that are available to discover and effectively test potential chemotherapeutic candidates.

Overview of **T. gondii** *Genetics*

The nuclear portion of the *T. gondii* genome is haploid for most of the parasite's life cycle, except for a brief diploid phase in the cat intestine prior to meiosis *(14)*. The genome is estimated to be 80–87 Mb, and genetic linkage analysis of approx 80 polymorphic loci defines eleven linkage groups with a total of 147 centimorgans (see ref. *15;* also summarized in ref. *16*). Because *T. gondii* chromosomes do not condense during meiosis, the karyotype was determined by pulsed-field gel electrophoretic *(PFGE)* analysis, which revealed 11 chromosomes designated by Roman numerals Ib, Ia, II to X, ranging in size from approx 1.9 Mb to greater than 10 Mb (the present limit that can be determined by PFGE) respectively *(17)*. The congruence of the linkage and karyotype analyses suggests that all of the chromosomes have been identified. Karyotype comparisons between strains show very little chromosomal size variation compared to other Apicomplexa such as *Plasmodium* spp. and are highly stable with passage, revealing no apparent changes in over 10 yr of continual passage *(17,18)*. Current and future genomic sequencing of *T. gondii* will refine our view of these data (J.W. Ajioka and D.S. Roos, *personal communication*).

A Primary Endosymbioses

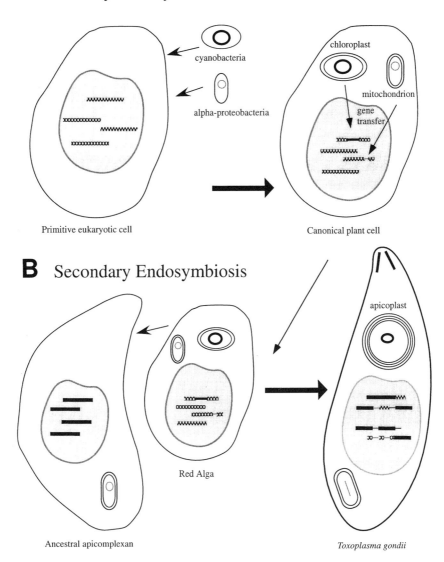

B Secondary Endosymbiosis

Fig. 1. Diagram of primary and secondary endosymbiotic events. (**A**) Primary endosymbioses; a prokaryotic cyanobacterium and alpha-proteobacterium are independently acquired via endosymbioses. The resulting eukaryotic cell contains organelles surrounded by two membranes, each containing its own genome. The process of gene transfer from the organellar genomes to the nuclear genome begins (indicated by insertion of thin gray and black lines into hatched eukaryotic chromosomes). (**B**) Secondary endosymbiosis; a eukaryotic cell containing a mitochondrion engulfs a eukaryotic algal cell. The algal nucleus is lost, but not before the transfer of numerous algal and organellar genes to the host nuclear genome (indicated by the insertion of hatched and linear elements into the thick black host chromosomes). The apicoplast, surrounded by four membranes, is the lone remnant of the algal cell. The transfer of organellar genes to the host nucleus continues. The mitochondrial genome is linearized.

Population genetic analyses have revealed that worldwide geographic isolates of *T. gondii* belong to one of three clonal lineages *(19,20)*. Although genetic exchange between the lineages occurs naturally and in deliberate crosses, the lineages—referred to as Types I, II, and III—are estimated to diverge by about 1% at the nucleotide level, and differ phenotypically and in host distribution *(20)*. Type I is a mouse virulent strain and does not readily participate in the sexual cycle, whereas Types II and III are non-virulent and retain the ability to complete the entire life cycle *(20,21)*.

The *T. gondii* nuclear DNA has a GC content of approx 55% compared to approx 20% for *Plasmodium* spp. *(10,11,22)*. Based on estimates from other apicomplexan parasites, we estimate that there are 6,000–8,000 nuclear-encoded genes, and cluster analysis of *T. gondii*. ESTs suggests that a significant proportion have been identified *(4,5)*. The genes examined to date appear to have a fairly conventional eukaryotic structure, in which the number and size of introns varies between genes, but may be typified by the gene encoding the microneme protein MIC2, which has a coding sequence of 2307 basepairs (bp) with three introns of 413, 167, respectively and 375 bp, *(23)*. Gene expression in *T. gondii* appears to be transcriptionally regulated, although conventional *cis*-acting eukaryotic promoters such as the TATA box or SP1 motif have not been observed. Upstream sequence analysis of several genes has identified a common, highly conserved T/AGAGACG heptanucleotide core element *(24–26)*, which that qualitatively acts like SP1 elements in determining transcriptional start sites in the absence of TATA promoter elements *(25,27)*.

T. gondii *Pathogenesis and the Need for New Drugs*

The parasitic protozoan *T. gondii* is a ubiquitous pathogen with the ability to infect virtually all warm-blooded animals *(28)*. Although *T. gondii* can invade and propagate in most nucleated cells, the usual disease pathology of the acute infection in immuno-competent hosts varies from asymptomatic to mild flu-like symptoms *(29)*. The major problems arise in hosts without effective immune defenses, such as transplacental fetal infections *(30)* or infection of immunocompromised AIDS patients *(31)*. *T. gondii* infection in the fetus is a major source of birth defects (e.g., brain damage, blindness), affecting up to 0.1% of live births in some locations *(32,33)*. Recrudescence of the latent cyst-form infection and the resulting life-threatening encephalitis appear in a significant proportion of AIDS patients *(31)*. Currently, no available drugs are effective against the latent form of the parasite, relegating AIDS patients to continuous prophylaxis with drugs used to treat the acute infection *(34)*. Along with the need to find new drugs to treat toxoplasmosis, *T. gondii* has emerged as the best model system for apicomplexan diseases such as malaria (*Plasmodium* spp.) and avian coccidiosis (*Eimeria* spp.) (*see* for example, articles in refs. *35* and *3*). The ability to culture *T. gondii* in vitro and development of molecular genetics and genomics allow investigations that are difficult or presently not possible in the other species. The exploitation of this taxonomic relationship between *T. gondii* and *P. falciparum* has already been successful in evaluating the natural selection of drug resistance in malaria *(36)*.

Nuclear-Encoded Chemotherapeutic Targets Present in the Cytosol

Some of the traditional drug targets and targets identified as a result of the recent discovery of genes of cyanobacterial and algal ancestry in the apicomplexan lineage appear to be nuclear-encoded, and function in the cytosol. Parasites, by definition, cannot exist as free-living organisms, and rely on the host for a variety of essential metabolites. *T. gondii*, like other protozoan parasites, have very limited mechanisms to salvage or synthesize nucleobases/nucleosides and aromatic amino acids *(37,38)*. The algal ancestry hypothesis stimulated both the search for *T. gondii* (and *Plasmodium* spp.) orthologs of plant enzymes in sequence databases and direct testing of known herbicides. Although the plant-like drug targets studied to date are nuclear-encoded, they belong to synthetic pathways or structural elements that may function either in the apicoplast or the cytosol of the parasite. The enzymes involved with fatty-acid synthesis localize to the apicoplast, and targets such as microtubules are likely to be primarily affected in the cytosol or nucleus *(39,40)*. Other targets such as enzymes in the shikimate pathway may function in either the apicoplast or cytoplasm, where the evolutionary origin of the pathway may provide vital clues to the site of activity *(41–43)*.

Purine Salvage and Subversive Substrates

Intracellular protozoan parasites such as *T. gondii* cannot synthesize purines *de novo* *(38)*, and depend upon salvage of host purines *(44,45)*. Subversive substrates such as adenine arabinoside (araA) have been the main working tools for defining purine metabolism in *T. gondii* (for recent review, *see* ref. *3*). These compounds have been invaluable for defining and characterizing these salvage pathways, but their structure-function relationships with specific enzymes may not be absolute predictors of therapeutic utility because the mechanism(s) of their toxicity may not correlate with the efficiency of the initial enzymatic reactions (*see* ref. *46*).

The parasitophorous vacuole allows free diffusion of small molecules on the order of 1.3 kDa *(47)*, and specific transporters move the nucleoside adenosine and the purine bases adenine, guanine, hypoxanthine, and xanthine across the plasma membrane *(48,49)*. Although *T. gondii* uses both nucleoside and nucleobase salvage, adenosine import and metabolism probably accounts for the majority of purine acquisition *(44)*. The conversion of araA into a toxic nucleotide suggests that adenosine is phosphorylated by adenosine kinase (AK) in the parasite cytoplasm *(50,51)*, and this hypothesis was confirmed by the molecular cloning of AK by insertional (knockout) mutagenesis and selection for resistance to araA *(52)*. Interestingly, two other loci were revealed in this screen, the parasite's main adenosine transporter and another that remains uncharacterized *(48,49)*. Similarly, the conversion of thioxanthine into a toxic nucleotide provides evidence that hypoxanthine-xanthine-guanine phosphoribosyltransferase (HXGPRT) phosphoribosylates hypoxanthine, xanthine, and guanine into IMP, XMP, and GMP, respectively *(53)*. Insertional mutagenesis and selection for resistance to thioxanthine led to the molecular cloning of HXGPRT *(54)*. The recovery of mutants with either a nonfunctional AK or HXGPRT indicates that the parasite can interconvert AMP and IMP, and that these purine salvage pathways are functionally redundant. Purine salvage appears to be limited to these pathways, given the inability to recover the AK/HXGPRT double mutant *(3)*.

The analysis of recombinant *T. gondii* AK protein highlights some important issues concerning the identification and development of subversive substrates as "lead" compounds, because toxicity may be largely caused by downstream metabolism of products from the initial enzymatic reaction *(46)*. Enzymatic activity and substrate recognition do not always correlate with differences in toxic effects on host and parasite. Like mammalian AK, the *T. gondii* enzyme appears to have strict specificity for adenonsine, and recognizes adenosine analogs, but kinetic studies show that K_m values for adenosine are much higher than for the human enzyme (1.9 μM and 41 nm, respectively *(46,55)*. This difference in the efficiency of substrate recognition extends to some subversive substrates. Curiously, araA is a very poor substrate for the *T. gondii* AK (K_m = 3.3 m*M*, K_{cat} =0.15 min^{-1}), yet has parasiticidal effects at low micromolar concentrations (IC$_{50}$ = 1.5 μM; *(46)*. This characterization of the parasite's AK underscores the requirement of in vivo screens and metabolic analyses for the development and understanding of subversive substrates for chemotherapy.

Pyrimidine Salvage, Synthesis, and Subversive Substrates

Enzymes for salvage or synthesis of pyrimidine nucleosides and precursors have long been considered as chemotherapeutic targets because the metabolic pathways are different between host and parasite. Pyrimidines in *T. gondii* can be generated either through uracil salvage or *de novo* synthesis of UMP *(37)*. The parasite uses uracil phosphoribosyl transferase (UPRT) to salvage uracil, an enzymatic function missing in the mammalian host. Since the parasite lacks thymidine kinase activity, the parasite depends upon thymidylate synthase (TS) conversion of UMP to TMP, and requires the folate cycle for the methyl donor. In contrast to the mammalian host, *T. gondii* and other protozoan parasites have the TS fused to dihydrofolate reductase (DHRF), and the DHFR is the target for currently used drugs such as trimethoprim, pyrimethamime, and cycloguanil. Dihydropteroate reductase, the enzyme that catalyzes the folate biosynthetic step immediately preceding DHFR-TS, is the target for sulfonamide drugs that are often used in combination with the DHFR inhibitors *(56)*.

Uracil salvaged through UPRT is the only mechanism available to *T. gondii* for utilizing preformed pyrimidines, as none of the pyrimidine nucleosides, nucleotides, or their deoxy counterparts can be incorporated by the parasite *(57)*. Despite the lack of UPRT activity in the mammalian host, compounds such as 5-fluorouracil (5-FU) which act as subversive substrates in *T. gondii* can also be highly toxic to the human host; thus, new prodrugs must be developed *(58)*. Like AK and HXGPRT, the *T. gondii* UPRT gene was cloned using the insertional mutagenesis/selection for subversive substrate 5-FU resistance strategy *(59)*. Crystal-structure analysis of the recombinant UPRT reveals that it belongs to the structural class I phosophoriboysl transferase (PRT) group of enzymes found in prokaryotes and lower eukaryotes, and is most similar to the *S. cerevisiae* UPRT *(60)*. Despite the general lack of sequence similarity between PRTs, the *T. gondii* UPRT shares the common PRTase core and phosphoribosyl pyrophosphate-binding motif with four short regions showing sequence identity with other UPRTs. The third conserved region, believed to participate in phosphate ion binding, also appears to be important in pyrimidine substrate discrimination. The C_β carbon atom of the Ala 168 residue in the third conserved region may constrain pyrimidine binding through steric hindrance. Both uracil and 5-FU form similar enzyme-substrate complexes, where the crystal structures suggest that the 5-fluoro group can rotate sufficiently to avoid steric clash with this C_β carbon atom. The failure of thymine (5-methyl group), 5-chloro, 5-bromo, and 5-iodouracil to bind supports this theory, as they have longer bond lengths and thus larger van der Waals radii. These results from the crystal-structure analysis and sequence comparisons to other UPRTs provide considerable insight into how UPRT substrate specificity is determined, and what may constrain the further development of prodrugs.

As noted previously, DHFR is the target for such widely used antiparasitic compounds as pyrimethamine and cyclguanil. Although the genes encoding *T. gondii* and *P. falciparum* DHFR-TS have been known for several years, crystallographic information is still lacking for these important bifunctional enzymes. Recombinant *T. gondii* DHFR-TS has been expressed in *E. coli, S. cerevisiae,* and transgenic parasites *(3,36,61)*. These studies have allowed the evolution of drug-resistant mutations in *P. falciparum* to be studied in detail *(61)*. A combination of in vitro and in vivo studies have also provided biochemical models that highlight the importance of several factors in drug sensitivity and resistance, including cofactor binding and the critical role of enzyme turnover (rather than Km) (M.G. Reynolds, L.M. Fohl & D.S. Roos, *unpublished results*).

The Shikimate Pathway

The requirement for folate precursors by *T. gondii* and other apicomplexans suggests that the shikimate pathway may be a good target for herbicidal attack because it is not present in mammalian hosts *(41)*. The shikimate pathway enzyme 5 enolpyruvyl shikimate 3-phosphate (EPSP) synthase is inhibited by the well-characterized herbicide glyphosate (N-(phosphonomethyl) glycine; RoundUp™, Zero™, Tumbleweed™), and the formation of EPSP with tachyzoite extracts and inhibition with glyphosate demonstrate the activity of this enzyme in *T. gondii*. 3.12 mM glyphosate inhibited *T. gondii* growth in HFF host cells and behaved synergistically with other anti-folate drugs pyrimethamine and sulfadiazine, increasing the survival rate of ND4 mice from a lethal challenge of RH strain tachyzoites *(41)*. This study also confirmed activity for chorismate synthase, the next enzyme in the shikimate pathway, and alignment of the full-length cDNA sequence from a putative *T. gondii* EST clone with other species confirmed the identity of the translation product and the existence of the pathway.

Although the shikimate pathway is localized to the plastid in plants, the enzymes are found in the cytosol in fungi *(62)*. The amino terminus of the translated chorismate synthase cDNA from *T. gondii* shows no evidence of a plastid-targeting leader sequence associated with known nuclear-encoded apicoplast proteins *(42)*. In addition, a phylogenetic analysis of chorsimate synthase from several species has revealed that the apicomplexan proteins are more closely related to fungal enzymes than to plastid representatives, and recent biochemical and immunological studies localize the *P. falciparum* chorismate synthase to the parasite cytosol *(63)*. These findings do not diminish the importance of the pathway as a drug target, and may actually prove useful in future therapy development, as the membranes surrounding the apicoplast could serve as barriers to potential antiparasitic compounds.

Microtubule Inhibition

Although microtubule disruption has long been exploited in herbicide development, it has only recently come to the fore as a possible therapeutic target in *T. gondii* and other apicomplexan parasites *(39,40)*.

Several dinitoraniline compounds that have been successfully developed to specifically disrupt polymerization of plant microtubules *(64,65)* have been shown to exhibit similar activity against green algae *(66,67)* and protozoan parasites *(68,69)*. The observation that these compounds also have activity against *T. gondii* grown in tissue culture is consistent with the phylogenetic analyses of α-tubulin and β-tubulin—both single-copy genes *(70)*—that group *T. gondii* with the plant and ciliate clade as opposed to the fungi/animal clade *(39)*. Oryzalin, ethalfluralin, and trifluralin all inhibited growth of tachyzoites at IC_{50} concentrations ranging from 100–300 *nm* without obviously affecting the human foreskin fibroblast (HFF) host cells at concentrations greater than 50 *μM*. The various cellular micotubule-based structures differed in their sensitivity to the drug, but spindle-pole body formation and cytokinesis appeared to be consistently abolished. Patterns of cross-resistance to oryzalin, ethalfluralin, and trifularlin suggest that resistance is a multigenic trait. Thus, each dinitroaniline may have different sites of action or different affinities to either tubulins or their associated proteins. The further development of dinitroanilines for systemic therapy will depend on the identification of compounds with greater solubility *(71)*.

Other microtubule-inhibiting drugs, such as like the diterpene compound paclitaxel (Taxol), generate unstable microtubules by inducing tubulin polymerization *(72)*. Treatment of *T. gondii* tachyzoites with 1 *μM* paclitaxel does not inhibit the parasite's ability to invade the host cell, but subsequent growth in the HFF host cell is severely inhibited as a result of impaired cytokinesis *(40)*. In contrast to the investigations with dinitroaniline compounds, paclitaxel was tested on the basis of that it has been approved by the FDA for use as anti-tumor agents *(73)* and have been shown to have some activity against protozoan parasites *(74)*. It is somewhat surprising that paclitaxel would have activity against the plant-like *T. gondii* microtubules, because the diterpene compound was isolated from the western yew *Taxus brevifolia (75)* and was most likely to have evolved as an anti-fungal or anti-herbivore agent.

For the further development of both dinitroaniline compounds and paclitaxel, elucidating the molecular basis for *T. gondii* sensitivity is vital. Although one oryzalin-resistant/paclitaxel hypersensitive mutant in the green algae *Chlamydamonas reinhardii* is correlated with a mutation in the α1-tubulin gene *(76)*, the *T. gondii* drug-resistant strains must be characterized to identify the full range of possible targets.

CHEMOTHERAPEUTIC TARGETS IN THE MITOCHONDRION

T. gondii cells contain a single mitochondrion. Like other Apicomplexans, the *T. gondii* tachyzoite mitochondrion maintains a membrane potential ($\Delta\Psi$) and some proteins required for electron transport, but is insensitive to the NADH-ubiquinone oxidoreductase inhibitor rotenone, indicating that this enzyme and complex I is absent or does not bind rotenone in these species *(77,78)*. Since apicomplexans probably generate pyrimidines primarily through *de novo* synthesis, it has been postulated that the main function of electron transport is to remove electrons generated by dihydroorotate dehydrogensase *(79,80)*. Although malarial parasites are not believed to use oxidative phosphorylation to generate adenosine triphosphate (ATP) *(81)*, the addition of malate and succinate to *T. gondii* permeabilized tachyzoites are able to stimulate adenosine 5′ diphosphate (ADP) phosphorylation, suggesting that the organelle can provide ATP as an energy source for this form of the parasite *(78)*. The addition of the NADH-linked substrates 3-oxoglutarate, glutamate, pyruvate, and isocitrate to this tachyzoite preparation do not stimulate ADP phosphorylation, confirming the theory that complex I is absent, and raising the possibility that the respiratory chain in *T. gondii* and other apicomplexans is distinct from the mammalian host. These data suggest a fumarate reductase respiratory model that bypasses complex I *(78)*.

At this time, the *T. gondii* mitochondrial genome has not been completely sequenced, but evidence including the complete sequence of the cytochrome b gene *(CYB) (82)* argues that the genome will be of similar size and composition to the linear 6-kb mitochondrial genomes of *Plasmodium* species *(83,84)*; J. Boothroyd, J. Feagin, *personal communication*. By homology, the *T. gondii* mitochondrial DNA will also encode the cytochrome oxidase c subunits I and III [COI, COIII], and the vast majority of mitochondrial proteins will be nuclear-encoded. In contrast to mammalian species, mitochondrial genomes in *Plasmodium* species appear to evolve at a much lower relative rate than their respective nuclear genomes *(85)*.

Atovaquone and Cytochrome B: A Model for a Mitochondrion-Encoded Drug Target

In the development of antimalarials, the hydroxynapthoquinone atovaquone (2-[trans-4-(4′-chlorophenyl)cyclohexyl]-3-hydroxy-1,4-hydroxynapthoquinone) or 566C80) has been shown to be a broad-spectrum antibiotic with activity against apicomplexans, including *Plasmodium* spp., *T. gondii*, and *Babesia (86–88)*. Atovaquone has held particular interest as an anti-toxoplasmosis drug, since it appears to have activity against the cyst form of the parasite, although at much greater concentration compared to activity against tachyzoites *(87,89)*. Structural features of the *Plasmodium* CYB suggest that this protein may be responsible for the parasite's susceptibility to 8-aminoquinolones and hydroxynapthoquinones, including atovaquone *(90)*—theory that is a consistent with the observation that the drug inhibits *T. gondii* respiration *(78)*. Characterization of atovaquone-resistant mutants in both *P. yoelli* and *T. gondii* correlate specific changes in CYB with resistance to the drug, where the mutations localize in the domain that binds ubiquinol *(82,91,92)*. A comparison of *P. yoelli* and *T. gondii* CYB structural models show that the two *T. gondii* amino-acid residues associated with atovaquone resistance, methionine 129 and isoleucine 254, have homologous counterparts in *P. yoelli*-resistant strains *(82,91)*, suggesting that mutations leading to resistance will be limited to a small number of specific changes.

Despite the intial efficacy of atovaquone, resistance to the drug develops relatively quickly when used as a single agent against both malaria and toxoplasmosis, probably because of the combination of frequent mutation and rapid dissemination of new sequence variants *(93,94)*. In the case of mitochondrial inhibitors like atovaquone, the block in electron transfer may increase the mutation rate though superoxide-generated free radicals and subsequent DNA damage *(91)*. The DNA damage includes formation of 8-oxo-guanine residues, which can basepair with A. Consistent with this proposition is the observation that 9 of the 11 *P. yoelli* and half of the *T. gondii* atovaquone-resistant mutants are A:T to G:C transversions *(82,91)*. A survey of mitochondrial DNA sequences from natural isolates of several *Plasmodium* species revealed a high degree of both inter- and intraspecific conservation *(85)*. These data indicate that there is significant selective pressure to maintain the integrity of the mitochondrial genome and/or that the mode of replication is not so error-prone as to generate a large number of selectively neutral mutations. The proposed rolling-circle mode of replication/frequent strand invasion in conjunction with the maintenance of 6–20 copies of the genome per mitochondrion *(95)* may allow the parasites to establish selectively advantageous mutations at the cellular level. Since mitochondrial genome recombination is likely to be negligible, selection probably acts on the genome as a single unit, whereas selection for an advantageous mutation at one locus would result in a "hitchhiking" effect for the remainder of the mitochondrial genome *(96)*. The predicted overall reduction in polymorphism in the population is consistent with the observation of only one nucleotide substitution in *CYB* gene sequences from five *P. falciparum* field isolates and the entire mitochondrial genome of two geographically separated isolates *(85)*. Given the similarities between *Plasmodium* spp. and *T. gondii* mitochondrial genomes and mitochondria-related physiology, drug-resistant mutations in *T. gondii* mitochondrion-encoded drug targets such as CYB probably occur via similar mechanisms. Although the spread of these *T. gondii* drug-resistant strains in the human population is unlikely (cannibalism is very rare), the long-term prophylaxis with drugs such as atovaquone in AIDS patients will be of limited use, unless they are used in combination with other drugs *(82)*.

Potential for Nuclear-Encoded Mitochondrial Chemotherapeutic Targets

Since the vast majority of mitochondrial proteins must be encoded in the nucleus, identification of these genes may reveal a wealth of potential drug targets. As with the nuclear-encoded apicoplast proteins, the ability to identify these proteins by secretion, organelle import, and expression elements from DNA sequence using computational methods will depend upon the evolution of organelle and nuclear interactions in the phylum. Although the *T. gondii* HSP60 mitochondrial chaperone has a classical 22 amino-acid mitochondrial targeting presequence *(97)*, the general lack of linear-sequence similarity between these sequences suggests that this feature alone will not be sufficient for computational data mining. Considering the likely evolutionary history of the Apicomplexa, plant studies may offer the most useful insight into how some of these genes may be identified.

Although it is not clear why the organelle-to-nucleus direction of gene transfer predominates, the transfer must involve a duplicate copy of a gene that is inserted into the nucleus; the acquisition of elements for nuclear expression; and the acquisition of targeting sequences for import into the organelle *(98,99)*. The expression and targeting sequences could possibly be random sequences that were fortuitously functional, or may be working units from pre-existing genes. For targeting sequences, an experiment in yeast showing that approximately 5–6% of random *E. coli* sequences will direct proteins for mitochondrial import *(100)*, whereas screens for sequences to promote transcription in plants seem to occur at a much lower frequency *(98)*. The latter observation argues that gaining appropriate gene expression sequences may be a more stringent process than for targeting sequences, suggesting that the acquisition of pre-existing sequences by mechanisms such as exon shuffling *(101)* would be a more effective mechanism. Analysis of the rice ribosomal protein S11 also supports this theory, as the two functional nuclear genes (as opposed to the mitochondrial pseudogene) appear to have acquired upstream sequences from two independent duplication events of nucleus-encoded mitochondrial proteins *(102)*. Sequence comparsions suggest that the 5′ upstream region and first exon/intron are duplicated from the *atpB* and *coxVb* genes for *rps11-1* and *rps11-2*, respectively. The maize *rps14* gene has achieved a similar result by alternative splicing after integration into the intron of the nucleus-encoded mitochondrial protein gene *sdh2 (103,104)*. Collectively, these studies suggest that identifying these nuclear-encoded genes by expression profiling (*see* for example Chapters 1 and 3) or comparison of upstream promoter sequences may be essential components to computational identification of nuclear-encoded mitochondrial proteins.

CHEMOTHERAPEUTIC TARGETS IN THE APICOPLAST

The 35-kb apicoplast genome of *T. gondii* contains an rRNA inverted repeat characteristic of chloroplast genomes; however, it appears to encode only a fraction of the genes observed in its chloroplast relatives. Analysis of the *T. gondii* apicoplast genome reveals a total of 33 tRNAs capable of translating all codons, 28 open reading frames (ORFs) (17 of which encode ribosomal proteins), *tuf*A, *clp, rpo*B, C1, C2 and ORF470 (*ycf*24). There are 5 ORFs of uncertain conservation and unknown function. The limited coding capacity of the 35-kb apicoplast DNA suggests that the vast majority of the organelle's proteins are encoded in the nucleus, where estimates of the number of apicoplast protein content ranges from 100–400 *(92)*; J. Kissinger, *unpublished results*). Computational methods for identifying these proteins/genes promise to be the most efficient approaches and have already proven to be useful. Identifying previously characterized chloroplast proteins by simply scanning the EST database (http://ParaDB.cis.upenn.edu/toxo/) revealed protein ortholog for apicoplast ribosomal subunits as well as components of a type II fatty-acid synthesis machinery *(105)*.

Although the apicoplast genome is severely limited in coding capacity when compared to those of other plastids, a cadre of pharmacological evidence indicates that proper maintenance of this DNA and production of apicoplast-encoded proteins are essential for parasite survival. Indeed, the recent recognition of the apicoplast and its genome provides a belated explanation for the long-recognized parasiticidal activity of numerous compounds historically defined as antibacterial agents *(9,106)*. Physiologically relevant concentrations of drugs directed against prokaryotic translation, transcription, and DNA replication are capable of inhibiting parasite growth. The unusual kinetics of parasite death following administration of these antibiotics is consistent with a common target. In all cases, extracellular parasites are resistant to drug treatment, and the intracellular growth rate is equivalent to untreated controls during invasion and replication within the initial host cell, even at drug concentrations >1000 × the IC_{50} *(107)*. It is only after the invasion of a subsequent host cell that replication rapidly declines and irrevocably ceases. This "delayed death" phenotype provides an important clue to the function of the apicoplast, suggesting that it is producing metabolites during its tenure in the first host cell that are critical for the establishment of a productive infectious cycle in the second *(107–109)*.

Plastid-Encoded Targets

A major portion of the apicoplast genome encodes factors devoted to the transcription and translation of its own ORFs. Both of these processes supply potential targets for chemotherapeutic intervention. The rifamycin class of antibiotics inhibits eubacterial RNA synthesis by strongly binding to the β-subunit of DNA-directed RNA polymerase (*rpoB* on the plastid genome) and preventing clearance of the nascent RNA chain *(110)*. Rifampin, primarily used in the treatment of tuberculosis, is effective against *Plasmodium spp* both in vitro and in vivo, and was shown to specifically arrest RNA synthesis from the apicoplast genome *(111)*. Although rifampin is ineffective against *T. gondii,* the analogs rifabutin and rifapentine are active in tissue culture as well as in murine models of toxoplasmosis *(112,113).*

Although several groups have demonstrated that transcription is active in the apicoplast *(111,114),* no direct proof exists that the plastid ORFs are in fact translated. Electron micrographs of apicoplast sections show that they contain particles that are analogous to prokaryotic 70S ribosomes *(8,13),* and plastid-specific nucleic-acid probes to density-gradient fractions confirm that *P. falciparum* has a minor subset of polysomes carrying plastid rRNAs and mRNAs *(115).* The most convincing evidence to date continues to be the observation that a wide variety of prokaryotic translation inhibitors are parasiticidal with some of the drugs including clindamycin and spiramycin, and are used clinically in the treatment of malaria and toxoplasmosis. Lincosamides (e.g., lincomycin, clindamycin) and macrolides (e.g., spiramycin, azithromycin) block protein synthesis by presumably interacting with the peptidyl-transferase domain of the plastid 23S rRNA *(116).* Thiopeptide antibiotics (e.g., thiostrepton or micrococcin), highly potent antimalarial compounds in vitro, also bind to the large subunit rRNA and inhibit functions linked to ribosomal GTP hydrolysis *(117–119).* In addition, antibiotics potentially directed against the plastid-encoded 16S rRNA (tetracycline and doxycycline) and elongation factor Tu (kirromycin and amythiamicin) are parasiticidal, but the targets of these antibiotics may reside in the mitochondria and require further characterization *(118,120,121).*

Nuclear-Encoded Proteins Targeted to the Apicoplast

Because the 35-kB circle primarily encodes housekeeping enzymes, the indispensable metabolic proteins that have forced retention of the plastid throughout apicomplexan evolution must be encoded in the nucleus and post-translationally imported into the organelle, as with chloroplasts and mitochondria. An extensive body of literature that characterizes the origin and biochemistry of plant and algal plastids provides a lengthy list of metabolic processes (and drug targets) that potentially reside within the apicoplast. The wealth of information received from sequencing of apicomplexan nuclear genomes, particularly that of *Plasmodium spp.,* has accelerated the discovery process for these proteins *(see 10,11).* In addition to a strong phylogenetic relationship to their prokaryotic precursors, these proteins harbor a distinct bipartite N-terminal extension *(7,105).* The extreme N-terminus encodes a classic hydrophobic-signal peptide targeting the nascent polypeptide to the secretory pathway. The rest of the extension resembles a chloroplast transit peptide, serving to import the protein through the additional plastid membranes. The N-terminal extensions of several nuclear-encoded apicoplast proteins are sufficient to target reporter molecules (such as green fluorescent protein (GFP)) to the apicoplast, providing convenient markers to follow plastid protein import and replication *(92,122).*

Plastid-Genome Maintenance and Post-Translational Modification

Plastid genomes, like those of their bacterial progenitors, are supercoiled DNA circles that require the action of DNA gyrase homologues (prokaryotic topoisomerase IIs) for proper gene expression, recombination, and replication *(123)*. DNA gyrase homologues are A_2B_2 tetramers that create a transient double-stranded break in the DNA during the enzymatic process. The quinolone antibiotics act as a "poison" to this step, locking the enzyme on the 5′ end of linear DNA. The fluoroquinolone ciprofloxacin, which kills apicomplexan parasites, specifically decreases the plastid-genome copy number in *T. gondii* and *P. falciparum* and also protects the 5′ end of the plastid genome from exonuclease digestion, strongly suggesting the presence of a gyrase-like activity in the apicoplast *(109,124,125)*. Both the A and B subunits of DNA gyrase homologues have been isolated from the *P. falciparum* and *P. yoelii* databases. They contain the bipartite N-terminal extension, which is indicative of an enzyme operating in the apicoplast, and the leaders of the *P. falciparum* proteins properly target a fluorescent reporter to the *T. gondii* plastid (M.J. Crawford, D.S. Roos, *unpublished results*).

Peptide deformylase is an iron-binding protein that removes the N-formyl group, which is placed on the initiator methionine of nascent eubacterial and plastid polypeptides *(126)*. This essential enzyme, for which a probable plastid-targeted homologue has been isolated from the *P. falciparum* genome, has received considerable attention as an unexploited candidate for novel antibacterial agents *(127)*. Peptidomimetic hydroxamic derivatives such as the antibiotic actinonin are potent deformylase inhibitors, which will be worth testing against apicomplexan parasites *(128)*.

Metabolic Pathways in the Apicoplast: Fatty Acid and Isoprene Biosynthesis

The first described nuclear-encoded plastid genes in *T. gondii* and *P. falciparum* were enzymes of a prokaryotic type II fatty-acid synthesis pathway *(105)*. This observation came as a surprise to many researchers, as Apicomplexans were originally believed to be incapable of *de novo* fatty-acid biosynthesis. Mining of the *P. falciparum* genome has revealed a complete plastid pathway for the conversion of acetyl-CoA to a long-chain fatty acid. The first step, the conversion of acetyl-CoA to malonyl-CoA by a plastid acetyl-CoA carboxylase, has been detected in *T. gondii* extracts, and is inhibitable by aryloxyphenoxypropionate herbicides, which also prevent parasite growth *(129,130)*. Compounds that prevent the condensation reactions (catalyzed by the plastid-targeted β-ketoacyl-ACP synthases) as well as the final reduction step (by enoyl-ACP reductase) during the cycle of fatty-acid synthesis have proven useful as parasiticidal agents *(105,131,132)*. In addition, *P. falciparum* extracts are able to synthesize fatty-acid synthesis from acetyl CoA to at least myristate (C14). This production is partially inhibited by the enoyl-ACP reductase inhibitor triclosan *(131)*.

Another metabolic pathway recently localized to the *P. falciparum* apicoplast is the non-mevalonate route of isoprene biosynthesis. Isoprenes, the precursors to thousands of compounds—including carotenoids, sterols, and modifying groups for ubiquinone and proteins—are synthesized through a mevalonic-acid intermediate in mammalian and yeast cells. However, chloroplasts and many bacteria rely on an incompletely elucidated pathway that includes deoxyxylulose 5-phosphate (DOXP) as an intermediate *(133)*. Fosmidomycin and FR900098, which target the apicoplast DOXP reductoisomerase, are potent antimalarial agents, with efficacy both in vitro and in the mouse model *(134)*.

Function of the Apicoplast

Although extensive pharmacological evidence has shown that processes carried out within the apicoplast are critical for parasite survival, the final nature and destination of the metabolites produced are currently unknown. Although the chloroplast fatty-acid synthase provides the entire supply of lipids for plants *(135)*, both *P. falciparum* and *T. gondii* have a robust capacity for scavenging fatty acids and would apparently not require a *de novo* biosynthetic pathway *(136)*. *T. gondii,* which is largely insensitive to DOXP reductoisomerase inhibitors, is capable of importing large amounts of serum and cholesterol, a primary end-product of isoprene units synthesized in other systems *(137)*. The apicoplast may produce specialized moieties based on fatty acid and iso-prene precursors that are required for parasite growth, particularly during the initial establishment of infection within the host cell. Despite the bevy of new drug targets provided by its discovery and initial characterization, the continued use of genetic, bio-chemical, and bioinformatic approaches is needed to unravel the contribution of this unusual and fascinating organelle to parasite survival (*see* Fig. 2).

COMPUTATIONAL APPROACHES TO THE IDENTIFICATION OF CHEMOTHERAPEUTIC TARGETS

One of the most important new tools to be added to the drug-target-discovery tool chest is the computer. The flood of sequence data for apicomplexan organisms has opened up a new research arena for those who are interested in mining this rich data resource *(138)*. There are currently several apicomplexan genome, EST, and genome survey sequence (GSS) sequencing projects underway from a diverse range of parasites (Table 1). The sequence data emerging from these projects, coupled with the *Arabidopsis, Synechocystis,* and numerous organellar genome-sequencing projects set the stage for data mining strategies based upon evolutionary comparisons (*see* Fig. 3).

In the search for chemotherapeutic targets within an evolutionary context, there are two main strategies to follow. One strategy discussed here is to look for genes of differ-ent evolutionary ancestry, e.g., those genes acquired during a horizontal transfer or via an endosymbiotic event. Such genes are usually recognizable by their stronger phylo-genetic affinity to a different group of organisms. The other strategy is to look for genes that are phylogenetically restricted in their distribution—for example, those genes that are only present in the Apicomplexa or within the Coccidia *(5)*. These genes also make excellent targets since they will not be present in the host organism.

Finally, it is worth mentioning that the most useful data mining approaches are those that are coupled to an experimental system. This coupling can validate the accuracy of a prediction but, of equal importance, it provides feedback on the accuracy of the algo-rithms employed and is very useful for making them better. Bioinformatics is still in its infancy, and much of the available data is "raw" and unannotated. Thus, it is essential to be able to test ones predictions or findings in vivo. In the case of *T. gondii,* we have an excellent experimental system to provide rapid biological validation of computa-tionally identified targets *(2,5)*.

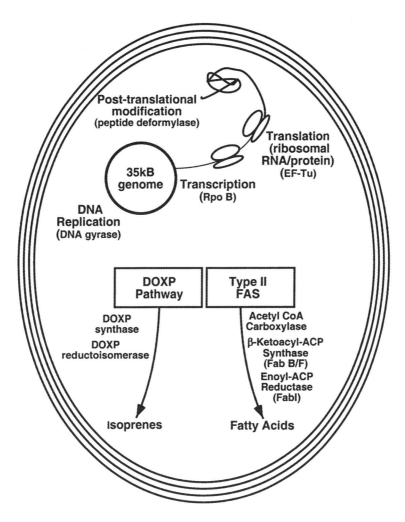

Fig. 2. Identified drug targets within the apicomplexan plastid. To date, five major processes within the apicoplast that can serve as potential drug tagets have been identified; genome replication, transcription, translation, isoprene biosynthesis, and fatty-acid biosynthesis.

Nuclear-Encoded Apicoplast Genes

Data mining of *T. gondii* EST [http://www.ParaDB.cis.upenn.edu/toxo/] and *P. falciparum* genomic sequences [http://plasmodb.org] has revealed a number of nuclear-encoded apicoplast genes *(7,105)*. The data mining strategy was multi-part and relied upon the detection of predicted proteins or ORFs that contained signal sequences, had N-terminal extensions relative to the mature protein and contained phylogenetic affinity to cyanobacterial genes *(3)*. Additionally, these data sources were searched for plastid genes that are known to have been transferred to the nuclear genome during the course of evolution in algae and plants *(139)*. Although a number of genes from this latter category, such as the genes involved in photosynthesis, have been lost in Apicomplexa, a surprising number have also been conserved and are being utilized in novel ways, such as the genes that encode ferredoxin and ferredoxin-NADP reductase.

Table 1
Apicomplexan Genomic/EST/GSS sequencing projects

Organism	Genome size	Type	Web access
Toxoplasma gondii ME49, RH	~80 Mb	EST	http://ParaDB.cis.upenn.edu/toxo/
Toxoplasma gondii ME49 B7		Genomic	http://www.sanger.ac.uk/Projects/T_gondii
Sarcocystis neurona Sn3		EST	http://ParaDB.cis.upenn.edu/sarco/
Neospora canium Nc-1		EST	http://ParaDB.cis.upenn.edu/neo/
Eimeria tenella LS18	~60 Mb	EST	http://genome.wustl.edu/est/eimeria_esthmpg.html and http://ParaDB.cis.upenn.edu/eim/
Cryptosporidium parvum I	~10 Mb	Genomic	http://www.parvum.mic.vcu.edu/
Cryptosporidium parvum II IOWA	10.4 Mb	Genomic	http://www.cbc.umn.edu/ResearchProjects/AGAC/Cp/
Cryptosporidium parvum II IOWA		GSS	http://medsfgh.ucsf.edu/id/CpTags/gss.html
Cryptosporidium parvum II IOWA		EST	http://medsfgh.ucsf.edu/id/CpTags/est.html
Plasmodium falciparum 3D7	25Mb	Genomic	http://PlasmoDB.org
Plasmodium falciparum 3D2		EST	http://parasite.vetmed.ufl.edu/falc.htm
Plasmodium falciparum 3D7		EST	http://133.11.149.55
Plasmodium falciparum HB3		GSS	http://parasite.vetmed.ufl.edu/falc.htm
Plasmodium yoelii 17XNL	25–30 Mb	Genomic	http://www.tigr.org/tdb/edb2/pya1/htmls
Plasmodium berghei ANKA	25–30 Mb	EST	http://parasite.vetmed.ufl.edu/berg.htm
		GSS	http://parasite.vetmed.ufl.edu/berg.htm
Plasmodium chabaudi	25–30 Mb	GSS	http://www.sanger.ac.uk/Projects/P_chabaudi
Plasmodium vivax Belem	35–40 Mb	GSS	http://parasite.vetmed.ufl.edu/viva.htm
Plasmodium vivax Salvador		GSS	http://parasite.vetmed.ufl.edu/viva.htm
Plasmodium vivax D10		YAC	http://www.sanger.ac.uk/Projects/P_vivax
Theileria annulata C9 Ankara	~10 Mb	Genomic	http://www.sanger.ac.uk/Projects/T_annulata
Theileria parva	~10 Mb	Genomic	http://www.tigr.org/tdb/e2k1/tpa1/
Babesia bovis	9.4 Mb	EST	http://www.sanger.ac.uk/Projects/B_bovis

270

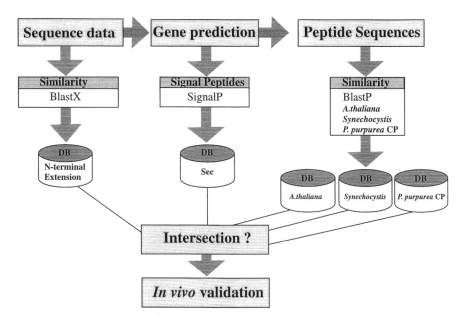

Fig. 3. Data-mining schema for discovering nuclear-encoded apicoplast genes. Apicomplexan sequence data (genomic, EST or GSS) is passed through a series of programs to detect similarity, predict genes, or predict signal peptides. The results of these various steps are saved as "mini-databases" each of which can be used as is, or in combination with other databases to reveal genes or proteins of interest. A nuclear-encoded apicoplast gene should have an N-terminal extension (relative to the mature protein), a signal sequence, and have significant cyanobacterial or chloroplast similarity. Putative candidate genes are then verified in vivo.

The products of these genes are normally associated with the terminal steps in photosystem I, but appear to be providing alternative electron transport functions in the apicoplast *(140)*.

Experimental validation of many of the computationally predicted nuclear-encoded plastid genes was performed using fluorescent reporter constructs. In the assay system, *T. gondii* parasites that had been transformed to express either a cyan or red fluorescent protein in their apicoplast were transformed with test constructs consisting of the N-terminus of computationally predicted proteins fused to a green fluorescent reporter protein *(105,108,130)*. Co-localization of the fluorescent reporters is used as in vivo verification of a predicted nuclear-encoded plastid protein.

Non-Apicoplast Nuclear-Encoded Genes of Other Evolutionary Origin

In addition to the large number of cyanobacterial genes that were transferred to the nuclear genome following the endosymbiotic events, there are a large number of algal nuclear genes that also appear to have been transferred. The completion of the *Arabidopsis thaliana* genome sequence combined with the data emerging from numerous other plant genome projects has facilitated the search for nuclear-encoded genes of plant (algal) origin. Some genes in this class are already known, such as the distinctly plant-like enolases of *T. gondii (141,142)*. Many new genes of plant (algal) ancestry have been discoved in *T. gondii* and *P. falciparum* using computational screens designed to detect genes with certain phylogenetic affinities (J.C Kissinger, D.S. Roos, *unpublished result*). It was necessary to use a screen based on phylogenetic affinity rather than known biochemical pathways, since in several instances a gene of algal ancestry has replaced its apicomplexan counterpart in a non "plant-specific" pathway.

A second class of genes with a different evolutionary origin are the nuclear-encoded mitochondrial targeted proteins of alpha-proteobacterial origin. As discussed here, these genes are more difficult to detect. However, if one casts a large phylogenetic net and looks for all genes of prokaryotic origin or similarity and then removes the class which is clearly of cyanobacterial origin or which clearly target to the apicoplast, one is left with several candidates, each of which can easily be experimentally verified in vivo via tagging with a fluorescent reporter.

CONCLUSION

Since all antibiotics work on the basis of evolutionary distance—i.e. large structural and/or functional differences between the host and pathogen—the development of antiprotozoal drugs compared to antibacterial drugs poses a particular problem because both host and pathogen are eukaryotes. In the quest for new drug targets, evolutionary genomic investigations and analyses of *T. gondii* have led to the view that Apicomplexans are genetic and biochemical chimeras. In particular, the discovery of the apicoplast and specific hypotheses related to a secondary endosymbiotic event has helped explain the action, behavior, and resistance to currently used drugs and opened up a wealth a of new drug targets related to plant and plastid functions. The rapid generation of genome sequence has produced a tidal wave of data for species ranging from bacterial pathogens to humans. However, it is important to consider that these data are not likely to have an immediate impact on drug discovery because target selection and validation continue to represent the real bottlenecks in the process *(143)*. For *T. gondii* and other Apicomplexan parasites, the process of target selection and validation is likely to be accelerated because both computational data-mining exercises and directed experiments will be based on hypotheses founded in our understanding of the evolutionary history of these species.

ACKNOWLEDGMENTS

We would like to thank the BBSRC (JWA), the NIH (DSR, JCK, MJC) the NSF (JCK) and the Burroughs Wellcome Fund (DSR) for their support.

REFERENCE

1. Roos DS, Donald RGK, Morrissette NS, Moulton ALC. Molecular tools for genetic dissection of the protozoan parasite *Toxoplasma gondii.* Methods Cell Biol 1994; 45:27–63.
2. Boothroyd JC, Black M, Kim K, Pfefferkorn ER, Seeber F, Sibley LD, Soldati D. Forward and reverse genetics in the study of the obligate intracellular parasite Toxoplasma gondii. Methods Mol Genet 1994; 3:1–29.
3. Roos DS, Darling JA, Reynolds MG, Hager KM, Striepen B, Kissinger JC. *Toxoplasma* as a model parasite: apicomplexan biochemistry, cell biology, molecular genetics ... and beyond. In: Tschudi C, Pearce E. (eds). Biology of Parasitism. Boston: Kluwer Press, 1999, pp. 143–167.
4. Wan KL, Blackwell JM, Ajioka JW. *Toxoplasma gondii* expressed sequence tags: Insight into tachyzoite gene expression. Mol Biochem Parasitol 1996; 75:179–186.

5. Ajioka JW, Boothroyd JC, Brunk BP, Hehl A, Hillier L, Manger ID, et al. Gene discovery by EST sequencing in *Toxoplasma gondii* reveals sequences restricted to the apicomplexa. Genome Res 1998; 8:18–28.

6. Wilson RJM, Wiliamson DH. Extrachromosomal DNA in the Apicomplexa. Microbiol Mol Biol Rev 1997; 61:1–16.

7. Roos DS, Crawford MJ, Donald RGK, Kissinger JC, Klimczak LJ, Striepen B. Origin, targeting, and function of the apicomplexan plastid. Curr Opin Microbiol 1999; 2:426–432.

8. Kohler S, Delwiche CF, Denny PW, Tilney LG, Webster P, Wilson RJM, et al. A plastid of probable green algal origin in apicomplexan parasites. Science 1997; 275:1485–1489.

9. McFadden GI, Roos DS. Apicomplexan plastids as drug targets. Trends Microbiol 1999; 7:328–333.

10. Gardner MJ, Tettelin H, Carucci DJ, Cummings LM, Aravind L, Koonin EV, et al. Chromosome 2 sequence of the human malaria parasite Plasmodium falciparum. Science 1998; 282:1126–1132.

11. Bowman S, Lawson D, Basham D, Brown D, Chillingworth T, Churcher CM, et al. The complete nucleotide sequence of chromosome 3 of Plasmodium falciparum. Nature 1999; 400:532–538.

12. Fast NM, Kissinger JC, Roos DS, Keeling PJ. Nuclear-encoded, plastid-targeted genes suggest a single common origin for apicomplexan and dinoflagellate plastids. Mol Biol Evol 2001; 18:418–426.

13. McFadden GI, Reith ME, Munholland J, LangUnnasch N. Plastid in human parasites. Nature 1996; 381:482.

14. Pferrerkorn LC, Pfefferkorn ER. *Toxoplasma gondii:* genetic recombination between drug resistant mutants. Experimental Parasitol 1980; 50:305–316.

15. Sibley LD, Leblanc AJ, Pfefferkorn ER, Boothroyd JC. Generation of a restriction fragment length polymorphism linkage map for *Toxoplasma gondii.* Genetics 1992; 132:1003–1015.

16. Ajioka JW, Fitzpatrick JM, Reitter CP. *Toxoplasma gondii* genomics: shedding light on pathogenesis and chemotherapy. Expert Reviews in Molecular Medicine 6 January, http://www-ermm.cbcu.cam.ac.uk/01002204h.htm. 2001.

17. Sibley LD, Boothroyd JC. Construction of a molecular karyotype for *Toxoplasma gondii.* Mol Biochem Parasitol 1992; 51:291–300.

18. Janse CJ. Chromosome size polymorphism and DNA rearrangements in *Plasmodium.* Parasitol Today 1993; 9:19–22.

19. Darde ML, Bouteille B, Pestrealexandre M. Isozyme analysis of 35 *Toxoplasma gondii* isolates and the biological and epidemiological implications. J Parasitol 1992; 78:786–794.

20. Howe DK, Sibley LD. *Toxoplasma gondii* comprises 3 clonal lineages: Correlation of parasite genotype with human disease. J Infect Dis 1995; 172:1561–1566.

21. Sibley LD, Boothroyd JC. Virulent strains of Toxoplasma gondii comprise a single clonal lineage. Nature 1992; 359:82–85.

22. Johnson AM. Comparison of dinucleotide frequency and codon usage in *Toxoplasma* and *Plasmodium:* evolutionary implications. J Mol Evol 1990; 30:383–387.

23. Wan KL, Carruthers VB, Sibley LD, Ajioka JW. Molecular characterization of an expressed sequence tag locus of *Toxoplasma gondii* encoding the micronemal protein MIC2. Mol Biochem Parasitol 1997; 84:203–214.

24. Soldati D, Boothroyd JC. A selector of transcription initiation in the protozoan parasite Toxoplasma gondii. Mol Cell Biol 1995; 15:87–93.

25. Mercier C, LefebvreVanHende S, Garber GE, Lecordier L, Capron A, Cesbron Delauw MF. Common cis-acting elements critical for the expression of several genes of *Toxoplasma gondii.* Mol Microbiol 1996; 21:421–428.

26. Nakaar V, Bermudes D, Peck KR, Joiner KA. Upstream elements required for expression of nucleoside triphosphate hydrolase genes of *Toxoplasma gondii*. Mol Biochem Parasitol 1998; 92:229–239.

27. Kadonaga JT, Jones KA, Tjian R. Promoter specific activation of RNA polymerase II transcription by SP1. Trends Biochem Sci 1986; 11:20–23.

28. Dubey JP. Toxoplasma, Hammondia, Besnotia, Sarcocystis and other tissue cyst forming coccida of man and animals. In: Kreier JP (ed). Parasitic Protozoa III. New York: Academic Press, 1997, pp. 101–237.

29. Remington JS, Krahenbuhl JL. Immunology of *Toxoplasma gondii*. Compr Immunol 1982; 9:327–371.

30. McLeod, R., Remington, J. S. Toxoplasmosis (Toxoplasma gondii). In: Nelson Textbook of Pediatrics, 16th edition, Behrman, R. E., Kliegman, R. M., Jensen, H., eds. Philadelphia: W.B. Saunders Company, pp. 1054–1062, 1999.

31. Luft BJ, Remington JS. Toxoplasmic encephalitis in AIDS patients. Clin Infect Dis 1992; 15:211–222.

32. Desmonts G, Couvreur J. Congenital toxoplasmosis: a prospective study of 378 pregnancies. N Engl J Med 1974; 290:1110–1116.

33. Jenum PA, Stray-Pedersen B, Melby KK, Kapperud G, Whitelaw A, Eskild A, Eng J. Incidence of *Toxoplasma gondii* infection in 35,940 pregnant women in Norway and pregnancy outcome for infected women. J Clin Microbiol 1998; 36:2900–2906.

34. Georgiev V. Management of toxoplasmosis. Drugs 1994; 48:179–188.

35. Ajioka JW. Analysis of apicomplexan parasites. Methods—A Companion to Methods in Enzymology 1997; 13:79–80.

36. Reynolds MG, Oh J, Roos DS. In vitro generation of novel pyrimethamine resistance mutations in the Toxoplasma gondii dihydrofolate reductase. Antimicrob Agents Chemother 2001; 45:1271–1277.

37. Schwartzman JD, Pfefferkorn ER. Pyrimidine synthesis by intracellular *Toxoplasma gondii*. J Parasitol 1981; 67:150–158.

38. Schwartzman JD, Pfefferkorn ER. *Toxoplasma gondii:* purine synthesis and salvage in mutant host cells and parasites. Exp Parasitol 1982; 53:77–86.

39. Stokkermans TJW, Schwartzman JD, Keenan K, Morrissette NS, Tilney LG, Roos DS. Inhibition of *Toxoplasma gondii* replication by dinitroaniline herbicides. Exp Parasitol 1996; 84:355–370.

40. Estes R, Vogel N, Mack D, McLeod R. Paclitaxel arrests growth of intracellular *Toxoplasma gondii*. Antimicrobial Agents and Chemotherapy 1998; 42:2036–2040.

41. Roberts F, Roberts CW, Johnson JJ, Kyle DE, Krell T, Coggins JR, et al. Evidence for the shikimate pathway in apicomplexan parasites. Nature 1998; 393:801–805.

42. Keeling PJ, Palmer JD, Donald RGK, Roos DS, Waller RF, McFadden GI. Shikimate pathway in apicomplexan parasites. Nature 1999; 397:219–220.

43. Roberts CW, Finnerty J, Johnson JJ, Roberts F, Kyle DE, Krell T, et al. Shikimate pathway in apicomplexan parasites—Reply. Nature 1999; 397:220.

44. Krug EC, Marr JJ, Berens RL. Purine metabolism in *Toxoplasma gondii*. J Biol Chem 1989; 264:10,601–10,607.

45. Ullman B, Carter D. Hypoxanthine-guanine phosphoribosyltransferase as a theraputic target in protozoal infections. Infectious Agents and Disease—Reviews Issues and Commentary 1995; 4:29–40.

46. Darling JA, Sullivan WJ, Carter D, Ullman B, Roos DS. Recombinant expression, purification, and characterization of *Toxoplasma gondii* adenosine kinase. Mol Biochem Parasitol 1999; 103:15–23.

47. Schwab JC, Beckers CJM, Joiner KA. The parasitophorous vacuole membrane surrounding intracellular *Toxoplasma gondii* functions as a molecular sieve. Proc Natl Acad Sci USA 1994; 91:509–513.

48. Schwab JC, Afifi MA, Pizzorno G, Handschumacher RE, Joiner KA. *Toxoplasma gondii* tachyzoites possess and unusual plasma membrane adenosine transporter. Mol Biochem Parasitol 1995; 70:59–69.

49. Chiang CW, Carter N, Sullivan WJ, Donald RGK, Roos DS, Naguib FNM, et al. The adenosine transporter of *Toxoplasma gondii*—Identification by insertional mutagenesis, cloning, and recombinant expression. J Biol Chem 1999; 274:35,255–35,261.

50. Pfefferkorn ER, Pfefferkorn LC. Arabinosyl nucleosides inhibit Toxoplasma gondii and allow the selection of resistant mutants. Exp Parasitol 1976; 44:26–35.

51. Pfefferkorn ER, Pfefferkorn LC. The biochemical basis for resistance to adenine arabinoside in a mutant of *Toxoplasma gondii*. J Parasitol 1978; 64:486–492.

52. Sullivan WJ, Chiang CW, Wilson CM, Naguib FNM, el Kouni MH, Donald RGK, et al. Insertional tagging and cloning of at least two loci associated with resistance to adenine arabinoside in *Toxoplasma gondii* and cloning of the adenosine kinase locus. Mol Biochem Parasitol 1999; 103:1–14.

53. Pfefferkorn ER, Borotz SE. Toxoplasma gondii: characterization of a mutant resistant to 6-thioxanthine. Exp Parasitol 1994; 79:374–382.

54. Donald RGK, Carter D, Ullman B, Roos DS. Insertional tagging, cloning and expression of the Toxoplasma gondii hypoxanthine-xanthine-guanine phosphoribosyltransferase gene: use as a selectable marker for stable transformation. J Biol Chem 1996; 271:14,010–14,019.

55. Spychala J, Datta NS, Takabayashi K, Datta M, Fox IH, Gribbin T, et al. Cloning of human adenosine kinase cDNA: sequence similarity to microbial ribokinases and fructokinases. Proc Natl Acad Sci USA 1996; 93:1232–1237.

56. Hitchings GH. In: Hitchings GH (ed). Inhibition of Folate Metabolism in Chemotherapy, Berlin: Springer-Verlag, 1983.

57. Pfefferkorn ER, Pfefferkorn LC. Characterization of a mutant resistant to 5-fluorodeoxyuridine. Exp Parasitol 1977; 42:44–45.

58. Carter D, Donald RGK, Roos DS, Ullman B. Expression, purification and characterization of uracil phosphoribosyltransferase from *Toxoplasma gondii*. Mol Biochem Parasitol 1997; 87:137–144.

59. Donald RGK, Roos DS. Insertional mutagenesis in a protozoan parasite: direct cloning of the uracil phosphoribosyl transferase gene from *Toxoplasma gondii*. Proc Natl Acad Sci USA 1995; 92:5749–5753.

60. Schumacher MA, Carter D, Scott DM, Roos DS, Ullman B, Brennan RG. Crystal structures of Toxoplasma gondii uracil phosphoribosyltransferase reveal the atomic basis of pyrimidine discrimination and prodrug binding. EMBO J 1998; 17:3219–3232.

61. Reynolds MG, Roos DS. A biochemical and genetic model for parasite resistance to antifolates—Toxoplasma gondii provides insights into pyrimethamine and cycloguanil resistance in Plasmodium falciparum. J Biol Chem 1998; 273:3461–3469.

62. Kishore GM, Shah DM. Amino acid biosynthesis inhibitors as herbicides. Annu Rev Biochem 1988; 57:627–663.

63. Fitzpatrick T, Ricken S, Lanzer M, Amrhein N, Macheroux P, Kappes B. Subcellular localization and characterization of chorismate synthase in the apicomplexan *Plasmodium falciparum*. Mol Microbiol 2001; 40:65–75.

64. Ashton FM, Crafts AS. Dinitroanilines. Mode of action of herbicides. New York: Wiley, 1981.

65. Bajer AS, Mole-Bajer J. Drugs with colchicine-like effects that specifically disassemble plant but not animal microtubules. Ann NY Acad Sci 1986; 466:767–784.

66. Hess FD, Bayer DE. Binding of the herbicide trifluralin to Chlamydomonas flagellar tubulin. J Cell Sci 1977; 24:351–360.

67. James SW, Lefebvre PA. Genetic interactions among *Chlamydomonas reinhardtii* mutations that confer resistance to anti-microtubule herbicides. Genetics 1992; 130:305–314.

68. Chan MMY, Fong D. Inhibition of leishmaniasis but not host macrophages by the anti-tubulin herbicide trifluralin. Science 1990; 249:924–926.

69. Kaidoh T, Nath J, Fujioka H, Okoye V, Aikawa M. Effect and localization of trifluralin in *Plasmodium falciparum* gametocytes: an electron-microscopic study. J Eukaryot Microbiol 1995; 42:61–64.

70. Nagel SD, Boothroyd JC. The alpha-tubulins and beta-tubulins of *Toxoplasma gondii* are encoded by single copy genes containing multiple introns. Mol Biochem Parasitol 1988; 29:261–273.

71. Palmer BD, Wilson WR, Cliffe S, Denny WA. Hypoxia-selective antitumor agents 5: synthesis of water-soluble nitroaniline mustards with selective cytotoxicity for hypoxic mammalian cells. J Med Chem 1992; 35:3214–3222.

72. Schiff PB, Fant J, Horwitz SB. Promotion of microtubule assembly in vitro by taxol. Nature 1979; 277:665–667.

73. Huizing MT, Misser VHS, Pieters RC, Huinink WWT, Veenhof CHN, Vermorken JB. Taxanes: a new class of antitumor agents. Cancer Investig 1995; 13:381–404.

74. Pouvelle B, Farley PJ, Long CA, Taraschi TF. Taxol arrests the development of blood-stage *Plasmodium falciparum* in vitro and *Plasmodium chabaudi adami* in malarial infected mice. J Clin Investig 1994; 94:413–417.

75. Wani M, Taylor HL, Wall ME. Plant antitumor agents VI: the isolation and structure of Taxol, a novel antileukemic and antitumor agent from *Taxus brevifolia*. J Am Chem Soc 1971; 93:2325–2327.

76. James SW, Silflow CD, Stroom P, Lefebvre PA. A mutation in the alpha-1-tubulin gene of *Chlamydomonas reinhardtii* confers resistance to antimicrotubule herbicides. J Cell Sci 1993; 106:209–218.

77. Srivastava IK, Rottenberg H, Vaidya AB. Atovaquone, a broad spectrum antiparasitic drug, collapses mitochondrial membrane potential in a malarial parasite. J Biol Chem 1997; 272:3961–3966.

78. Vercesi AE, Rodrigues CO, Uyemura SA, Zhong L, Moreno SNJ. Respiration and oxidative phosphorylation in the apicomplexan parasite *Toxoplasma gondii*. J Biol Chem 1998; 273:31,040–31,047.

79. Gero AM, Brown GV, O'Sullivan WJ. Pyrimidine de novo synthesis during the life-cycle of the intraerythrocytic stage of *Plasmodium falciparum*. J Parasitol 1984; 70:536–541.

80. Prapunwattana P, O'Sullivan WJ, Yuthavong Y. Depression of *Plasmodium falciparum* dihydroorotate dehydrogenase activity in in vitro culture by tetracycline. Mol Biochem Parasitol 1988; 27:119–124.

81. Scheibel LW. Plasmodial metabolism and related organellar function during various stages of the life-cycle: carbohydrates. In: Wernsdorfer WH, McGregor I. Malaria: principles and practice of malariology(1). New York: Churchill Livingston, 1988, pp. 171–217.

82. McFadden DC, Tomavo S, Berry EA, Boothroyd JC. Characterization of cytochrome b from *Toxoplasma gondii* and Q(o) domain mutations as a mechanism of atovaquone-resistance. Mol Biochem Parasitol 2000; 108:1–12.

83. Feagin JE. The 6-kb element of *Plasmodium falciparum* encodes mitochondrial cytochrome genes. Mol Biochem Parasitol 1992; 52:145–148.

84. Feagin JE. The extrachromosomal DNAs of Apicomplexan parasites. Annu Rev Microbiol 1994; 48:81–104.

85. McIntosh MT, Srivastava R, Vaidya AB. Divergent evolutionary constraints on mitochondrial and nuclear genomes of malaria parasites. Mol Biochem Parasitol 1998; 95:69–80.

86. Fowler RE, Sinden RE, Pudney M. Inhibitory activity of the antimalarial atovaquone (566C80) against ookinetes, oocysts and sporozoites of *Plasmodium berghi*. J Parasitol 1995; 81:452–458.

87. Araujo FG, Huskinson J, Remington JS. Remarkable in vitro and in vivo activities of the hydroxynapthoquinone 566C80 against tachyzoites and tissue cysts of Toxoplasma gondii. Antimicrob Agents Chemother 1991; 35:293–299.

88. Pudney M, Gray JS. Therapeutic efficacy of atovaquone against the bovine intraerythrocytic parasite, *Babesia divergens.* J Parasitol 1997; 83:307–310.

89. Ferguson DJP, Huskinsonmark J, Araujo FG, Remington JS. An ultrastructural study of the effect of treatment with atovaquone in brains of mice chronically infected with the ME49 strain of *Toxoplasma gondii.* Int J Exp Pathol 1994; 75:111–116.

90. Vaidya AB, Lashgari MS, Pologe LG, Morrisey J. Structural features of Plasmodium cytochrome b that may underlie susceptibility fo 8-aminoquinolines and hydroxynaptho-quinones. Mol Biochem Parasitol 1993; 58:33–42.

91. Srivastava IK, Morrisey JM, Darrouzet E, Daldal F, Vaidya AB. Resistance mutations reveal the atovaquone-binding domain of cytochrome b in malaria parasites. Mol Microbiol 1999; 33:704–711.

92. Waller RF, Reed MB, Cowman AF, McFadden GI. Protein trafficking to the plastid of *Plasmodium falciparum* is via the secretory pathway. EMBO J 2000; 19:1794–1802.

93. Torres RA, Weinberg W, Stansell J, Leoung G, Kovacs J, Rogers M, et al. Atovaquone for salvage treatment and suppression of toxoplasmic encephalitis in patients with AIDS. Clin Infect Dis 1997; 24:422–429.

94. Chiodini PL, Conlon CP, Hutchinson DBA, Farquhar JA, Hall AP, Peto TEA, et al. Evaluation of atovaquone in the treatment of patients with uncomplicated *Plasmodium falciparum* malaria. J Antimicrob Chemother 1995; 36:1073–1078.

95. Preiser PR, Wilson RJM, Moore PW, McCready S, Hajibagheri MAN, Blight KJ, et al. Recombination associated with replication of malarial mitochondrial DNA. EMBO J 1996; 15:684–693.

96. Maynard Smith J, Haigh J. The hitchhiking effect of a favourable gene. Genet Res 1974; 23:23–35.

97. Toursel C, Dzierszinski F, Bernigaud A, Mortuaire M, Tomavo S. Molecular cloning, organellar targeting and developmental expression of mitochondrial chaperone HSP60 in Toxoplasma gondii. Mol Biochem Parasitol 2000; 111:319–332.

98. Martin W, Herrmann RG. Gene transfer from organelles to the nucleus: How much, what happens, and why? Plant Physiol 1998; 118:9–17.

99. Blanchard JL, Lynch M. Organellar genes—why do they end up in the nucleus? Trends Genet 2000; 16:315–320.

100. Baker A, Schatz G. Sequences from a prokaryotic genome or the mouse dihydrofolate-reductase gene can restore the import of a truncated precursor protein into yeast mitochondria. Proc Natl Acad Sci USA 1987; 84:3117–3121.

101. Long MY, DeSouza SJ, Rosenberg C, Gilbert W. Exon shuffling and the origin of the mitochondrial targeting function in plant cytochrome c1 precursor. Proc Natl Acad Sci USA 1996; 93:7727–7731.

102. Kadowaki KI, Kubo N, Ozawa K, Hirai A. Targeting presequence acquisition after mitochondrial gene transfer to the nucleus occurs by duplication of existing targeting signals. EMBO J 1996; 15:6652–6661.

103. Figueroa P, Gomez I, Holuigue L, Araya A, Jordana X. Transfer of rps14 from the mitochondrion to the nucleus in maize implied integration within a gene encoding the iran-sulphur subunit of succinate dehydrogenase and expression by alternative splicing. Plant J 1999; 18:601–609.

104. Kubo N, Harada K, Hirai A, Kadowaki K. A single nuclear transcript encoding mitochondrial RPS14 and SDHB of rice is processed by alternative splicing: common use of the same mitochondrial targeting signal for different proteins. Proc Natl Acad Sci USA 1999; 96:9207–9211.

105. Waller RF, Keeling PJ, Donald RGK, Striepen B, Handman E, Lang-Unnasch N, et al. Nuclear-encoded proteins target to the plastid in *Toxoplasma gondii* and *Plasmodium falciparum*. Proc Natl Acad Sci USA 1998; 95:12,352–12,357.

106. Geary TG, Divo AA, Jensen JB. Stage specific actions of antimalarial drugs on *Plasmodium falciparum* in culture. Am J Trop Med Hyg 1989; 40:240–244.

107. Fichera ME, Bhopale MK, Roos DS. In vitro assays elucidate peculiar kinetics of clindamycin action against *Toxoplasma gondii*. Antimicrob Agents Chemother 1995; 39:1530–1537.

108. He CY, Shaw MK, Pletcher CH, Striepen B, Tilney LG, Roos DS. A plastid segregation defect in the protozoan parasite Toxoplasma gondii. EMBO J 2001; 20:330–339.

109. Fichera ME, Roos DS. A plastid organelle as a drug target in apicomplexan parasites. Nature 1997; 390:407–409.

110. Lal R, Lal S. Recent trends in rifamycin research. Bioessays 1994; 16:211–216.

111. McConkey GA, Rogers MJ, McCutchan TF. Inhibition of Plasmodium falciparum protein synthesis—Targeting the plastid-like organelle with thiostrepton. J Biol Chem 1997; 272:2046–2049.

112. Araujo FG, Silfer T, Remington JS. Rifabutin is active in murine models of toxoplasmosis. Antimicrob Agents Chemother 1994; 38:570–575.

113. Araujo FG, Khan AA, Remington JS. Rifapentine is active in vitro and in vivo against *Toxoplasma gondii*. Antimicrob Agents Chemother 1996; 40:1335–1337.

114. Preiser P, Williamson DH, Wilson RJM. Transfer-RNA genes transcribed from the plastid-like DNA of *Plasmodium falciparum*. Nucleic Acids Res 1995; 23:4329–4336.

115. Roy A, Cox RA, Williamson DH, Wilson RJMI. Protein synthesis in the plastid of *Plasmodium falciparum*. Protist 1999; 150:183–188.

116. Douthwaite S, Voldborg B, Hansen LH, Rosendahl G, Vester B. Recognition determinants for proteins and antibiotics within 23S rRNA. Biochem Cell Biol-Biochimie et Biologie Cellulaire 1995; 73:1179–1185.

117. Rogers MJ, Bukhman YV, McCutchan TF, Draper DE. Interaction of thiostrepton with an RNA fragment derived from the plastid-encoded ribosomal RNA of the malaria parasite. RNA-A Publication of the RNA Society 1997; 3:815–820.

118. Clough B, Strath M, Preiser P, Denny P, Wilson I. Thiostrepton binds to malarial plastid rRNA. FEBS Lett 1997; 406:123–125.

119. Rogers MJ, Cundliffe E, McCutchan TF. The antibiotic micrococcin is a potent inhibitor of growth and protein synthesis in the malaria parasite. Antimicrob Agents Chemother 1998; 42:715–716.

120. Beckers CJM, Roos DS, Donald RGK, Luft BJ, Schwab JC, Joiner KA. Inhibition of cytoplasmic and organellar protein synthesis in *Toxoplasma gondii:* implications for the target of macrolide antibiotics. J Clin Investig 1995; 95:367–376.

121. Budimulja AS, Syafruddin Tapchaisri P, Wilairat P, Marzuki S. The sensitivity of *Plasmodium* protein synthesis to prokaryotic ribosomal inhibitors. Mol Biochem Parasitol 1997; 84:137–141.

122. DeRocher A, Hagen CB, Froehlich JE, Feagin JE, Parsons M. Analysis of targeting sequences demonstrates that trafficking to the *Toxoplasma gondii* plastid branches off the secretory system. J Cell Sci 2000; 113:3969–3977.

123. Drlica K, Zhao XL. DNA gyrase, topoisomerase IV, and the 4-quinolones. Microbiol Mol Biol Rev 1997; 61:377–.

124. Weissig V, Vetro-Widenhouse TS, Rowe TC. Topoisomerase II inhibitors induce cleavage of nuclear and 35- kb plastid DNAs in the malarial parasite Plasmodium falciparum. DNA Cell Biol 1997; 16:1483–1492.

125. Gozalbes R, Brun-Pascaud M, Garcia-Domenech R, Galvez J, Girard PM, Doucet JP, et al. Anti-*Toxoplasma* activities of 24 quinolones and fluoroquinolones in vitro: prediction of activ-

ity by molecular topology and virtual computational techniques. Antimicrob Agents Chemother 2000; 44:2771–2776.

126. Giglione C, Pierre M, Meinnel T. Peptide deformylase as a target for new generation, broad spectrum antimicrobial agents. Mol Microbiol 2000; 36:1197–1205.

127. Meinnel T. Peptide deformylase of eukaryotic protists: a target for new antiparasitic agents? Parasitol Today 2000; 16:165–168.

128. Chen DZ, Patel DV, Hackbarth CJ, Wang W, Dreyer G, Young DC, et al. Actinonin, a naturally occurring antibacterial agent, is a potent deformylase inhibitor. Biochemistry 2000; 39:1256–1262.

129. Zuther E, Johnson JJ, Haselkorn R, McLeod R, Gornicki P. Growth of *Toxoplasma gondii* is inhibited by aryloxyphenoxypropionate herbicides targeting acetyl-CoA carboxylase. Proc Natl Acad Sci USA 1999; 96:13,387–13,392.

130. Jelenska J, Crawford MJ, Harb OS, Zuther E, Haselkorn R, Roos DS, et al. Subcellular localization of acetyl-CoA carboxylase in the apicomplexan parasite *Toxoplasma gondii*. Proc Natl Acad Sci USA 2001; 98:2723–2728.

131. Surolia N, Surolia A. Triclosan offers protection against blood stages of malaria by inhibiting enoyl-ACP reductase of *Plasmodium falciparum*. Nat Med 2001; 7:167–173.

132. McLeod R, Muench SP, Rafferty JB, Kyle DE, Mui EJ, Kirisits MJ, et al. Triclosan inhibits the growth of *Plasmodium falciparum* and Toxoplasma gondii by inhibition of apicomplexan Fab I. Int J Parasitol 2001; 31:109–113.

133. Eisenreich W, Rohdich F, Bacher A. Deoxyxylulose phosphate pathway to terpenoids. Trends Plant Sci 2001; 6:78–84.

134. Jomaa H, Wiesner J, Sanderbrand S, Altincicek B, Weidemeyer C, Hintz M, et al. Inhibitors of the nonmevalonate pathway of isoprenoid biosynthesis as antimalarial drugs. Science 1999; 285:1573–1576.

135. Somerville C, BJ. Plant lipids: metabolism, mutants, and membranes. Science 1991; 252:80–87.

136. Vial HJ, Eldin P, Martin D, Gannoun L, Calas M, Ancelin ML. Transport of phospholipid synthesis precursors and lipid trafficking into malaria-infected. Novartis Foundation Symposia 1999; 226:74–83.

137. Coppens I, Sinai AP, Joiner KA. Toxoplasma gondii exploits host low-density lipoprotein receptor-mediated endocytosis for cholesterol acquisition. J Cell Biol 2000; 149:167–180.

138. Tarleton RI, Kissinger JC. Parasite genomics: current status and future Prospects. Curr Opin Immunol 2001; 13:395–402.

139. Martin W, Stoebe B, Goremykin V, Hansmann S, Hasegawa M, Kowallik KV. Gene transfer to the nucleus and the evolution of chloroplasts. Nature 1998; 393:162–165.

140. Vollmer M, Thomsen N, Wiek S, Seeber F. Apicomplexan parasites possess distinct nuclear-encoded, but apicoplast-localized, plant-type ferredoxin-NADP(+) reductase and ferredoxin. J Biol Chem 2001; 276:5483–5490.

141. Dzierszinski F, Popescu O, Toursel C, Slomianny C, Yahiaoui B, Tomavo S. The protozoan parasite Toxoplasma gondii expresses two functional plant-like glycolytic enzymes – Implications for evolutionary origin of apicomplexans. J Biol Chem 1999; 274:24,888–24,895.

142. Read M, Hicks KE, Sims PFG, Hyde JE. Molecular characterization of the enolase gene from the human malaria parasite *Plasmodium falciparum:* evidence for ancestry within a photosynthetic lineage. Eur J Biochem 1994; 220:513–520.

143. Hefti F. From genes to effective drugs for neurological and psychiatric diseases. Trends Pharmacol Sci 2001; 22:159–160.

18

The Molecular Biology and Pathogenicity of *Entamoeba histolytica*

Barbara J. Mann and Brendan J. Loftus

INTRODUCTION

In October 2000, The Institute of Genomic Research (TIGR) received funding from the National Institutes of Health to sequence approximately 99% of the *Entamoeba histolytica* genome. There are many questions regarding the pathogenicity and biology of *E. histolytica* that will be fully addressed by the genome project. Practical applications, such as new diagnostic agents, vaccine candidates, and potential new drug targets, may also be revealed. This chapter updates the latest knowledge regarding these aspects of this parasite and indicates those areas in which the genome project is likely to have a particular impact.

EPIDEMIOLOGY

E. histolytica causes amebiasis, a potentially deadly diarrheal disease that is estimated to infect 50 million people and cause 70,000–100,000 deaths each year *(1)*. Amebiasis is endemic in most developing countries. For example, a serological survey of the population of Mexico in 1989 revealed that 8.4% of the sera were positive for *E. histolytica* antibodies *(2)*. In an urban slum in Northeastern Brazil, 24.7% seropositivity and 10.6% intestinal colonization were found *(3,4)*. Studies in Bangladesh indicate that more than 50% of the children have had prior exposure to the disease *(5)*. In the United States and other developed countries, most cases are imported from immigrants from or travelers to endemic areas. The last major outbreak in the United States was at the Chicago World's Fair in 1933 *(6)*. Over 1000 cases of amebiasis were reported, which caused nearly 100 deaths. The source of the outbreak was determined to be a cross-connection of water and sewer pipes at two adjacent hotels. Contaminated water supplies were probably the source of an outbreak in 1998 in Tbilisi, Georgia. A total of 177-cases of amebiasis were reported over a 6-mo time period *(7)*. During this same period, 600–700 breakdowns of the water and sewer system were reported.

CLINICAL MANIFESTATIONS OF AMEBIASIS

In most individuals, infection with *E. histolytica* is symptomless, yet approximately 10% will develop invasive symptomatic disease *(8)*. Individuals who are at

From: *Pathogen Genomics: Impact on Human Health*
Edited by: K. J. Shaw © Humana Press Inc., Totowa, NJ

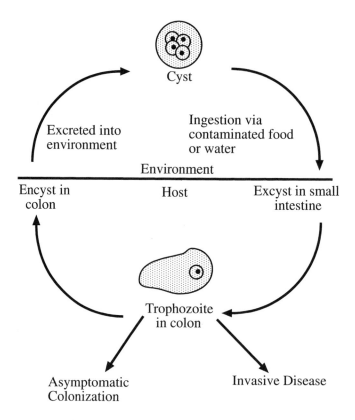

Fig. 1. Life-cycle of *Entamoeba histolytica*

increased risk include the very young and old, pregnant women, people treated with corticosteroids, and the malnourished. No increased severity of disease or frequency has been observed in individuals with acquired immunodeficiency syndrome (AIDS) *(9)*. Amebic dysentery is most commonly associated with bloody diarrhea, abdominal pain and tenderness, and tenesmus. In contrast to bacillary dysentery, which has an abrupt onset and limited duration, amebic colitis usually develops gradually over a period of several weeks, and persists. Weight loss is often observed, but fever is relatively rare. Although the incidence of amebic colitis is equally split between males and females, amebic liver abscess is ten times more common in adult males than in women or children. The most commonly observed symptoms of liver abscess are fever, cough, and abdominal and right upper-quadrant pain, which can occur acute or subacutely. Most patients do not have concomitant amebic colitis, but may have a history of recent colitis. Abscesses can also form at other sites such as the pericardium or pleural cavity by extension from the liver, or by hematogenous spread to the brain.

LIFE CYCLE OF *E. histolytica*

E. histolytica is spread by a fecal-oral route (Fig. 1). Environmentally persistent cysts are shed in the feces of infected individuals. New infections occur when fecally contaminated food or water is consumed. The ingested cyst excysts in the small intestine then divides to form the invasive trophozoite form of the parasite. Trophozoites colonize the large bowel, where they can remain for up to 6 mo or more, although most are eliminated within 12 mo *(10)*. Trophozoites can encyst and be excreted to start a new round of infection, and in some cases may invade through the intestinal epithelium and form abscesses in other tissues. The most common extraintestinal site is the liver. The environmental or parasite factors that control the parasite's development or invasiveness are largely unknown.

The Cyst

The cyst form of the parasite has been difficult to study because viable cysts are not readily formed in culture. The majority of the information on encystation and excystation of *Entamoeba* species comes from the study of the *E. invadens,* a species of ameba that infects reptiles *(11)*. Unlike *E. histolytica, E. invadens* can be made to encyst in culture by osmotic shock, glucose deprivation, or the addition of the kinetoplastid *Crithidia fasciculata* to the culture medium *(12)*. Encystation of *E. invadens* is a galactose- and N-acetyl glucosamine-mediated event, because addition of either of these sugars inhibits encystation *(12)*. An abundant cyst-wall protein designated "jacob" that has five cysteine-rich chitin-binding domains has been purified from *E. invadens* cysts *(13)*. This protein is able to binding both chitin and galactose residues, and may form a bridge upon which the cyst wall forms. It has been difficult to determine how similar encystation and the cyst structure of *E. invadens* are to *E. histolytica.* Cross-hybridization of DNA probes and monoclonal antibodies (MAbs) have not been very successful. The genome project should provide an excellent opportunity to look for homologues of cyst-specific *E. invadens* genes and to identify new genes and strategies that may be involved in cyst formation and development.

THE GENOME

Chromosomes

There are many unresolved questions regarding the organization and composition of the *E. histolytica* genome. Estimates of chromosome number range from 5–6 to 12–16 per nucleus by light and electron microscopy *(14,15)*. Chromosome spreads are difficult because the nuclear membrane apparently remains intact during mitosis *(16)*. The chromosomes of *E. histolytica* have been difficult to resolve by pulsed-field gel electrophoresis (PFGE); however, Willhoeft and Tannich have used a rotating-field electrophoresis system to establish a karyotype for the HM1-IMSS strain *(17)* (Fig. 2). Thirty-one to thirty-five chromosomal-sized DNA, ranging in size from 0.3 to 2.2 Mb, were identified. These investigators also established 14 independent linkage groups by hybridizing with probes from 68 independent cDNA clones. Single-copy genes hybridized to as many as four different bands, suggesting a ploidy of 4n. Some of the homologous chromosomes were vastly different in size, differing by as much as 1 Mb. By adding up the sizes of the largest band in each linkage group, a maximum genome-size estimate of 20 Mb was made. The genome sequence will clarify issues regarding chromosome number, ploidy, and size differences among homologues as well as telomeres, which have not been identified by conventional methods.

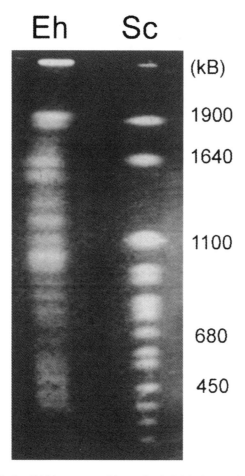

Fig. 2. Total *E. histolytica* DNA separated by pulsed-field electrophoresis. DNA from *E.histolytica* was run in lane Eh. DNA from *Saccharomyces cerevisiae* was run in lane Sc. The gel was stained with ethidum bromide. Molecular size markers in kilobases (kb) are indicated to the right of the gel. "Reprinted from Molec. Biochem. Parasitol. volume 99, Willhoeft and Tannich, The electrophoretic karyotype of *Entamoeba histolytica,* p. 44, (1999) with permission from Elsevier Science."

Episomes

E. histolytica also has circular episomes ranging in size from 4–50 kb *(18)*. Seventy-eight percent of these circles (or roughly 200 copies per genome) are the 25-kb episome that contains rRNA genes. In *E. histolytica,* rRNA genes are located exclusively on an episome. Early data from the TIGR genome project indicates that, as predicted, the rDNA episome comprises approximately 15% of the genomic DNA. The coding capacity of other episomes has not been studied.

Gene Organization

Gene organization has been studied in a few cases. From these few examples, it appears that coding regions appear to be fairly densely packed, with 0.45–2.1 kb between genes *(19–21)*. There is one example of overlapping genes. The 3′ end of the *pak* gene overlaps with the adjacent 5′ end of the *mcm3* gene by 40 basepairs (bp) *(22)*. Thus far, introns are rare, and only four have been identified *(17,23–25)*. These amebic introns are less than 100 bp, and have recognizable branch-point and *cis*-splicing sites. Intergene regions have identifiable elements that have been shown to play a role in influencing gene expression *(19,26–32)*.

The core promoter consists of an initiator element (INR) overlapping the start of transcription, a "TATA"-like box at -30 and a third unique element, located at variable distances between TATA and INR that has been designated "GAAC" *(19,26)*. A "GAAC"-like element has been identified in the core promoter region of at least 12 *E. histolytica* genes *(28)*. Mutations in the "GAAC", TATA, and/or INR sequences influence the level and also the initiation site of transcription *(26)*. Untranslated 5′ leader sequences tend to be short (5–21 bases), but longer leaders have been identified (up to 265 bp) *(22,23,33)*. There is no evidence of transsplicing or polycistronic messages, as are found in trypanosomatids.

Genetic Manipulation of Amebae

Genetic manipulation of *E. histolytica* has made significant strides in the past 10 years. Stable DNA transformation is possible with several different selectable markers *(34–36)*. Expression of transfected genes can be regulated using tetracycline-inducible promoters *(37,38)*. Gene knockouts by homologous recombination have not been achieved thus far; and transfected DNA appears to be maintained episomally *(39)*. However, since the ploidy may be as high as 4n, this is probably not a useful approach for gene knockouts. Anti-sense RNA has been used in several instances to reduce the expression of a targeted gene *(40–42)*. The only report of DNA integration involves the use of pantropic retroviral vectors *(43)*.

GENOMIC-SEQUENCING STRATEGY

TIGR will sequence the genome of *E. histolytica* strain HM1:IMSS. This strain was isolated from a patient with amebic dysentery at the Hospital General, Centro Medico Nacional in Mexico DF in 1967 *(44)*. HM1:IMSS is the primary strain used by investigators for studies of virulence, biochemistry, and molecular biology. It forms liver abscesses in animal models, and is cytotoxic to host cells.

Sequencing of the *E. histolytica* genome at TIGR will be carried out using the shotgun sequencing approach, which has been used to completely sequence more than 30 microbial genomes (http://www.tigr.org/tdb/). The construction of random genomic libraries is one of the most critical steps in sequencing a genome by the random shotgun sequencing approach. In addition to the usual requirements for a low background of nonrecombinant and chimeric clones, the random genomic library must be representative of the entire genome, with a relatively tight insert size range, few clones with no inserts, and no clones with chimeric inserts. Of course, this randomness of genome representation is affected by factors intrinsic to the genome being sequenced, such as unstable or unclonable genes. To address these problems, a new streamlined library construction protocol using three new vectors has been developed:(1) pHOS1, a pUC-derived vector with a copy number of 200, (2) pHOS2, a pBR-based vector with a copy number of 25, and (3) pHOS3, a BAC-based vector with a copy number of 1. All three vectors have been modified by insertion of a BstXI restriction site into the multiple cloning site and removal of strong promoters (such as lacZ) oriented toward the cloning site. Inserts with *BstXI*-adaptor modified ends will only ligate to the vector, which facilitates the preparation of libraries with <2% no insert and chimeric clones. A BAC library will also be constructed and used to help to assemble the contigs and fill gaps in the sequence.

Each clone is sequenced from both ends and assembled into contiguous fragments using the TIGR Assembler *(45,46)*. TIGR Assembler simultaneously clusters and assembles fragments of the genome using a best-match-first strategy. The previous version of TIGR Assembler worked by establishing a seed contig and exhausting the sequence list until no more sequences would extend the contig. It then proceeded to establish a second contig, and repeated the process until all possible contigs were built. Although this method was effective in finding all possible contigs, performance was improved dramatically in the Version 2 TIGR Assembler, which establishes many seed contigs simultaneously. Each new sequence is checked against established contigs; if it does not match any of them, it is used as the seed for a new contig. The major enhancements in Version 2 include incorporation of sequence quality values, simultaneous assembly of multiple contigs, improved pairwise comparison, variable stringency parameters, jump-start parameters, semi-automation of several steps in closure, and editing of the sequence.

Assembly of Larger Genomes with Improvements to TIGR Assembler

TIGR is making improvements to the TIGR Assembler program and in its computational resources in order to handle significantly larger genomes than have been assembled in the past. The main limitation is memory: the program requires approximately one gigabyte per Mb of assembled sequence. Using the current TIGR assembler the 8.5-Mb *Theileria parva* genome from 8X shotgun data and the 20-Mb chromosome 2 of *Arabodpsis thaliana* have been assembled from BAC sequence data. TIGR's current high-end server, a Compaq Alpha ES40 with 16 gigabytes of RAM, can assemble this genome is less than 36 h. The maximum genome size for this machine is approx 16 Mb at 8X coverage. A new version of TIGR Assembler reduces memory usage by 33%, raising the maximum genome size to 23 Mb. TIGR's assembly team is currently developing a new version of the assembler that will handle genomes up to 150 Mb; initial release is scheduled for September 2001. This new version will also make greater use of clone-mate information, and will be able to handle an unlimited number of different clone insert sizes.

In the first year of operation of the *E. histolytica* genome project, over 79,000 sequences have been deposited in Genbank. These sequences can be accessed at the TIGR website (www.tigr.org/tdb/edb2/enta/htmls/). The genome should be completed before the end of 2003. An *Entamoeba* homepage that contains other information about the organism can be found at www.Lshtm.ac.uk/mp/bcu/enta/homef.htm.

PATHOGENICITY OF *E. histolytica*

Invasion of the intestinal mucosa by *E. histolytica* leads to the formation of characteristic flask-shaped ulcers (Fig.3). Subsequent migration from colonic lesions to other sites is believed to occur by hematogenous spread. A key feature of tissue invasion and pathogenicity is the ability of the organism to adhere to, lyse, and phagocytose intestinal epithelium and other host tissues.

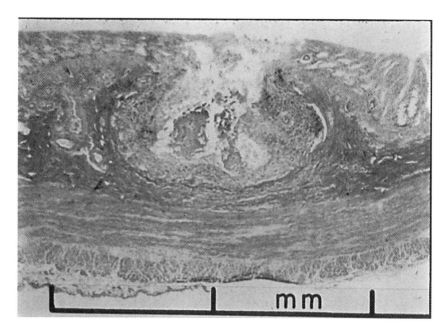

Fig. 3. Flask-shaped ulcer caused by *E. histolytica* trophozoites in the colonic epithelium. From the collection of Harrison Juniper.

Cytotoxic Activity of E. histolytica

The lytic activity of *E. histolytica* is striking. In less than 1 min after contact, target cells undergo membrane blebbing, loss of cytoplasmic granules, and disruption of membrane integrity (Fig.4). Amebae are capable of killing a variety of host cells, including macrophages, T lymphocytes, and neutrophils as well as colonic epithelial cells *(47)*. Killing is contact-dependent and extracellular. Target-cell death can occur by both apoptotic and necrotic mechanisms. DNA fragmentation and activation of caspase 3 is observed in target cells after contact with target cells *(48,49)*. Apoptotic cells have been observed in association with amebic colitis in a mouse model using TUNEL staining *(48,50)*. Apoptotic cells have also been observed in a mouse model of amebic liver abscess *(51)*. In this model, apoptotic cell death occurs even in mice lacking the Fas/Fas ligand or the tumor necrosis factor (TNF)-receptor pathways, indicating that alternative mechanisms for apoptotic cell death are used. Necrosis has been observed as the primary mechanism of cell death in the Jurkat and HL-60 cell line *(52)*. The molecular mechanisms employed by the parasite and host that result in host-cell death have not yet been defined. Several virulence factors of *E. histolytica* have been characterized that contribute to tissue invasion and cell death. The best-characterized include pore-forming "amoebapore" proteins, a novel galactose/N-acetyl-D-galactosamine (Gal/GalNAc) inhibitable lectin, and a family of cysteine proteases.

Amoebapores

Amoebapores are a family of unique pore-forming proteins that are capable of forming ion channels in lipid membranes and depolarizing the membranes of target

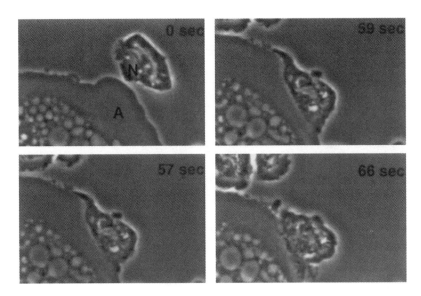

Fig. 4. Frames from cinemicroscopy of *E. histolytica* killing human neutrophils. The upper left frame shows a neutrophil approaching an ameba (only a section is visible in the lower left section of each frame). (Magnification X2000) The complete time-lapse video can be viewed at http://www.med.virginia.edu/som-cl/internal/petri-mann/amebamovie.html. "Reprinted from Crit. Rev. Clin. Lab. Sci. volume 33, Petri, "Recent advances in Amebiasis (1996), p. 12, with permission from CRC Press, INC."

cells (53–55). Amoebapores are small peptides that are 77 amino acids in length, and contain 6 cysteine residues that form three intramolecular disulfide bonds *(56)*. Three isoforms—A,B, and C—share 35–57% identity. These peptides also share significant similarity with NK lysin, an effector molecule of porcine cytotoxic lymphocytes *(57)*. When amoebapore proteins are incubated with membranes, they tend to form higher mol-wt complexes that, based on crosslinking studies, are driven by peptide-peptide interactions *(58)*. This type of assembly is consistent with the barrel-stave model proposed for other pore-forming proteins in which peptide monomers oligomerize after insertion and form a water-filled channel through which ions and other small molecules can pass.

Purified amoebapores are capable of killing eukaryotic cells at high concentrations, and may play a role in cell death *(59)*. However, Leippe and colleagues have proposed that the major function of amoebapore proteins may be to kill ingested bacteria that serve as a nutrient source for the ameba *(59,60)*. *E. histolytica* is a very active phagocytic cell capable of ingesting bacteria, host cells, and erythrocytes. Purified amoebapore protein has been shown to kill gram-positive bacteria, and also gram-negative organisms, although higher concentrations of amoebapore proteins are needed *(61)*. Amoebapore proteins are concentrated in cytoplasmic granules of ameba and are not constitutively expressed into media *(62)*. Thus, the amoebapore proteins, concentrated in the granules, could deliver a highly potent hit to ingested cells.

Anti-sense technology has been used to investigate the role of amoebapores in cytotoxicity *(63)*. When plasmid constructs—which express an anti-sense transcript of

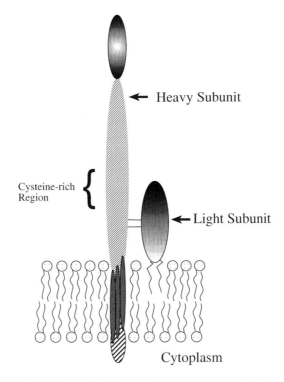

Fig. 5. Schematic diagram of the Gal/GalNAc lectin.

amoebapore A, the most abundant amoebapore—are introduced into ameba, the amoebapore mRNA is inhibited up to 60% and a marked inhibition of amebic cytotoxic activity against eukaryotic and bacterial cells is observed, indicating a role for amoebapores in these activities. No other membranolytic molecules of *E. histolytica* have been identified biochemically. However, the genome project should be useful for determining if there are other potential peptides that may function in this capacity.

Gal/GalNAc Lectin

An essential step in the cytolytic process is adherence to the host or target cells. Early investigations of amebic adherence to target cells revealed that pretreatment of amebae with galactose or GalNAc blocked both amebic adherence to and cytolysis of target cells *(64,65)*. A Gal/GalNAc inhibitable lectin was first purified by galactose affinity columns *(65)*. It is glycosylated, and in its native state it migrates as a 260-Kd protein on SDS-polyacrylamide gels. Upon reduction with beta-mercaptoethanol, the Gal/GalNAc lectin dissociates into heavy 170-Kd and 31–35-Kd light subunits *(66)*. The heavy subunit of the Gal/GalNAc lectin consists of a large extracellular domain that can be divided into putative domains based on amino-acid composition, a single transmembrane-spanning domain and a short cytoplasmic domain (Fig.5). The light subunit is associated with the membrane by a glycerol phosphatidyl inositol anchor. There are several isoforms of each subunit that are encoded by 5–6 genes *(67)*. The heavy subunit isoforms are 89–95% identical, and the light subunit forms average about 80% identity with each other. Studies have not revealed whether the different isoforms or specific pairings of subunits have any functional differences. Neither the heavy or the light subunit shares any amino-acid similarity with the carbohydrate-binding domains that are found in C- or S-types lectins *(68)*, but a carbohydrate-binding activity has been identified in the cysteine-rich region of the heavy subunit *(69,70)*. The derived amino acids of both subunits do not share any significant similarities with any other known proteins in the database, although some limited regions of similarities have been proposed.

MAbs produced against the native lectin have been useful for studying both the structure and function of the lectin. Some anti-lectin MAbs block amebic adherence to target cells and also cytolysis *(71)*. However, some of the lectin-specific MAbs enhance rather than inhibit amebic adherence to target cells. Interestingly, enhanced cytolysis is not observed with these "enhancing" MAbs, but in fact a slight decrease *(72)*. These results suggest that the Gal/GalNAc lectin may undergo conformational changes associated with ligand binding, and further implies that the lectin may be involved in signal transduction. This hypothesis is supported by studies that overexpressed only the cytoplasmic-domain portion of the heavy subunit, which is the only part of the protein in contact with the cytoplasm *(73)*. Overexpression of the cytoplasmic tail results in decreased adherence to target cells. This effect can be abrogated by expressing a mutated version of cytoplasmic-domain peptide. These results imply that there are factors in the cytoplasm that associate with the lectin tail to increase the affinity of the lectin for its ligand. This is analogous to mammalian and avian integrin molecules, which signal via their cytoplasmic tails. The cytoplasmic domain of the lectin shares some sequence similarity with the β-integrins *(73)*. Mutation of conserved residues that have been shown to be important in integrin signaling are also important in lectin-mediated signaling *(74)*.

Cysteine Proteinases

Amebic cysteine proteinases, which belong to the papain superfamily, are initially produced as preproenzymes, and have substrate specificity similar to cathepsin B *(75)*. Six genes that encode amebic cysteine proteinases have been identified by screening genomic libraries *(76–77)*. These genes encode products that share 40–85% identity with each other. Three of the proteinases are apparently responsible for more than 90% of the activity in vitro, and the other three are either poorly expressed or not expressed *(76)*. Most of the proteinases are constitutively secreted into culture medium; however, one (CP5) is associated with the membrane *(78)*. There has been some controversy regarding the number and size of amebic cysteine proteinases, with reports of proteinases ranging from 16 to 197 Kd in size. All of the proteinases for which a gene has been identified encode mature proteins of approx 30 Kd *(76)*. Although two of the higher mol-wt proteins have been identified as products of two of the cloned genes, the knowledge of the complete genome should help to identify all genes that encode cysteine proteinases *(79)*.

Cysteine proteinases secreted by *E. histolytica* are believed to primarily facilitate the penetration of the intestinal mucosa and tissue invasion by amebic trophozoites *(75)*. Amebae exhibit cytopathic effects on tissue-culture monolayers and disrupt basement membranes, presumably by degrading extracellular matrix (ECM) proteins such as fibronectin, laminin, and collagen *(80–84)*. The ability of amebic cysteine proteinases to degrade IgA, IgG, and complement anaphylatoxins C3a and C5a may also contribute to dampening host immune responses to the parasite *(85–86)*. Cysteine proteinases have been shown to be important for the disease process in vivo. Severe combined immunodeficient (SCID) mice, treated with E64, a cysteine proteinase inhibitor, develop smaller amebic liver abscesses than controls *(87)*. Cysteine proteinases also appear to play a role in the inflammatory response. An E. histolytica-infected human intestinal xenograft, implanted in a SCID mouse, produce lower cytokines levels of IL-1β and IL-8, and less inflammation and damage to the intestinal barrier when grafts are infected with amebae that express cysteine proteinase antisense RNA. Amebic cysteine proteinases have an IL-1β converting enzyme activity (ICE) and may be major contributors to inflammatory effects by activating IL-β *(87)*.

E. histolytica/E. dispar

Entamoeba histolytica was first identified in 1875 as "Amoeba coli" by Fedor Losch in St. Petersburg Russia in the stools of a Russian man with dysentery *(88)*. However, Losch attributed the dysentery to bacteria rather than amebae. It was in the classic work of Councilman and Lafleur in 1891, working in Baltimore, Maryland that identified *E. histolytica* in a bacteriologically sterile liver abscess *(89)*. Although *E. histolytica* was widely accepted as a pathogen, there was a disconnection between the prevalence of the parasite and the amount of active disease. In 1925, Emile Brumpt postulated that *E. histolytica* was actually two separate yet morphologically identical species, pathogenic *E. histolytica* and nonpathogenic *E. dispar (90)*. Although the Brumpt hypothesis fit the epidemiology of the disease, it was not widely accepted. Instead, *E. histolytica* was classified as having pathogenic and nonpathogenic zymodemes. Zymodeme classification is based on the pattern of electrophoretic mobilities of several isoenzymes on starch gels *(91)*. This work was pioneered by Sargeaunt, who identified more than 20 different patterns of isoenzymes or zymodemes *(92)*. Pathogenic strains of *E. histolytica* make up nine of these zymodemes, and isolates exhibiting the other 11 nonpathogenic zymodemes have never been associated with disease. It was also recognized that approximately 90% of *E. histolytica* infections were comprised of ameba with non-pathogenic zymodemes.

As the ability to apply molecular techniques to the study of *E. histolytica* became possible, genetic differences among pathogenic and nonpathogenic zymodemes began to be reported *(93,94)*. A comparison of homologous clones isolated from strains with pathogenic and nonpathogenic zymodemes were found to be 10% different at the nucleic-acid level *(93)*. Perhaps the most compelling evidence for recognizing separate species was that the ribosomal RNA genes of pathogenic and nonpathogenic strains were found to be distinct sequences *(94)*. Genetic differences were also supported by the existence of a number of MAbs that were specific for pathogenic zymodemes and not nonpathogenic, and vice-versa *(71,95–97)*. In 1997, a panel of experts in the field of amebiasis convened by the World Health Organization, the Pan American Health Organization, and UNESCO agreed to recognize two species—*E. histolytica,* the causative agent of amebiasis, and *E. dispar,* a commensal organism that has never been associated with disease.

Although these two organisms are now recognized as separate species, the basis for differences in pathogenicity remains somewhat of an enigma. Both *E. histolytica* and *E. dispar* can adhere to and lyse target and host cells via a Gal/GalNAc lectin, although the level of cytotoxicity is decreased in *E. dispar (98–100)*. The heavy and the light subunits of the Gal/GalNAc lectin of *E. dispar* have at least 86% and 79% amino-acid identity to the *E. histolytica* lectin *(99–101)*. A homolog of amoebapore A has been found in *E. dispar,* but its specific activity is only 30% of *E. histolytica* amoebapore A, despite a 95% identity of the primary structure *(102). E. dispar* contains only four of the six identified genes that encode cysteine proteinases *(76)*. Most notably, *E. dispar* lacks CP5, the cysteine proteinase that comprises over 90% of the cysteine proteinase activity of *E. histolytica.* More recently, a pseudogene for CP5 has been identified in *E. dispar (21)*. Interestingly, this pseudogene is found in the same genetic location as in *E. dispar.* A complete conservation of gene order was found between the two species at this particular locus. This suggests that genomes of *E. histolytica and E. dispar* are syntenic. The synteny of these two species provides an exciting opportunity for discovering the basis of pathogenicity of *E. histolytica.* Because the two species share a high identity, microarrays hybridized with *E. dispar* DNA could reveal any large deletions or even rearrangements if an ordered array is used. Hybridizations with *E. dispar* cDNA could reveal differences in gene expression, or possibly regulatory changes by comparing cDNA isolated from different growth conditions.

DIAGNOSIS

The traditional method for diagnosis and detection of intestinal infection with *E. histolytica* is microscopic examination of stools. This method is insensitive, requires considerable expertise, and is complicated by the inability to distinguish pathogenic *E. histolytica* from its morphologically similar but nonpathogenic relative *Entamoeba dispar.* Microscopy is only 33–66% sensitive compared to the gold standard of culture *(103)*. Specific diagnostic tests that can distinguish between *E. histolytica* and *E. dispar* are important, since *E. dispar* infection does not require treatment. In addition, the epidemiology of *E. histolytica* must be evaluated, since many older studies relied solely on microscopy for identification. Diagnosis of amebic liver abscess presents it own challenge, since symptoms can vary widely and ultrasound or computer tomography images do not reliably distinguish between a bacterial or amebic abscess. Several ELISA antigen detection kits are commercially available *(104–106),* and *E. histolytica-*specific PCR primers have been identified that are useful for epidemiological studies *(107–108)*. Genome analysis may reveal new tools for molecular and ELISA detection methods.

ELISA Antigen Detection

Antigen detection by ELISA is a useful method for diagnosis and detection because it is a simple, fast and reliable technique. There are three commercially available detection kits; the *E. histolytica* kit®, ProSpecT® ELISA, and Merlin Optimum S ELISA *(103–106)*. Only the *E. histolytica* kit® distinguishes *E. histolytica* from *E. dispar.* Antigen detection is most useful for stool specimens, and has a reported sensitivity of greater than 90% *(103)*. This sensitivity is comparable to isoenzyme analysis or PCR techniques *(104)*. The *E. histolytica* kit® has also been used to detect antigen in sera.

(109). Nearly 100% of liver abscess patients had antigen in their sera before chemotherapy was administered. Antigen was also detectable in sera in some colitis cases, but antigen detection in the stool appears to be a more sensitive method for diagnosis intestinal colonization. Antibody detection is not as useful for diagnosis because it cannot distinguish current from prior infections *(110)*.

PCR Detection

PCR methods have been particularly useful for discriminating strains of *E. histolytica* as well as other *Entamoeba* species. Unlike isoenzyme (zymodeme) analysis, PCR does not require culturing the organism. *E. histolytica* DNA has been successfully amplified from stool and liver pus *(111–113)*. The serine-rich protein gene (SREHP) and a strain-specific gene have shown extensive polymorphism among isolates from different geographic regions *(114)*. These two markers identified 16 different patterns among 18 isolates that were stable over time, animal passage, and axenization. Primers derived from these genes and others should be useful in characterizing the molecular epidemiology of both endemic and epidemic occurrences of disease.

TREATMENT

Metronidazole is the drug of choice to treat amebiasis *(115)*. It is more than 90% effective in treating both intestinal and tissue infections. Although some carcinogenic effects of metronidazole have been reported in animals and mutagenesis in bacteria, no association has been reported in humans. Drug-resistant amebae have been produced in the laboratory, but no naturally occurring drug resistance has been reported in human populations. It is recommended that metronidazole should be used with a luminal agent, since metronidazole is not effective against cysts. Paromomycin diiodohyroxyquin, diloxanide furoate, and iodoquniol are the most frequently prescribed luminal agents.

VACCINE

Despite the availability of effective treatment with metronidazole, significant levels of morbidity and mortality associated with amebiasis still persist. Since there are no intermediate hosts and humans are the only epidemiologically significant reservoir of the parasite, an effective vaccine that could eliminate *E. histolytica* as a cause of human disease is theoretically possible. The genome project should be useful for identifying potential vaccine candidates. One possible approach would be to search the genome for putative surface-exposed proteins, a method used with the genome of *Neisseria meningitidis (116)*. The genes encoding putative surface proteins were cloned and expressed in *E. coli,* purified, and then used to immunize mice. The immune sera was then tested for bacteriocidal activity as a means of identifying antigens with protective potential.

Immunity to Amebiasis

Although there are numerous examples of immunity to amebiasis in animal models of amebic liver abscess *(117–119),* only limited data exists on immunity to amebiasis in humans. Anecdotal reports suggest that recurrence after invasive amebiasis is rare. A chart review in Mexico of 1021 amebic liver abscess patients revealed that only three patients had a reoccurrence over a 5-yr period *(120)*. There is data suggesting that both humoral and cell-mediated responses contribute to immunity. Secretory IgA and serum antibodies to *E. histolytica* develop during human infection *(110,121)*. Although no conclusive role for antibody-mediated protection has been made in humans, several animal studies have produced supportive data. For instance, passive transfer of anti-*E. histolytica* antibodies to SCID mice protect against amebic liver abscess formation *(117)*. Reports of exacerbated disease in patients who have received corticosteroids suggest a role for cell-mediated responses; however, there is no apparent increase in the incidence or severity of amebiasis in AIDS patients *(122,123)*. Lymphocytes from patients cured of amebic liver abscess exhibit amebicidal activities in vitro in response to amebic antigen *(124–126)*. In the gerbil model of amebic liver abscess, interventions that depress cellular immune responses such as corticosteroids, splenectomy, or neonatal thymectomy also result in exacerbated hepatic abscesses *(127–129)*. Controlled human studies are needed to fully characterize the nature of protective immunity.

Vaccine Candidates

Total *E. histolytica* antigen is an effective vaccine in animal models against amebiasis, yet this is an expensive and somewhat impractical type of vaccine *(127)*. Subunit vaccines are an attractive alternative because of the possibility of producing large amounts at a lower cost and perhaps fewer side effects. Several proteins have been tested as vaccines, but the two most promising vaccine candidates are SREHP and the Gal/GalNAc lectin.

Gal/GalNAc Lectin

The Gal/GalNAc lectin is a logical vaccine candidate because of its critical role in pathogenicity. It is also an antigenically conserved protein, that has been found on isolates from a variety of geographic regions *(130)*. The lectin is antigenic. Both humoral and cell-mediated immune responses to the Gal/GalNAc lectin have been found in patients with amebiasis *(124,130)*.

In one of the first lectin vaccine studies, gerbils were parenterally immunized with the native lectin, which consists of both heavy and light subunits. Complete protection was observed in 67% of the animals *(131)*. However, it was noted that the abscesses in the immunized animals that were not protected were significantly larger than controls. Subsequently, immunization with recombinantly expressed portions of the cysteine-rich region of the heavy subunit (*see* Fig. 5) have been shown to produce approximately the same amount of protection as the native lectin, and no increase in abscess size has been observed in unprotected animals *(132–136)*. Lotter et al. found that immunization with the amino-terminal cysteine-poor region of the heavy subunit did not protect, and that abscess sizes were increased compared to controls *(137)*. These results suggest that the amino-terminal region of the heavy subunit may have contributed to the larger abscesses in the initial vaccine trial with the native lectin.

SREHP

SREHP is a phosphorylated surface protein that is apparently lipid-linked to the membrane *(138,139)*. As its name implies, it has a high percentage of serine residues (52 of 233), and contains multiple octapeptide and dodecappetide amino-acid repeats. It is a conserved antigen in *E. histolytica,* but the number of peptide repeats can vary in different isolates. Its role in the ameba has not been clearly established, although high-titer specific antiserum inhibits adherence to target cells. SREHP has been shown to be an effective immunogen in animal models of amebiasis. Passive transfer of anti-SREHP antibodies, as well as parenteral immunization with recombinant SREHP, produces protection in animal models *(140)*. Some of the immunization trials with an SREHP-maltose-binding protein fusion have produced 100% protection in a gerbil model of amebic liver abscess *(141)*.

Oral immunization with attenuated strains of *Salmonella* that express SREHP or the Gal/GalNAc have also been an effective route of vaccination. Mice and gerbils orally immunized with *S. typhimurium* expressing SREHP produced specific sIgA and IgG *(142)*. When gerbils were challenged, only 22% of immunized animals developed liver abscesses compared to 100% of controls. SREHP has also been expressed in *S. typhi* *(143)*. Oral immunization with *S. dublin* expressing the Gal/GalNAc lectin resulted in a significant reduction in abscess sizes in immunized animals, but there was no significant reduction in the number of animals with abscesses *(133)*. An oral vaccine for amebiasis may be an effective type of vaccine for this enteric disease. It is striking that although the models used in these oral immunization trials examined systemic disease, protection was still possible through an oral route of vaccination.

CONCLUSION

Many questions will be solved or addressed when the complete genome sequence of *E. histolytica* becomes available. Basic knowledge of the genome organization and chromosome structure should become apparent. New information should be provided about the cyst and parasite development. The identification of new virulence factors and the ability to identify new markers for isolate and strain identification should help with the understanding of pathogenicity and epidemiology. As the other genomes emerge upon the scene, phylogenetic relationships and genetic exchanges may become more apparent and may provide a further understanding of the interactions of pathogens and hosts.

REFERENCES

1. World Health Organization. The world health report—bridging the gaps. World Health Forum 1995; 16:377–385.
2. Caballero-Salcedo A, Viveros-Rogel M, Salvatierra B, et al. Seroepidemiology of amebiasis in Mexico. Am J Trop Med Hyg 1994; 50:412–419.
3. Braga LL, Lima AA, Sears CL, et al. Seroepidemiology of *Entamoeba histolytica* in a slum in northeastern Brazil. Am J Trop Med Hyg 1996; 55:693–697.
4. Braga LL, Mendonca Y, Paiva CA, Sales A, Cavalcante AL, Mann BJ. Seropositivity for and intestinal colonization with *Entamoeba histolytica* and *Entamoeba dispar* in individuals in northeastern Brazil. J Clin Microbiol 1998; 36:3044–3045.
5. Haque R, Ali IM, Petri WA, Jr. Prevalence and immune response to *Entamoeba histolytica* infection in preschool children in Bangladesh. Am J Trop Med Hyg 1999; 60:1031–1034.
6. National Institutes of Health. Epidemic amebic dysentery: the Chicago outbreak of 1933. NIH Bulletin 1936; Mar:166.
7. Kreidl P, Imnadze P, Baidoshvili L, Greco D. Investigation of an outbreak of amoebiasis in Georgia. Surveillance 1999; 4:103–106.
8. Reed SL. Clinical manifestations and diagnosis. In: Ravdin JI (ed). Amebiasis, London, Imperial College Press, 2000, pp. 113–126.

9. Seeto RK, Rockey DC. Amebic liver abscess: epidemiology, clinical features, and outcome. West J Med 1999; 170:104–109.

10. Gathiram V, Jackson TF. A longitudinal study of asymptomatic carriers of pathogenic zymodemes of *Entamoeba histolytica*. S Afr Med J 1987; 72:669–672.

11. Eichinger D. Encystation of Entamoeba parasites. Bioessays 1997; 19:633–639.

12. Cho J, Eichinger D. *Crithidia fasciculata* induces encystation of *Entamoeba invadens* in a galactose-dependent manner. J Parasitol 1998; 84:705–710.

13. Frisardi M, Ghosh SK, Field J, et al. The most abundant glycoprotein of amebic cyst walls (Jacob) is a lectin with five Cys-rich, chitin-binding domains. Infect Immun 2000; 68:4319–4324.

14. Orozco E, Baez-Camargo M, Gamboa L, Flores E, Valdes J, Hernandez F. Molecular karyotype of related clones of *Entamoeba histolytica*. Mol Biochem Parasitol 1993; 59:29–40.

15. Petter R, Rozenblatt S, Schechtman D, Wellems TE, Mirelman D. Electrophoretic karyotype and chromosome assignments for a pathogenic and a nonpathogenic strain of *Entamoeba histolytica*. Infect Immun 1993; 61:3574–3577.

16. Willhoeft U, Tannich E. Fluorescence microscopy and fluorescence in situ hybridization of *Entamoeba histolytica* nuclei to analyze mitosis and the localization of repetitive DNA. Mol Biochem Parasitol 2000; 105:291–296.

17. Willhoeft U, Tannich E. The electrophoretic karyotype of *Entamoeba histolytica*. Mol Biochem Parasitol 1999; 99:41–53.

18. Dhar SK, Choudhury NR, Bhattacharaya A, Bhattacharya S. A multitude of circular DNAs exist in the nucleus of *Entamoeba histolytica*. Mol Biochem Parasitol 1995; 70:203–206.

19. Bruchhaus I, Leippe M, Lioutas C, Tannich E. Unusual gene organization in the protozoan parasite *Entamoeba histolytica*. DNA Cell Biol 1993; 12:925–933.

20. Petter R, Rozenblatt S, Nuchamowitz Y, Mirelman D. Linkage between actin and ribosomal protein L21 genes in *Entamoeba histolytica*. Mol Biochem Parasitol 1992; 56:329–333.

21. Willhoeft U, Hamann L, Tannich E. A DNA sequence corresponding to the gene encoding cysteine proteinase 5 in *Entamoeba histolytica* is present and positionally conserved but highly degenerated in *Entamoeba dispar*. Infect Immun 1999; 67:5925–5929.

22. Gangopadhyay SS, Ray SS, Sinha P, Lohia A. Unusual genome organization in *Entamoeba histolytica* leads to two overlapping transcripts. Mol Biochem Parasitol 1997; 89:73–83.

23. Urban B, Blasig C, Forster B, Hamelmann C, Horstmann RD. Putative serine/threonine protein kinase expressed in complement-resistant forms of *Entamoeba histolytica*. Mol Biochem Parasitol 1996; 80:171–178.

24. Plaimauer B, Ortner S, Wiedermann G, Scheiner O, Duchene M. An intron-containing gene coding for a novel 39-kilodalton antigen of *Entamoeba histolytica*. Mol Biochem Parasitol 1994; 66:181–185.

25. Lohia A, Samuelson J. Cloning of the Eh cdc2 gene from *Entamoeba histolytica* encoding a protein kinase p34cdc2 homologue. Gene 1993; 127:203–207.

26. Singh U, Purdy J, Mann BJ, Petri WA, Jr. Three conserved cis-acting sequences in the core promoter control gene expression in the protozoan parasite *Entamoeba histolytica*. Arch Med Res 1997:41–42.

27. Bruchhaus I, Tannich E. Induction of the iron-containing superoxide dismutase in *Entamoeba histolytica* by a superoxide anion-generating system or by iron chelation. Mol Biochem Parasitol 1994; 67:281–288.

28. Purdy JE, Pho LT, Mann BJ, Petri WA, Jr. Upstream regulatory elements controlling expression of the *Entamoeba histolytica* lectin. Mol Biochem Parasitol 1996; 78:91–103.

29. Ortiz D, del Carmen Dominguez-Robles M, Villegas-Sepulveda N, Meza I. Actin induction during PMA and cAMP-dependent signal pathway activation in *Entamoeba histolytica* trophozoites. Cellular Microbiol 2000; 2:391–400.

30. Gilchrist CA, Purdy J, Mann BJ, Petri WA, Jr. Control of gene expression in *Entamoeba histolytica* by a cis-acting upstream regulatory element. Arch Med Res 1997:39–40.

31. Hidalgo ME, Orozco E. Structural characterization of the *Entamoeba histolytica* enolase gene promoter. Arch Med Res 1997:46–48.

32. Schaenman JM, Driscoll PC, Hockensmith JW, Mann BJ, Petri WA, Jr. An upstream regulatory element containing two nine basepair repeats regulates expression of the *Entamoeba histolytica* hg15 lectin gene. Mol Biochem Parasitol 1998; 94:309–313.

33. De Meester F, Bracha R, Huber M, Keren Z, Rozenblatt S, Mirelman D. Cloning and characterization of an unusual elongation factor-1 alpha cDNA from *Entamoeba histolytica*. Mol Biochem Parasitol 1991; 44:23–32.

34. Vines RR, Purdy JE, Ragland BD, Samuelson J, Mann BJ, Petri WA, Jr. Stable episomal transfection of *Entamoeba histolytica*. Mol Biochem Parasitol 1995; 71:265–267.

35. Hamann L, Nickel R, Tannich E. Transfection and continuous expression of heterologous genes in the protozoan parasite *Entamoeba histolytica*. Proc Natl Acad Sci USA 1995; 92:8975–8979.

36. Ramakrishnan G, Rogers J, Mann BJ, Petri WA. New tools for genetic analysis of *Entamoeba histolytica:* blasticidin S deaminase and green fluorescence protein. Parasitol Int 2001; 50:47–50.

37. Hamann L, Buss H, Tannich E. Tetracycline-controlled gene expression in *Entamoeba histolytica*. Mol Biochem Parasitol 1997; 84:83–91.

38. Ramakrishnan G, Vines RR, Mann BJ, Petri WA, Jr. A tetracycline-inducible gene expression system in *Entamoeba histolytica*. Mol Biochem Parasitol 1997; 84:93–100.

39. Dhar SK, Vines RR, Bhattacharya S, Petri WA, Jr. Ribosomal DNA fragments enhance the stability of transfected DNA in *Entamoeba histolytica* . J Eukaryot Microbiol 1998; 45:656–660.

40. Ankri S, Stolarsky T, Mirelman D. Antisense inhibition of expression of cysteine proteinases does not affect *Entamoeba histolytica* cytopathic or haemolytic activity but inhibits phagocytosis. Mol Microbiol 1998; 28:777–785.

41. Ankri S, Padilla-Vaca F, Stolarsky T, Koole L, Katz U, Mirelman D. Antisense inhibition of expression of the light subunit (35 kDa) of the Gal/GalNac lectin complex inhibits *Entamoeba histolytica* virulence. Mol Microbiol 1999; 33:327–337.

42. Ankri S, Stolarsky T, Bracha R, Padilla-Vaca F, Mirelman D. Antisense inhibition of expression of cysteine proteinases affects *Entamoeba histolytica*-induced formation of liver abscess in hamsters. Infect Immun 1999; 67:421–422.

43. Que X, Kim D, Alagon A, et al. Pantropic retroviral vectors mediate gene transfer and expression in *Entamoeba histolytica*. Mol Biochem Parasitol 1999; 99:237–245.

44. Kazuko-Kawashima P, Tanimoto-Weki M, De la Torre M, Gonzalez-Sanchez SM. [Comparative study of pathogenic and nonpathogenic *E. histolytica* strains with light microscopy and immunofluorescent reactions]. [Spanish]. Arch Investig Med (Suppl 1973) 1:11–16.

45. Fraser CM, Caskems S, Huang WM, et al. Genomic sequences of a Lyme disease spirochaete, *Borrelia burgdorferi*. Nature 1997; 390:580–586.

46. Gardner MJ, Tettelin H, Carucci DJ, Cummings LM. Chromosome 2 sequence of the human malaria parasite *Plasmodium falciparum*. Science 1998; 282:1126–1132.

47. Ravdin JI, Guerrant RL. Role of adherence in cytopathogenic mechanisms of *Entamoeba histolytica*. Study with mammalian tissue culture cells and human erythrocytes. J Clin Investig 1981; 68:1305–1313.

48. Huston CD, Houpt ER, Mann BJ, Hahn CS, Petri WA. Caspase 3-dependent killing of host cells by the parasite *Entamoeba histolytica*. Cell Microbiol 2000; 2:617–625.

49. Ragland BD, Ashley LS, Vaux DL, Petri WA, Jr. *Entamoeba histolytica*: target cells killed by trophozoites undergo DNA fragmentation which is not blocked by Bcl-2. Exp Parasitol 1994; 79:460–467.

50. Huston CD, Mann BJ, Hahn CS, Petri WA. Role of host caspases in cell killing by *Entamoeba histolytica*. Arch Med Res 2000; 31:S216–S217.

51. Seydel KB, Stanley SL, Jr. *Entamoeba histolytica* induces host cell death in amebic liver abscess by a non-Fas-dependent, non-tumor necrosis factor alpha-dependent pathway of apoptosis. Infect Immun 1998; 66:2980–2983.

52. Berninghausen O, Leippe M. Necrosis versus apoptosis as the mechanism of target cell death induced by *Entamoeba histolytica*. Infect Immun 1997; 65:3615–3621.

53. Lynch EC, Rosenberg IM, Gitler C. An ion-channel forming protein produced by *Entamoeba histolytica*. EMBO J 1982; 1:801–804.

54. Rosenberg I, Bach D, Loew LM, Gitler C. Isolation, characterization and partial purification of a transferable membrane channel (amoebapore) produced by *Entamoeba histolytica*. Mol Biochem Parasitol 1989; 33:237–247.

55. Young JD, Young TM, Lu LP, Unkeless JC, Cohn ZA. Characterization of a membrane pore-forming protein from *Entamoeba histolytica*. J Exp Med 1982; 156:1677–1690.

56. Leippe M, Andra J, Nickel R, Tannich E, Muller-Eberhard HJ. Amoebapores, a family of membranolytic peptides from cytoplasmic granules of *Entamoeba histolytica*: isolation, primary structure, and pore formation in bacterial cytoplasmic membranes. Mol Microbiol 1994; 14:895–904.

57. Dandekar T, Leippe M. Molecular modeling of amoebapore and NK-lysin: a four-alpha-helix bundle motif of cytolytic peptides from distantly related organisms. Fold Des 1997; 2:47–52.

58. Andra J, Leippe M. Pore-forming peptide of *Entamoeba histolytica*: significance of positively charged amino acid residues for its mode of action. FEBS Lett 1994; 354:97–102.

59. Leippe M, Muller-Eberhard HJ. The pore-forming peptide of *Entamoeba histolytica*, the protozoan parasite causing human amoebiasis. Toxicology 1994; 87:5–18.

60. Leippe M. Amoebapores. Parasitol Today 1997; 13:178–183.

61. Leippe M, Andra J, Muller-Eberhard HJ. Cytolytic and antibacterial activity of synthetic peptides derived from amoebapore, the pore-forming peptide of *Entamoeba histolytica*. Proc Natl Acad Sci USA 1994; 91:2602–2606.

62. Leippe M, Sievertsen HJ, Tannich E, Horstmann RD. Spontaneous release of cysteine proteinases but not of pore-forming peptides by viable *Entamoeba histolytica*. Parasitology 1995; 111:569–574.

63. Bracha R, Nuchamowitz Y, Leippe M, Mirelman D. Antisense inhibition of amoebapore expression in *Entamoeba histolytica* causes a decrease in amoebic virulence. Mol Microbiol 1999; 34:463–472.

64. Guerrant RL, Brush J, Ravdin JI, Sullivan JA, Mandell GL. Interaction between *Entamoeba histolytica* and human polymorphonuclear neutrophils. J Infect Dis 1981; 143:83–93.

65. Petri WA, Jr, Ravdin JI. Cytopathogenicity of *Entamoeba histolytica*: the role of amebic adherence and contact-dependent cytolysis in pathogenesis. Eur J Epidemiol 1987; 3:123–136.

66. Petri WA, Jr, Chapman MD, Snodgrass T, Mann BJ, Broman J, Ravdin JI. Subunit structure of the galactose and N-acetyl-D-galactosamine-inhibitable adherence lectin of *Entamoeba histolytica*. J Biol Chem 1989; 264:3007–3012.

67. Ramakrishnan G, Ragland BD, Purdy JE, Mann BJ. Physical mapping and expression of gene families encoding the N-acetyl D-galactosamine adherence lectin of *Entamoeba histolytica*. Mol Microbiol 1996; 19:91–100.

68. Drickamer K. Making a fitting choice: common aspects of sugar-binding sites in plant and animal lectins. Structure 1997; 5:465–468.

69. Dodson JM, Lenkowski PW, Jr, Eubanks AC, et al. Infection and immunity mediated by the carbohydrate recognition domain of the *Entamoeba histolytica* Gal/GalNAc lectin. J Infect Dis 1999; 179:460–466.

70. Pillai DR, Wan PS, Yau YC, Ravdin JI, Kain KC. The cysteine-rich region of the *Entamoeba histolytica* adherence lectin (170-kilodalton subunit) is sufficient for high-affinity Gal/GalNAc-specific binding in vitro. Infect Immun 1999; 67:3836–3841.

71. Petri WA, Jr, Snodgrass TL, Jackson TF, et al. Monoclonal antibodies directed against the galactose-binding lectin of *Entamoeba histolytica* enhance adherence. J Immunol 1990; 144:4803–4809.

72. Saffer LD, Petri WAJR. Role of the galactose lectin of *Entamoeba histolytica* in adherence-dependent killing of mammalian cells. Infect Immun 1991; 59:4681–4683.

73. Vines RR, Ramakrishnan G, Rogers JB, Lockhart LA, Mann BJ, Petri WA, Jr. Regulation of adherence and virulence by the *Entamoeba histolytica* lectin cytoplasmic domain, which contains a beta2 integrin motif. Mol Biol Cell 1998; 9:2069–2079.

74. Peter K, O'Toole TE. Modulation of cell adhesion by changes in αLβ2(LFA-1, CD11a/CD18)) cytoplasmic domain/cytoskeleton interaction. J Exp Med 1995; 181:315–326.

75. Que X, Reed SL. Cysteine proteinases and the pathogenesis of amebiasis. Clin Microbiol Rev 2000; 13:196–206.

76. Bruchhaus I, Jacobs T, Leippe M, Tannich E. *Entamoeba histolytica* and *Entamoeba dispar:* differences in numbers and expression of cysteine proteinase genes. Mol Microbiol 1996; 22:255–263.

77. Reed S, Bouvier J, Sikes Pollack A, et al. Cloning of a virulence factor of *Entamoeba histolytica*. Pathogenic strains possess a unique cysteine proteinase gene. J Clin Investig 1993; 91:1532–1540.

78. Jacobs T, Bruchhaus I, Dandekar T, Tannich E, Leippe M. Isolation and molecular characterization of a surface-bound proteinase of *Entamoeba histolytica*. Mol Microbiol 1998; 27:269–276.

79. Hellberg A, Nickel R, Lotter H, Tannich E, Bruchhaus I. Overexpression of cysteine proteinase 2 in *Entamoeba histolytica* or *Entamoeba dispar* increases amoeba-induced monolayer destruction in vitro but does not augment amoebic liver abscess formation in gerbils. Cell Microbiol 2001; 3:13–20.

80. Keene WE, Hidalgo ME, Orozco E, McKerrow JH. *Entamoeba histolytica*: correlation of the cytopathic effect of virulent trophozoites with secretion of a cysteine proteinase. Exp Parasitol 1990; 71:199–206.

81. Bracha R, Mirelman D. Virulence of *Entamoeba histolytica* trophozoites. Effects of bacteria, microaerobic conditions, and metronidazole. J Exp Med 1984; 160:353–368.

82. Luaces AL, Barrett AJ. Affinity purification and biochemical characterization of histolysin, the major cysteine proteinase of *Entamoeba histolytica*. Biochem J 1988; 250:903–909.

83. Schulte W, Scholze H. Action of the major protease from *Entamoeba histolytica* on proteins of the extracellular matrix. J Protozool 1989; 36:538–543.

84. Li E, Yang WG, Zhang T, Stanley SL, Jr. Interaction of laminin with *Entamoeba histolytica* cysteine proteinases and its effect on amebic pathogenesis. Infect Immun 1995; 63:4150–4153.

85. Tran VQ, Herdman DS, Torian BE, Reed SL. The neutral cysteine proteinase of *Entamoeba histolytica* degrades IgG and prevents its binding. J Infect Dis 1998; 177:508–511.

86. Reed SL, Ember JA, Herdman DS, DiScipio RG, Hugli TE, Gigli I. The extracellular neutral cysteine proteinase of *Entamoeba histolytica* degrades anaphylatoxins C3a and C5a. J Immunol 1995; 155:266–274.

87. Stanley SL, Jr, Zhang T, Rubin D, Li E. Role of the *Entamoeba histolytica* cysteine proteinase in amebic liver abscess formation in severe combined immunodeficient mice. Infect Immun 1995; 63:1587–1590.

88. Losch FD. Massenhafte entwickelung von ameoben in Dickdarm. Arch Pathol Anat 1875; 65:196–211.

89. Councilman WT, Lafleur HA. Amoebic dysentery. Johns Hopkins Hospital Bulletin 1891; 2:395–548.

90. Brumpt E. Etude sommaire de l' "*Entamoeba dispar*"n. sp. Amibe a kystes quadrinuclees, parasite de l'homme. Bull Acad Med (Paris) 1925; 94:943–952.

91. Sargeaunt PG, Williams JE. Electrophoretic isoenzyme patterns of *Entamoeba histolytica* and *Entamoeba coli*. Trans R Soc Trop Med Hyg 1978; 72:164–166.

92. Sargeaunt PG, Jackson TF, Wiffen SR, Bhojnani R. Biological evidence of genetic exchange in *Entamoeba histolytica*. Trans R Soc Trop Med Hyg 1988; 82:862–867.

93. Tannich E, Horstmann RD, Knobloch J, Arnold HH. Genomic DNA differences between pathogenic and nonpathogenic *Entamoeba histolytica*. Proc Natl Acad Sci USA 1989; 86:5118–5122.

94. Clark CG, Diamond LS. Ribosomal RNA genes of 'pathogenic' and 'nonpathogenic' *Entamoeba histolytica* are distinct. Mol Biochem Parasitol 1991; 49:297–302.

95. Bracha R, Nuchamowitz Y, Mirelman D. Molecular cloning of a 30-kilodalton lysine-rich surface antigen from a nonpathogenic *Entamoeba histolytica* strain and its expression in a pathogenic strain. Infect Immun 1995; 63:917–925.

96. Tachibana H, Kobayashi S, Kaneda Y, Takeuchi T, Fujiwara T. Preparation of a monoclonal antibody specific for *Entamoeba dispar* and its ability to distinguish *E. dispar* from *E. histolytica*. Clin Diagn Lab Immunol 1997; 4:409–414.

97. Tachibana H, Kobayashi S, Kato Y, Nagakura K, Kaneda Y, Takeuchi T. Identification of a pathogenic isolate-specific 30,000-Mr antigen of *Entamoeba histolytica* by using a monoclonal antibody. Infect Immun 1990; 58:955–960.

98. Burchard GD, Bilke R. Adherence of pathogenic and non-pathogenic *Entamoeba histolytica* strains to neutrophils. Parasitol Res 1992; 78:146–153.

99. Dodson JM, Clark CG, Lockhart LA, Leo BM, Schroeder JW, Mann BJ. Comparison of adherence, cytotoxicity, and Gal/GalNAc lectin gene structure in *Entamoeba histolytica* and *Entamoeba dispar*. Parasitol Int 1997; 46:225–235.

100. Espinosa-Cantellano M, Gonzales-Robles A, Chavez B, et al. *Entamoeba dispar*: ultrastructure, surface properties and cytopathic effect. J Euk Microbiol 1998; 45:265–272.

101. Pillai DR, Britten D, Ackers JP, Ravdin JI, Kain KC. A gene homologous to hgl2 of *Entamoeba histolytica* is present and expressed in *Entamoeba dispar*. Mol Biochem Parasitol 1997; 87:101–105.

102. Leippe M, Bahr E, Tannich E, Horstmann RD. Comparison of pore-forming peptides from pathogenic and nonpathogenic *Entamoeba histolytica*. Mol Biochem Parasitol 1993; 59:101–109.

103. Haque R, Neville LM, Hahn P, Petri WA, Jr. Rapid diagnosis of *Entamoeba* infection by using *Entamoeba* and *Entamoeba histolytica* stool antigen detection kits. J Clin Microbiol 1995; 33:2558–2561.

104. Haque R, Ali IK, Akther S, Petri WA, Jr. Comparison of PCR, isoenzyme analysis, and antigen detection for diagnosis of *Entamoeba histolytica* infection. J Clin Microbiol 1998; 36:449–452.

105. Ong SJ, Cheng MY, Liu KH, Horng CB. Use of the ProSpecT microplate enzyme immunoassay for the detection of pathogenic and non-pathogenic *Entamoeba histolytica* in faecal specimens. Trans R Soc Trop Med Hyg 1996; 90:248–249.

106. Mirelman D, Nuchamowitz Y, Stolarsky T. Comparison of use of enzyme-linked immunosorbent assay-based kits and PCR amplification of rRNA genes for simultaneous detection of *Entamoeba histolytica* and *E. dispar*. J Clin Microbiol 1997; 35:2405–2407.

107. Acuna-Soto R, Samuelson J, De Girolami P, et al. Application of the polymerase chain reaction to the epidemiology of pathogenic and nonpathogenic *Entamoeba histolytica*. Am J Trop Med Hyg 1993; 48:58–70.

108. Jetter A, Walderich B, Britten D, et al. An epidemiological study of *Entamoeba histolytica* and *E. dispar* infection in eastern Turkey using a colorimetric polymerase chain reaction. Arch Med Res 1997:319–321.

109. Haque H, Mollah NU, Ali IKM, et al. Diagnosis of amebic liver abscess and intestinal infection with the TechLab *Entamoeba histolytica* II antigen detection and antibody tests. J Clin Microbiol 2000; 38:3235–3239.

110. Ravdin JI, Jackson TF, Petri WA, Jr, et al. Association of serum antibodies to adherence lectin with invasive amebiasis and asymptomatic infection with pathogenic *Entamoeba histolytica*. J Infect Dis 1990; 162:768–772.

111. Katzwinkel-Wladarsch S, Loscher T, Rinder H. Direct amplification and differentiation of pathogenic and nonpathogenic *Entamoeba histolytica* DNA from stool specimens. Am J Trop Med Hyg 1994; 51:115–118.

112. Haque R, Kress K, Wood S, et al. Diagnosis of pathogenic *Entamoeba histolytica* infection using a stool ELISA based on monoclonal antibodies to the galactose-specific adhesin. J Infect Dis 1993; 167:247–249.

113. Aguirre A, Molina S, Blotkamp C, et al. Diagnosis of *Entamoeba histolytica* and *Entamoeba dispar* in clinical specimens by PCR-SHELA. Arch Med Res 1997:282–284.

114. Clark CG, Diamond LS. *Entamoeba histolytica*: a method for isolate identification. Exp Parasitol 1993; 77:450–455.

115. Pillai DR, Keytsone JS, Kain KC. Treatment. In: Ravdin JI (ed). Amebiasis. London: Imperial College Press, 2000, pp. 127–136.

116. Pizza M, Scarlato V, Masignani V, et al. Identification of vaccine candidates against serogroup B meningococcus by whole-genome sequencing. Science 2000; 287:1816–1822.

117. Seydel KB, Braun KL, Zhang T, Jackson TF, Stanley SL, Jr. Protection against amebic liver abscess formation in the severe combined immunodeficient mouse by human anti-amebic antibodies. Am J Trop Med Hyg 1996; 55:330–332.

118. Campbell D, Gaucher D, Chadee K. Serum from *Entamoeba histolytica*-infected gerbils selectively suppresses T cell proliferation by inhibiting interleukin-2 production. J Infect Dis 1999; 179:1495–501.

119. Krupp IM. Experimental induction of protective immunity to amebic infection. Arch Invest Med(mex) 1974; 2:415–422.

120. De Leon A. [Delayed prognosis in amebic hepatic abscess]. Arch Invest Med(mex) 1970; 1:205–206.

121. Kelsall BL, Jackson TG, Gathiram V, et al. Secretory immunoglobulin A antibodies to the galactose-inhibitable adherence protein in the saliva of patients with amebic liver disease. Am J Trop Med Hyg 1994; 51:454–459.

122. Jessurun J, Barron-Rodriguez LP, Fernandez-Tinoco G, Hernandez-Avila M. The prevalence of invasive amebiasis is not increased in patients with AIDS. Aids 1992; 6:307–309.

123. Cimerman S, Cimerman B, Lewi DS. Enteric parasites and AIDS. Sao Paulo Med Revista Paulista de Medicina 1999; 117:266–273.

124. Schain DC, Salata RA, Ravdin JI. Human T-lymphocyte proliferation, lymphokine production, and amebicidal activity elicited by the galactose-inhibitable adherence protein of *Entamoeba histolytica*. Infect Immun 1992; 60:2143–2146.

125. Salata RA, Murray HW, Rubin BY, Ravdin JI. The role of gamma interferon in the generation of human macrophages cytotoxic for *Entamoeba histolytica* trophozoites. Am J Trop Med Hyg 1987; 37:72–78.

126. Salata RA, Cox JG, Ravdin JI. The interaction of human T-lymphocytes and *Entamoeba histolytica*: killing of virulent amoebae by lectin-dependent lymphocytes. Parasite Immunol 1987; 9:249–261.

127. Ghadirian E, Meerovitch E, Hartmann DP. Protection against amebic liver abscess in hamsters by means of immunization with amebic antigen and some of its fractions. Am J Trop Med Hyg 1980; 29:779–784.

128. Ghadirian E, Meerovitch E. Effect of splenectomy on the size of amoebic liver abscesses and metastatic foci in hamsters. Infect Immun 1981; 31:571–573.

129. Ghadirian E, Kongshavn PA. The effect of splenectomy on resistance of mice to *Entamoeba histolytica* infection. Parasite Immunol 1985; 7:479–487.

130. Petri WA, Jr, Broman J, Healy G, Quinn T, Ravdin JI. Antigenic stability and immunodominance of the Gal/GalNAc adherence lectin of *Entamoeba histolytica*. Am J Med Sci 1989; 297:163–165.

131. Petri WA, Jr, Ravdin JI. Protection of gerbils from amebic liver abscess by immunization with the galactose-specific adherence lectin of *Entamoeba histolytica*. Infect Immun 1991; 59:97–101.

132. Beving DE, Soong CJ, Ravdin JI. Oral immunization with a recombinant cysteine-rich section of the *Entamoeba histolytica* galactose-inhibitable lectin elicits an intestinal secretory immunoglobulin A response that has in vitro adherence inhibition activity. Infect Immun 1473; 64:1473–1476.

133. Mann BJ, Burkholder BV, Lockhart LA. Protection in a gerbil model of amebiasis by oral immunization with *Salmonella* expressing the galactose/N-acetyl D-galactosamine inhibitable lectin of *Entamoeba histolytica*. Vaccine 1997; 15:659–663.

134. Zhang T, Stanley SL, Jr. Protection of gerbils from amebic liver abscess by immunization with a recombinant protein derived from the 170-kilodalton surface adhesin of *Entamoeba histolytica*. Infect Immun 1994; 62:2605–2608.

135. Soong CJ, Kain KC, Abd-Alla M, Jackson TF, Ravdin JI. A recombinant cysteine-rich section of the *Entamoeba histolytica* galactose-inhibitable lectin is efficacious as a subunit vaccine in the gerbil model of amebic liver abscess. J Infect Dis 1995; 171:645–651.

136. Campbell D, Mann BJ, Chadee K. A subunit vaccine candidate region of the *Entamoeba histolytica* galactose-adherence lectin promotes interleukin-12 gene transcription and protein production in human macrophages. Eur J Immunol 2000; 30:423–430.

137. Lotter H, Zhang T, Seydel KB, Stanley SL, Jr, Tannich E. Identification of an epitope on the *Entamoeba histolytica* 170-kD lectin conferring antibody-mediated protection against invasive amebiasis. J Exp Med 1793; 185:1793–1801.

138. Stanley SL, Jr, Becker A, Kunz-Jenkins C, Foster L, Li E. Cloning and expression of a membrane antigen of *Entamoeba histolytica* possessing multiple tandem repeats. Proc Natl Acad Sci USA 1990; 87:4976–4980.

139. Stanley SL, Jr, Tian K, Koester JP, Li E. The serine-rich *Entamoeba histolytica* protein is a phosphorylated membrane protein containing O-linked terminal N-acetylglucosamine residues. J Biol Chem 1995; 270:4121–4126.

140. Seydel KB, Braun KL, Zhang TH, Jackson TFHG, Stanley SL. Protection against amebic liver absess formation in the severe combined immunodeficient mouse by human anti-amebic antibodies. Am J Trop Med Hyg 1996; 55:330–332.

141. Zhang T, Cieslak PR, Stanley SL, Jr. Protection of gerbils from amebic liver abscess by immunization with a recombinant *Entamoeba histolytica* antigen. Infect Immun 1166; 62:1166–1170.

142. Zhang T, Stanley SL, Jr. Oral immunization with an attenuated vaccine strain of *Salmonella typhimurium* expressing the serine-rich *Entamoeba histolytica* protein induces an antiamebic immune response and protects gerbils from amebic liver abscess. Infect Immun 1526; 64:1526–1531.

143. Zhang T, Stanley SL, Jr. Expression of the serine rich *Entamoeba histolytica* protein (SREHP) in the avirulent vaccine strain *Salmonella typhi* TY2 chi 4297 (delta cya delta crp delta asd): safety and immunogenicity in mice. Vaccine 1319; 15:1319–1322.

Index

A

Acquired immune deficiency, *see* Human immunodeficiency virus
AFLP, *see* Epidemiology
AIDS, *see* Human immunodeficiency virus
Allylamines, *see* Fungal infections
Amebiasis, *see* Entamoeba histolytica
Amoebapores, 287–289
Amplified fragment length polymorphism, *see* Epidemiology
Animal models, *see* Gene therapy; *Borrelia*
Antibacterial drug discovery, *see* Drug discovery
Antifungal agents, *see* Fungal infections
Antifungal targets,
   C. neoformans, 203
   characteristics, 156, 173, 174, 203
   common, 156, 202, 216–218
   proteomics, 206
Antisense, 204
Antiviral therapeutic identification, *see* Drug discovery
Apicomplexan parasite, *see* Toxoplasma gondii
Apicoplast, *see* Toxoplasma gondii
Apoptosis, 287
ART, *see* Human immunodeficiency virus
Arthroconidium, *see* Coccidiodes immitis
Aspergillus nidulans (*see also* Essentiality; EST function; Fungal infections), 219–222

Assays,
   biochemical, 92
   cell-based, 63, 92
   direct binding, 64
   indirect binding, 64
   virtual screening, 92
Atovaquone, see Toxoplasma gondii
Attenuation, *see* BCG vaccine
AUR1, see IPC synthase
Aureobasidin A, *see* Fungal infections
Azoles, *see* Fungal infections

B

Bacille Calmette-Guerin, *see* BCG vaccine
Bacterial genome, *see* DNA sequencing
Basidium, 198
BCG vaccine, 69, 75–79
Binding assays, *see* Assays
Bioinformatics, 84, 87
Biopsy, HPV, 30
Borrelia,
   animal models (*see also* Plasminogen), 141, 142
   burgdorferi, 134
   characteristics, 134, 135
   decorin-binding protein, 139, 140, 144, 145
   genetic tools, 137
   genome sequence, 136, 137
   host-parasite interaction, 139
   infectivity, 138
   innate response, 140
   integral membrane proteins, 145
   Lyme disease, 134, 135

From: *Infectious Disease: Pathogen Genomics*
Edited by: K. J. Shaw © Humana Press Inc., Totowa, NJ

outer surface protein
    OspA, 143, 144
    OspC, 144
phylogeny, 135, 136
plasmids, 136, 138
relapsing fever, 133
spirochetemia, 134
spread, 140
tissue tropism, 141, 142

C

Calcium-binding protein, *see Histo
    plasma capsulatum*
Candida, see Fungal infections
Caspofungin, *see* Fungal infections
Catalase, *see Histoplasma capsulatum*
cDNA synthesis, *see* Microarray
Cell cycle control, viral, 5
Cell wall *(see also* Fungi),
    Cryptocococcus neoformans, 202, 203
    Histoplasma capsulatum, 241
    inhibitors, 203
    anchoring, 252
Ciprofloxacin, 107
Coccidioides immitis (see also DNA se-
    quencing; Fungal infections),
    dissemination, 247
    genome structure, 251, 252
    geographic distribution, 248, 249
    mycology, 249, 250
    spherule
        growth, 250
        segmentation, 251, 252
    taxonomy, 251
    vaccine candidates, 252, 253
Coccidioidomycosis, *see Coccidioides
    immitis;* Fungal infections
Comparative genomics, 55, 72, 90, 207,
    218–222
Coregulation, 60, 61, 186
Cryptococcosis *(see also* Fungal infec-
    tions), 168, 197
Cryptococcus neoformans (see also DNA
    sequencing; Fungal infections),
    animal models, 199, 200
    biology of, 198, 199
    mating type, 201
    melanin, 201

phopholipase B, 202
polysaccharide capsule, 201
transcriptome analysis, 207, 208
urease, 202
virulence, 200–202, 209
Cyanobacteria, 256
CYP51 gene *(see also* Resistance),
    175–177
Cyst *(see also Entamoeba histolytica),* 283
Cysteine proteases, *see Entamoeba
    histolytica*

D

Data mining, 269-271
Dbp, *see Borrelia*
Diagnostics,
    PCR-based, 4
    viral DNA microarrays, 3, 4
Dimorphism, *see Histoplasma capsulatum*
DNA sequencing,
    apicoplast genome *(see also Toxo-
        plasma gondii),* 265
    Apicomplexan genomes, 268–272
    bacterial genome, 53–55, 85–87,
        97–98, 114–115
    Borrelia genome, 136, 137
    Coccidiodes immitis genome, 251, 252
    Cryptococcus neoformans genome,
        204–206
    Entamoeba histolytica genome, 283–286
    expressed sequence tags (EST), 218,
        219, 252
    filamentous fungi, 218
    fungal, 157
    Histoplasma capsulatum genome, 233,
        234, 242
    mycobacterial genome, 70-72
    Toxoplasma gondii genome, 256, 258,
        270
DNA viruses,
    herpesviruses, 2
    HPV, 25
Drug discovery,
    genomic scale, 162, 163
    target identification, 89, 202-204
    target validation, 56, 89, 91, 103, 107,
        161
    viral, 4

Drug resistance, *see* Resistance
Dysentery, 282

E
Early genes, *see* Human
    papillomavirus
Endosymbioses, 256
Entamoeba dispar, 291, 292
Entamoeba histolytica (see also DNA sequenc-
    ing), 287–289
    clinical manifestations, 281, 282
    cysteine proteases, 290, 291
    cytotoxic activity, 287
    diagnosis, 292, 293
    Gal/GalNAc Lectin, 289, 290
    immunity, 293, 294
    life cycle, 282, 283
    pathogenicity, 286
    promoter, 285
    treatment, 293
    vaccine, 293–295
Epidemiology,
    amplified fragment length polymor-
      phism, 117
    data analysis, 124, 125
    interrelationships, 113, 115
    multi-locus sequence typing, 122,
      123
    pulsed-field gel electrophoresis,
      116–119
    random chromosomal analysis, 116
    repetitive sequence distribution analysis,
      116
    restriction fragment length polymor-
      phisms, 116, 117
    sequence analysis, 123, 124
    single-locus sequence typing, 121,
      122
Ergosterol biosynthesis, 159, 184, 185,
    197, 206, 216, 217
Essential functions,
    broad specificity, 90, 104
    fungal, 222–225
    viral, 4, 5
Essentiality,
    evaluation, 56, 91, 104, 203, 204
    genetic footprinting, 56
    in vivo, 57

signature-tagged mutagenesis, 57
EST, *see* Expressed sequence tags
Expressed sequence tags, *see species;*
    DNA sequencing

F
Fatty acid synthase, 225
5-FC, *see* Fungal infections
Flucytosine, *see* Fungal infections
Fluor, *see* Microarray
Fungal cell biology, 159
Fungal infections *(see also species),*
    aureobasidin A, 174
    azoles, 170–173, 175–178, 197, 198,
      217
    caspofungin, 170, 173
    flucytosine, 169, 170, 217
    griseofulvin, 170, 171, 217
    incidence, 167, 168, 197–199, 216, 231,
      247, 248
    polyenes, 170, 171, 217
    terbinafine, 170, 173, 217
    treatment, 155, 169–173, 197, 216
Fungi *(see also* Knock-out; Gene func-
    tion), 160
    gene expression, 158
    genome comparisons, 157, 181,182
    in vivo target validation *(see also*
      Drug Discovery), 161

G
Gal/GalNAc Lectin, *see Entamoeba*
    histolytica
Gene chips, *see* Microarray
Gene disruption, *see* Knock-out
Gene function,
    antisense, 208, 209
    confirmation, 59
    gene-expression profiling, 60, 61, 106,
      107
    linkage, 59, 60
    mutant approaches, 88
Gene therapy,
    animal models, 43
    clinical trials, 44, 45
    drug resistance, 44, 45
Gene-expression profile, 61
Genetic footprinting, *see* Essentiality

Genome comparisons, *see* DNA
    sequencing; Drug discovery;
    Fungi
Genome sequencing, *see* DNA sequencing
Glucan, 241, 242
Glucan synthase, 203
Griseofulvin, *see* Fungal infections

H
Haploid, 199, 251, 256
HCMV, *see* Human cytomegalovirus
Herpes simplex virus, 3
Herpesviruses,
    asymptomatic, 2
    gene expression, 2
    host adaptation, 2
    human cytomegalovirus, 3
    Kaposi's sarcoma-associated herpesvi-
        rus, 3
    temporally regulated, 2, 3
Histoplasma capsulatum (see also DNA
    sequencing; Knock-out),
    calcium-binding protein, 240
    catalase, 241
    cell wall composition, 241
    dimorphism, 231, 232, 234–239
    PMA1, 240, 241
    quorum sensing, 242
    sideophores, 240
    transformation, 236
    URA5, 240
Histoplasmosis (see also Fungal infec-
    tions), 231
HIV, *see* Human immunodeficiency
    virus
Host-cell pathways,
    cell cycle, 5
    gene expression profiles
        anti-inflammatory, 6
        pro-inflammatory, 6
    Golgi-protease furin, 5
    HCMV replication, 5
    HIV infection, 15
    interferon-stimulated genes, 6
    lytic infection, 7
    prostaglandin synthesis, 7
    ubiquitin, 5
    viral budding, 5
    viral induction, 6, 7

Host-parasite interaction, *see Borrelia*
HPV, *see* Human papillomavirus
HSV, *see* Herpes simplex virus
Human cytomegalovirus,
    gene-expression, 3
    microarray, 3
    replication, 5
    virion RNAs, 3
Human immunodeficiency virus,
    AIDS, 14
    apoptosis, 15
    bioinformatic analysis, 15
    budding, 5
    cellular pathways, 5
    disease manifestation, 14, 15
    gene therapy, *see* Gene therapy
    host entry, 14
    opportunistic fungal infection, 197
    pathogenesis, 14, 40
    target cell depletion, 15
    treatment, 39–40
    zinc finger proteins, *see* Zinc finger
        proteins
Human papillomavirus,
    biopsy, 30
    classification, 25, 26
    early genes, 26–28
    gene expression, 26
    genome, 26
    hyperproliferation, 25, 28
    interferon response, 32
    late genes, 26
    modulation of host immune
        response, 32
    pathogenesis, 25
    related symptoms, 25, 26
    tissue-culture, 30
    transformation, 28
    treatment, 29
    warts, 25
Hybridization, *see* Microarray

I
Imidazoles, *see* Fungal infections
Infectivity, *see Borrelia*
Innate response, *see Borrelia*
Interferon stimulated genes, 6
IPC synthase, 174, 175
Isoniazid, 107

Isoprenoid biosynthesis, 59

K
Kaposi's sarcoma-associated herpes
　　virus, 3
Karyotype, 256, 283
Keratinocytes,
　　differentiation, 32-33
　　HPV tissue culture, 30
　　microarray analysis, 31
Knock-out,
　　bacterial, 56, 91
　　drug-inhibition, 4
　　fungal, 158, 302
　　Histoplasma capsulatum, 236, 237
　　Toxoplasma gondii, 259
　　viral mutant, 4
KSHV, *see* Kaposi's sarcoma-associated
　　herpesvirus

L
Late genes, *see* Human papillomavirus
Latent infection, 31
Lectin, *see* Entamoeba histolytica
Ligand binding assays, *see* Assays
Linear chromosome, *see* Borrelia
Linear plasmids, *see* Borrelia
Lyme disease, *see* Borrelia

M
Mating type, *see* Cryptococcus
　　neoformans, 201
Mechanism of action, 61, 107, 108, 183, 206
Microarray (see also Coregulation),
　　Affymetrix GeneChips, 13, 14
　　bacterial RNA extraction, 99
　　cDNA synthesis, 99, 100
　　co-expression, 105
　　data analysis, 102, 103
　　fabrication, 98, 99
　　fingerprint, 4, 183–186
　　fluor, 101
　　fungal, 159, 160
　　Histoplasma capsulatum, 242
　　HPV gene expression, 33
　　HPV pathogenesis, 29-33
　　hybridization, 100-102
　　mechanism of action, *see* Mechanism
　　　　of action

mechanism of resistance, *see* Resis-
　　tance
oligonucleotide array, 98, 99
random primers, 100
target selection, 103, 182
validation, 104, 105
viral (*see also* Host-cell pathways), 5
　　diagnostics, 3, 4
　　drug discovery, 3, 4
　　drug inhibition, 3
　　human cytomegalovirus, 3
　　Kaposi's sarcoma-associated
　　　　herpesvirus, 3
　　pharmacogenomics, 3, 4
　　temporally regulated, 2, 3
Microbial genomes, *see* bacterial genome
Microbial physiology, 88, 89
Mitochondrion targets, *see* Toxoplasma
　　gondii
MLST, *see* Epidemiology
Mode of action, *see* Mechanism of action
Mold to yeast (M-Y), 232, 235, 237–239
Multi-locus sequence typing, *see* Epidemi-
　　ology
Mutant generation, *see* Gene Function
Mutant, *see* Knock-out
Mycobacterium tuberculosis,
　　attenuated strains (*see also* BCG vac-
　　　　cine), 73
　　genomic variability, 74–75
　　polymorphic loci, 72
　　RFLP, 73
　　vaccination (*see also* BCG vaccine), 69,
　　　　70
Mycoses (*see also* Fungal infections), 167,
　　172

N
NNRTI, *see* Human immunodeficiency
　　virus
Nonessential targets, 64, 65
NRTI, *see* Human immunodeficiency
　　virus

O
Oligonucleotide array, *see* Microarray
Opportunistic pathogen, 197, 199
Organelle, 256

OspA, *see Borrelia*
Outer surface protein, *see Borrelia*

P
Paclitaxel, 262
Parasite, 259
Pathogenicity (*see also species*), 64, 65
Peptide deformylase, 267
PFGE, *see* Epidemiology
Phagolysosomes, *see Histoplasma capsulatum*
Pharmacogenomics, viral biology, 4
PI, *see* Human immunodeficiency virus treatment
Plasmids, *see Borrelia*
Plasminogen, 142, 143
Plastid, *see Toxoplasma gondii*
Ploidy, 233, 234
Pneumocystis carinii, see Fungal infections
Polyenes, *see* Fungal infections
Polymorphic loci, *see Mycobacterium tuberculosis*
Proteomics, bacterial, 62
Proteomics, fungal, 206, 207
Pulsed-field gel electrophoresis, *see* Epidemiology

R
Random primers, *see* Microarray
Randomly amplified polymorphic DNA, *see* Epidemiology
RAPD, *see* Epidemiology
Relapsing fever, *see Borrelia*
Resistance, bacterial, 83, 108
Resistance, fungal,
    decreased drug accumulation, 178
    transporters, 179–181
Restriction fragment length polymorphism (*see also* Epidemiology), 73, 233
RF, *see Borrelia*
RFLP, *see* Epidemiology
Ribozyme,
    cleavage activity, 41, 42
    design, 41
    hammerhead, 41
RNA, bacterial, 99

S
Saccharomyces cerevisiae, 156, 157
Screens, *see* Assays
Shotgun sequencing, 285
Siderophores, *see Histoplasma capsulatum*
Signal transduction pathway, 201
Signature-tagged mutagenesis (*see also* Essentiality), 57, 161, 209
Single-locus sequence typing, *see* Epidemiology
SLST, *see* Epidemiology
Spherule, *see Coccidiodes immitis*
Spirochetemia, *see Borrelia*
Subversive substrates (*see also Toxoplasma gondii*), 259–261

T
Target identification, *see* Drug Discovery
Target selection, *see* Microarray; Fungi
Target validation, *see* Drug Discovery
Targeting sequences, 264
Targets, organism specific (*see also* Drug discovery; *species*), 93
Taxol, *see* paclitaxel
Terbinafine, *see* Fungal infections
Tetracycline-responsive promoter, 161
TIGR assembler, 286
Toxoplasma gondii,
    algal gene transfer, 271, 272
    apicoplast
        chemotherapeutic targets, 265, 266
        function, 268
        targeting sequences, 266
    atovaquone, 263
    evolution, 256
    fatty acid biosynthesis, 267
    genetics, 256, 258
    isoprene biosynthesis, 267, 268
    microtubule, 261, 262
    mitochondrion, 262-265
    pathogenesis, 258, 259
    plastid genome, 267
    plastid-encoded targets, 265, 266
    population genetic analyses, 258
    purine salvage, 259, 260
    pyrimidine salvage, 260, 261
    shikimate pathway, 261

Toxoplasmosis, *see Toxoplasma gondii*
Transformation (*see also Histoplasma capsulatum; Cryptococcus neoformans*), tumorigenesis, 6, 28
Transporters (*see also* Fungal infections), 179–181
Treatment, *see specific infections*
Triazoles, *see* Fungal infections
Trophozoite (*see also Entamoeba histolytica*), 283

U
Unknown function, *see* Assays; Gene function
Uracil salvage, 260, 261

V
Vaccine, (*see also species; Borrelia*), 143–146
  C. immitis candidate, 252, 253
  E. histolytica candidate, 294, 295
Viral chips, *see* Microarray
Virtual screening, *see* Assays
Virulence (*see also species*), 64, 161, 162
Virus DNA Arrays, *see* Microarray

W
Warts, *see* Human papillomavirus

Z
Zinc finger proteins, modulation during HIV infection, 15